ADVANCES IN ABDOMINAL SURGERY 2002

ADVANCES IN ABDOMINAL SURGERY 2002

Edited by

Attilio Maria Farinon
Professor of Surgery and Chairman,
Department of Surgery,
University of Rome "Tor Vergata",
Rome, Italy

A survey of researches funded by the Italian Ministry of the University and of Scientific and Technological Research

KLUWER ACADEMIC PUBLISHERS
DORDRECHT / BOSTON / LONDON

A C.I.P. Catalogue record for this book is available from the Library of Congress

ISBN 1-4020-0907-0

Published by Kluwer Academic Publishers,
P.O. Box 17, 3300 AA Dordrecht, The Netherlands.

Sold and distributed in North, Central and South America
by Kluwer Academic Publishers,
101 Philip Drive, Norwell, MA 02061, U.S.A.

In all other countries, sold and distributed
by Kluwer Academic Publishers,
P.O. Box 322, 3300 AH Dordrecht, The Netherlands.

Printed on acid-free paper

Printed in the Netherlands.

Dedication

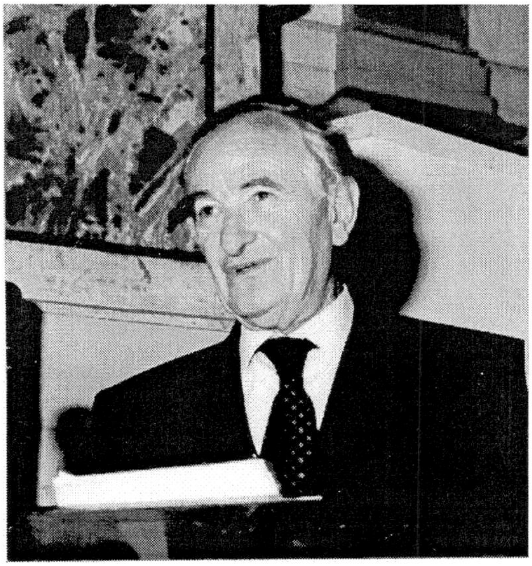

To the memory of Professor Everardo Zanella for his distinguished contribution to surgical sciences.

Contents

SECTION V: MINIMALLY-INVASIVE SURGERY

SECTION VI: TRANSPLANTATION

List of contributors

L. Albarello
Department of Pathology, University of Insubria, Varese, Italy

D. F. Altomare
Department of Emergency and Organ Transplantation, Section of General Surgery and Liver Transplantation, University of Bari, Bari, Italy

E. Ancona
Department of Medical and Surgical Sciences, 4th Surgical Clinic, University of Padua, Padua, Italy

V. Arsena
3rd Department of Surgery, S. Gerardo Hospital Monza, University of Milan, Bicocca, Italy

G. Ausili Cefaro
Institute of Radiology, Catholic University of the Sacred Heart, Rome, Italy

M. Bacosi
Liver Pathophysiology Laboratory, Department of Clinical Sciences, University of Rome "La Sapienza", Rome, Italy

E. Baggio
Department of Surgical and Gastroenterological Sciences, University of Verona, Verona, Italy

G. Batignani
Department of Clinical Physiopathology, Surgical Unit, University of Florence, Florence, Italy

V. Beltrami
Department of Surgical Sciences, University of Rome "La Sapienza", Rome, Italy

A. Benevento
Department of Surgery, University of Insubria, Varese, Italy

A. Bertolotti
Department of Surgical Sciences, University of Rome "La Sapienza", Rome, Italy

U. Boggi
Department of Surgery and Organ Transplantation, University of Pisa, Pisa, Italy

L. Boni
Department of Surgery, University of Insubria, Varese, Italy

L. Bortolasi
Department of Surgery, University of Verona, Verona, Italy

M. Bosco
Institute of Anesthesiology, Catholic University of the Sacred Heart, Rome, Italy

A. S. Boselli
Department of Surgery of Parma Hospital, University of Parma, Parma, Italy

G. Branca
Institute of Microbiology, Catholic University of the Sacred Heart, Rome, Italy

F. Brivio
3rd Department of Surgery, S. Gerardo Hospital Monza, University of Milan, Bicocca, Italy

C. Capella
Department of Pathology, University of Insubria, Varese, Italy

C. U. Casciani
Department of Surgery, University of Rome "Tor Vergata", Rome, Italy

G. Catalano
Department of Surgery and Organ Transplantation, University of Pisa, Pisa, Italy

S. Cipriani
Department of Surgery, University of Rome "Tor Vergata", Rome, Italy

L. Codello
Department of Surgery and Oncology, 2nd Surgical Clinics, University of Padua, Padua, Italy

F. Consorti
Department of Surgical Sciences, University of Rome "La Sapienza", Rome, Italy

A. Conti
Department of Surgery and Anesthesiology, 1st Surgical Clinic, University of Bologna, Bologna, Italy

V. Corso
3rd Department of Surgery, S. Gerardo Hospital Monza, University of Milan, Bicocca, Italy

M. Costantini
Department of Medical and Surgical Sciences, 4th Surgical Clinic, University of Padua, Padua, Italy

M. Costantino
Department of Medical and Surgical Sciences, IVth Surgical Clinics, University of Padua, Padua, Italy

R. Costi
Department of Surgery of Parma Hospital, University of Parma, Parma, Italy

A. Covotta
Department of Surgical Sciences, University of Rome "La Sapienza", Rome, Italy

F. Crosta
Institute of Surgical Sciences, University of Ancona, Ancona, Italy

M. Del Chiaro
Department of Surgery and Organ Transplantation, University of Pisa, Pisa, Italy

S. Del Prato
Department of Endocrinology and Metabolism, Section of Metabolism, University of Pisa, Pisa, Italy

P. Del Rio
Department of Surgery, University of Parma, Parma, Italy

A. De Sanctis
Institute of Surgical Sciences, University of Ancona, Ancona, Italy

P. De Sole
Institute of Physiology, Catholic University of the Sacred Heart, Rome, Italy

S. D'Innocenzo
Liver Pathophysiology Laboratory, Department of Clinical Sciences, University of Rome "La Sapienza", Rome, Italy

G. L. Dionigi
Department of Surgery, University of Insubria, Varese, Italy

R. Dionigi
Department of Surgery, University of Insubria, Varese, Italy

G. Fadda
Institute of Microbiology, Catholic University of the Sacred Heart, Rome, Italy

A. M. Farinon
Department of Surgery, University of Rome "Tor Vergata", Rome, Italy

L. Fattori
3rd Department of Surgery, S. Gerardo Hospital Monza, University of Milan, Bicocca, Italy

F. Feliciotti
Institute of Surgical Sciences, University of Ancona, Ancona, Italy

M. Foletto
Department of Surgery and Oncology, 2nd Surgical Clinics, University of Padua, Padua, Italy

M. Gallinella Muzi
Department of Surgery, University of Rome "Tor Vergata", Rome, Italy

A. Garcea
Department of Clinical Physiopathology, Surgical Unit, University of Florence, Florence, Italy

A. L. Gaspari
Department of Surgery, University of Rome "Tor Vergata", Rome, Italy

P. Gazzella
Institute of Microbiology, Catholic University of the Sacred Heart, Rome, Italy

E. Giarnieri
Department of Experimental Medicine and Pathology, University of Rome "La Sapienza", Rome, Italy

I. Giovannini
Institute of Surgical Pathology, Catholic University of the Sacred Heart, Rome, Italy

F. Giuliante
Institute of Surgical Pathology, Catholic University of the Sacred Heart, Rome, Italy

M. Grande
Department of Surgery, University of Rome "Tor Vergata", Rome, Italy

V. M. Greco
Department of Surgery and Anesthesiology, 1st Surgical Clinics, University of Bologna, Bologna, Italy

M. Guerrieri
Institute of Surgical Sciences, University of Ancona, Ancona, Italy

A. Guglielmi
Department of Emergency and Organ Transplantation, Section of General Surgery and Liver Transplantation, University of Bari, Bari, Italy

C. Iacono
Department of Surgery, University of Verona, Verona, Italy

F. Leone
Institute of Microbiology, Catholic University of the Sacred Heart, Rome, Italy

E. Lezoche
2nd Surgical Clinic, University of Rome "La Sapienza", Rome, Italy

M. Lise
Department of Surgery and Oncology, 2nd Surgical Clinics, University of Padua, Padua, Italy

L. Luzzatto
Department of Surgical Sciences, University of Rome "La Sapienza", Rome, Italy

S. Manfrida
Institute of Radiology, Catholic University of the Sacred Heart, Rome, Italy

P. Marchetti
Department of Endocrinology and Metabolism, Section of Metabolism, University of Pisa, Pisa, Italy

G. Marmiroli
Institute of Radiology, Catholic University of the Sacred Heart, Rome, Italy

D. Marrano
Department of Surgery and Anesthesiology, 1st Surgical Clinics, University of Bologna, Bologna, Italy

N. Marrano
Department of Surgery and Anesthesiology, 1st Surgical Clinic, University of Bologna, Bologna, Italy

V. Mazzarella
CNR Institute, Rome, Italy

P. Mazzella
Institute of Microbiology, Catholic of University of the Sacred Heart, Rome, Italy

C. Meloni
CNR Institute, Rome, Italy

V. Memeo
Department of Emergency and Organ Transplantation, Section of General Surgery and Liver Transplantation, University of Bari, Bari, Italy

G. Midiri
Department of Surgical Sciences, University of Rome "La Sapienza", Rome, Italy

L. Miglioresi
Liver Pathophysiology Laboratory, Department of Clinical Sciences, University of Rome "La Sapienza", Rome, Italy

S. Mocellin
Department of Surgery and Oncology, 2nd Surgical Clinic, University of Padua, Padua, Italy

D. Molena
Department of Medical and Surgical Sciences, 4th Surgical Clinics, University of Padua, Padua, Italy

I. Monaci
Department of Clinical Physiopathology, Surgical Unit, University of Florence, Florence, Italy

C. Montana
Department of Surgical Sciences, University of Rome "La Sapienza", Rome, Italy

E. Montresor
Department of Surgery, University of Verona, Verona, Italy

C. Moretto
Department of Surgery and Organ Transplantation, University of Pisa, Pisa, Italy

F. Mosca
Department of Surgery and Organ Transplantation, University of Pisa, Pisa, Italy

L. Nardone
Institute of Radiology, Catholic University of the Sacred Heart, Rome, Italy

A. Nespoli
3rd Department of Surgery, S. Gerardo Hospital Monza, University of Milan, Bicocca, Italy

L. Nespoli
3rd Department of Surgery, S. Gerardo Hospital Monza, University of Milan, Bicocca, Italy

L. Nicoletti
Department of Medical and Surgical Sciences, IVth Surgical Clinics, University of Padua, Padua, Italy

D. Nitti
Department of Surgery and Oncology, 2nd Surgical Clinics, University of Padua, Padua, Italy

G. Nuzzo
Institute of Surgical Pathology, Catholic University of the Sacred Heart, Rome, Italy

A. M. Paganini
Institute of Surgical Sciences, University of Ancona, Ancona, Italy

M. Petrolino
Department of Emergency and Organ Transplantation, Section of General Surgery and Liver Transplantation, University of Bari, Bari, Italy

M. Piantelli
Institute of Pathology, Catholic University of the Sacred Heart, Rome, Italy

A. Pietrabissa
Department of Surgery and Organ Transplantation, University of Pisa, Pisa, Italy

P. Pilati
Department of Surgery and Oncology, 2nd Surgical Clinics, University of Padua, Padua, Italy

L. Pinciroli
Department of Surgery and Oncology, 2nd Surgical Clinics, University of Padua, Padua, Italy

F. Pisani
Department of Surgery, University of Rome "Tor Vergata", Rome, Italy

S. Pollicita
Department of Surgery, University of Rome "Tor Vergata, Rome, Italy

G. Portale
Department of Medical and Surgical Sciences, 4th Surgical Clinics, University of Padua, Padua, Italy

G. L. Ricci
Liver Pathophysiology Laboratory, Department of Clinical Sciences, University of Rome "La Sapienza", Rome, Italy

M. Rinaldi
Department of Emergency and Organ Transplantation, Section of General Surgery and Liver Transplantation, University of Bari, Bari, Italy

C. Rizzetto
Department of Medical and Surgical Sciences, IVth Surgical Clinics, University of Padua, Padua, Italy

L. Roncoroni
Department of Surgery of Parma Hospital, University of Parma, Parma, Italy

C. R. Rossi
Department of Surgery and Oncology, 2nd Surgical Clinics, University of Padua, Padua, Italy

F. Rulli
Department of Surgery, University of Rome "Tor Vergata", Rome, Italy

F. Russo
Liver Pathophysiology Laboratory, Department of Clinical Sciences, University of Rome "La Sapienza", Rome, Italy

G. Salvi
Institute of Radiology, Catholic University of the Sacred Heart, Rome, Italy

L. Sarli
Department of Surgery, University of Parma, Parma, Italy

M. Seccia
Department of Surgery, University of Pisa, Pisa, Italy

G. Serio
Department of Surgery, University of Verona, Verona, Italy

G. Sgobba
Department of Surgery, University of Parma, Parma, Italy

M. Sianesi
Department of Surgery, University of Parma, Parma, Italy

G. S. Sica
Department of Surgery, University of Rome "Tor Vergata", Rome, Italy

T. Spanu
Institute of Microbiology, Catholic University of the Sacred Heart, Rome, Italy

G. Splendiani
Department of Surgery, University of Rome "Tor Vergata", Rome, Italy

I. Stroppa
Department of Surgery, University of Rome "Tor Vergata", Rome, Italy

A. Tamburini
Institute of Surgical Sciences, University of Ancona, Ancona, Italy

G. Tisone
Department of Surgery, University of Rome "Tor Vergata", Rome, Italy

F. Tonelli
Department of Clinical Physiopathology, Surgical Unit, University of Florence, Florence, Italy

M. Totis
3rd Department of Surgery, S. Gerardo Hospital Monza, University of Milan, Bicocca, Italy

M. Valerio
3rd Department of Surgery, S. Gerardo Hospital Monza, University of Milan, Bicocca, Italy

A. Vecchione
Department of Experimental Medicine and Pathology, University of Rome "La Sapienza", Rome, Italy

R. Vecchioni
Department of Surgical and Gastroenterological Sciences, University of Verona, Verona, Italy

A. Veglia
Department of Emergency and Organ Transplantation, Section of General Surgery and Liver Transplantation, University of Bari, Bari, Italy

M. Vellone
Institute of Surgical Pathology, Catholic University of the Sacred Heart, Rome, Italy

A. Villani
Institute of Anesthesiology, Catholic University of the Sacred Heart, Rome, Italy

V. Violi
Department of Surgery of Parma Hospital, University of Parma, Parma, Italy

F. Vistoli
Department of Surgery and Organ Transplantation, University of Pisa, Pisa, Italy

G. Zaninotto
Department of Medical and Surgical Sciences, 4th Surgical Clinic, University of Padua, Padua, Italy

C. Zardini
Department of Surgical and Gastroenterological Sciences, University of Verona, Verona, Italy

Foreword

The sudden death of Professor Everardo Zanella occurred when the project of editing a second volume of "Advances in adominal surgery" represented his main interest.

He was so proud of the warm approbation that the first volume, edited 1999, earned by italian academic surgical community.

I worked so intimately and for so many years with him that the final tasks of editing this volume were immediately taken on by me, convinced that my views could not vastly differ from those that he would have expressed.

I truly hope that this book will be a fitting tribute to the memory of Professor Everardo Zanella, a man who contributed greatly to the education and practice of surgery.

ATTILIO MARIA FARINON
Professor of General Surgery
University of Rome "Tor Vergata"

Scientific Secretariat

F.RULLI, M.LAZZARI
Department of Surgery
University of Rome "Tor Vergata"
Rome, Italy

Acknowledgments

We are indebted with Mrs. W. Rubertelli for secretarial assistance, and with Mrs. M. A. Smith for english revision.

SECTION I

SURGICAL INFECTIONS

CHAPTER 1

IN VITRO ANTIMICROBIAL ACTIVITIES OF β-LACTAMS, AMINOGLYCOSIDES, QUINOLONES, GLYCOPEPTIDES AND TRIMETHOPRIM-SULFAMETHOXAZOLE AGAINST GRAM-NEGATIVE AND GRAM-POSITIVE BACTERIA ISOLATED FROM PATIENTS WITH INTRAABDOMINAL INFECTIONS.

Giovanna Branca, Teresa Spanu, Fiammetta Leone, Patrizia Mazzella, Giovanni Fadda

Institute of Microbiology, Catholic University of the Sacred Heart, Rome, Italy

Abstract

Objective To determine the *in vitro* activity of β-Lactams Aminoglycosides, fluoroquinolones, glycopeptides, and trimethoprim-sulfamethoxazole against Gram-negative and Gram-positive organisms isolated from patients with intraabdominal infections

Design Observational study from 1999 to 2000

Setting Surgery wards

Results *Escherichia coli, Pseudomonas aeruginosa, Staphylococcus aureus, Staphylococcus epidermidis, Enterococcus faecalis, Bacteroides fragilis, Enterococcus faecium, Proteus mirabilis, Enterobacter cloacae, Klebsiella pneumoniae* and *Citrobacter freundii* were the most frequently isolated organisms (Tab. 1). The activities of antimicrobial agents were species dependent. Of *Staphylococcus aureus* 50% were a methicillin resistant strain. For enterococci, ampicillin resistance was significantly more prevalent for *Enterococcus faecium* than for *E. faecalis*. One strain of *E. faecalis* resistant to vancomycin was isolated.

Among Gram-negative rods, β-lactams activity varied considerably. Overall meropenem, ceftazidime, piperacillin and piperacillin-tazobactam had the broadest spectrum of activity against all bacteria except *Stenotrophomonas maltophilia* isolates. Ciprofloxacin was active against most Gram-negative bacteria, but was inactive against most strains of *Acinetobacter calcoaceticus-baumanni complex* and *S.maltophilia*. In vitro both amikacin and gentamycin were active against most species, amikacin was always more active than gentamycin. Trimethoprim-sulphamethoxazole was active against most *Enterobacteriaceae*, but was inactive against most strains of *P.aeruginosa, P. mirabilis* and *Acinetobacter* spp.

Conclusions Data documenting antibiotic susceptibility against the most frequent isolates organisms that can cause infections are reviewed here. In our study many pathogens responsible for intraabdominal infections were resistant to many antimicrobial agents used for therapy. These

A.M. *Farinon (ed.), Advances in Abdominal Surgery 2002*, 3-12.

problems underline the need for continued and timely surveillance of resistance among bacteria responsible for surgical infections. The selection of the most effective therapy minimizes the risk of surgical site infection.

Keywords
Antimicrobial resistance, Intraabdominal infections

INTRODUCTION

Infections of intraabdominal organs are an important cause of illness worldwide. The pathogenesis of intraabdominal infections is determined by several factors including bacterial factors which influence the transition from contamination to infection [2]. The species and number of bacteria present at surgical site correlate with postpoperative wound infection. When microorganisms cultured from intraabdominal wound infections are resistant to the profile antimicrobial therapy, the incidence of postoperative infections is singnificantly increased [5]. Timely and appropiate antimicrobial therapy is an essential component of the management of infection. Therefore, it is of great concern that pathogens responsible for these infections have become resistant to many antimicrobial agents.

Our aims was to evaluate the activity of β-lactams, aminoglycosides, fluoroquinolones, glycopeptides, macrolides and trimethoprim-sulfamethoxazole against microorganisms isolated from patients with intaabdominal infections from 1999 to 2000.

MATERIALS AND METHODS

Organisms

The microorganisms studied included 1242 strains isolated from patients with infections following abdominal surgery at the University Hospital "A. Gemelli" in Rome. Specimens were placed in a suitable transport container (Portagerm Bio Merieux) and promptly transported to the Microbiological Laboratory. All clinical samples were plated onto sheep blood agar, chocolate agar, Mac Conkey agar for Gram-negative bacteria, sheep blood agar with colistin and nalidixic acid for Gram-positive cocci, Mannitol salt agar for

Staphylococcus spp, Shaedler blood agar for anaerobes. All media were immediately incubated in aerobic and anaerobic conditions at 36°C. Identification was obtained by standard methods (Vitek system).

Antimicrobial susceptibility tests

The minimum inibitory concentrations (MICs) of penicillin, ampicillin, amoxicillin-clavulanic acid, cephalotin, cephotetan, ceftazidime, piperacillin, piperacillin-tazobactam, imipenem, meropenem, amikacin, gentamicin, ciproflofloxacin, trimethoprim-sulfamethoxazole, clarithromycin , rifampin, vancomycin, and teicoplanin were determined by a standardized broth microdilution method. Selection of the appropriate antimicrobial agents to be tested was dependent on clinical efficacy, on prevalence of resistance and on bacterial species. Quality control strains and breakpoint for defining susceptibility were used according to the National Committee for Clinical Laboratory Standards.

RESULTS AND DISCUSSION

Antimicrobial resistance in the hospital setting has emerged as an important variable that influences patient outcomes. Both antibiotic resistant Gram-negative bacteria and Gram-positive cocci are reported as being important causes of hospital acquired infections.

In our study , we have evaluated antimicrobial susceptibility against 1442 microorganisms isolated from patients who underwent abdominal surgery at University Hospital "A. Gemelli" from 1999 to 2000 (Tab.1).

Pseudomonas aeruginosa, Escherichia coli, Staphylococcus aureus, Staphylococcus epidermidis, Enterococcus faecalis, Bacteroides fragilis, Klebsiella pneumoniae, Enterococcus faecium, Proteus mirabili were the most frequently isolated organisms.

E. coli, P. aeruginosa, K. pneumoniae, Enterobacter spp, *P. mirabilis* and *Citrobacter freundii* were the most frequently isolated Gram-negative bacteria.The most prevalent Gram-positive cocci was *Staphylococcus aureus* followed by *Enterococcus* spp, coagulase-negative *Staphylococcus* spp. Another gram positive organism was *Streptococcus* spp. Anaerobic flora account for 7.8% of all strains.

Results of MIC susceptibility are shown in Table 2. Gram negative non fermentative rods and Enterobacteriaceae are important pathogens of serious infections in hospitalized patients. New epidemiological patterns are being observed for multidrug-resistant nosocomial organisms [4]. The emergence of multi drug resistance is becoming increasingly apparent. Among the β-lactams studied imipenem and ceftazidime yielded the highest activity against Gram-negative non fermentative isolates followed by piperacillin-tazobactam [7]. In the present study tazobactam enhaced the activity of piperacillin against *P. aeruginosa* isolates. Amikacin was the most active aminoglycoside against *P. aeruginosa*; most strains of *Acinetobacter* spp were resistant. The fluoroquinolones, primarily ciprofloxacin have been reported to be active against Gram-negative bacteria. In our study we reported high resistance rates among *P. aeruginosa* and *Acinetobacter* spp isolates.

Stenotrophomonas maltophilia exibited the species antimicrobial susceptibility pattern typical of this organism, including susceptibility to trimethoprim-sulfametoxazole and a high level of resistance to meropenem. Ceftazidime was active against 67% of *S. maltophilia* isolates.

The increasing use of broader-spectrum cephalosporins in the 1990s has become one of the major factors responsible for the high rate of selection of extended-spectrum study 27% *K. pneumoniae*, 6% *E. coli*, 32% *P. mirabilis* had extended spectrum β-lactamases (ESBLs) [3]. Furthermore, high rates of multiple β-lactamase(ESBL) producing microorganisms have been shown by *Citrobacter* spp, *Enterobacter* spp and *Morganella morganii* isolates.

Carbapenems or fluoroquinolones are considered as being a reliable therapeutic treatment for postoperative infections caused by these microorganisms.

In our study all *Enterobacteriaceae* were susceptible to Imipenem and Meropenem.

The Gram-positive cocci have re-emerged worldwide as important pathogens in recent years. *Staphylococcus aureus*, coagulase-negative *Staphylococcus* spp, account for approximately one third of all intraabdominal infections. The importance of methicillin-resistant *S. aureus* (MRSA) as a nosocomial pathogen is now well established [1].

In our study no strain with reduced susceptibility to vancomycin were isolated during the time of the study. In the present study *Enterococcus* spp accounts for 12.88%. Resistance of *Enterococcus faecium* isolates to ampicillin is relatively high (61%). 5% of *E. faecium* isolates were resistant to vancomycin. Our data are in accordance with previous reports, which showed the extensive resistance of Gram-negative and Gram-positive microorganisms. Moreover, the activity of different antimicrobial agents are species dependent. Therefore no single antimicrobial agent is adequate to take care of all patients with intraabdominal infections. Appropriate therapy is an essential component of more effective management of intraabdominal infections [6]. Rapid identification of ethiologic pathogens and their antibiotic susceptibility profiles, could help reduce the administration of inadequate treatment. Further studies are needed to speed up microbiological identification, including molecular techniques, DNA amplification , use of monoclonal antibodies to bacterial antigens and application of PCR to detect antimicrobial susceptibility. Rapid provision of such information could have a significant impact on patient management in terms of appropriate antibiotic prescription and treatment outcome.

Table 1. Gram-negative and Gram-positive bacteria Isolated from patients with intraabdominal infection at University Hospital "Agostino Gemelli" from 1999 to 2000

Organism	**N. (%)**	**isolated**
Gram-negative		
Pseudomonas aeruginosa	186	(14.97)
Stenotrophomonas maltophilia	13	(1.04)
Acinetobacter spp	19	(1.52)
Enterobacter cloacae	40	(3.22)
Enterobacter aerogenes	12	(0.96)
Escherichia coli	185	(14.89)
Citrobacter freundii	37	(2.97)
Klebsiella pneumoniae	55	(4.42)
Serratia marcescens	11	(0.88)
Morganella morganii	23	(1.85)
Proteus mirabilis	41	(3.30)
Proteus vulgaris	4	(0.32)
Providencia stuartii	3	(0.24)
Gram-positive		
Staphylococcus aureus	167	(13.44)
Staphylococcus epidermidis	126	(10.14)
Staphylococcus haemolyticus	16	(1.28)
Enterococcus faecalis	105	(8.45)
Enterococcus faecium	50	(4.02)
Enterococcus durans	5	(0.40)
Streptococcus agalactiae	15	(1.20)
Streptococcus constellatus	4	(0.32)
Anaerobes		Su
Bacteroides fragilis	78	(6.28)
Bacteroides vulgatus	5	(0.40)
Fusobacterium nucleatus	3	(0.24)
Prevotella bivia	1	(0.08)
Peptostreptococcus magnum	1	(0.08)
Clostridium perfrigens	9	(0.72)
LIEVITI	28	(2.25)

Table 2. Susceptibilities of Gram-negative and Gram-positive bacteria

Organism	Antimicrobial Agent	CMI 50 (µg/ml)	CMI90 (µg/ml)	S%	I%	R%
Pseudomonas aeruginosa	Amikacin	<=16	>=64	58	19	23
	Amoxi./Clavu.	>=32	>=32		1	99
	Ampicillin	>=32	>=32			100
	Cefotaxime	>=64	>=64	6	24	70
	Cefotetan	>=64	>=32			100
	Ceftazidime	16	>=32	42	10	48
	Ciprofloxacin	2	>=4	51	3	46
	Gentamicin	4	>=16	49	4	47
	Imipenem	4	>=16	50	20	30
	Meropenen	8	>=16	32	20	48
	Piperacillin	32	>=128	56		44
	Piperacillin./Tazobac.	32	>=128	71		29
	Trimetho/Sulfa.	>=4/76	>=4/76	3		97
S. maltophilia	Amikacin	32	32	33	67	
	Amoxi./Clavu.	>=32	>=32	11		89
	Ampicillin	>=32	>= 32	11		89
	Cefotaxime	>=64	> = 64	22	22	56
	Cefotetan	16	>=32	67	22	11
	Ceftazidime	16	>=32	44	11	55
	Ciprofloxacin	>=4	>=4	11	11	78
	Gentamicin	<=4	>=16	55	11	34
	Imipenem	>=16	>=16	7		93
	Meropenem	>=16	>016	11		89
	Piperacillin	>=128	>=128	25		75
	Piperacillin/Tazobact.	64	>=128	56		44
	Trimetho/Sulfa.	<=0.5/9.5	>=4/75	79		21
Acinetobacter spp	Amoxi./Clavu.	>=32	>=32	27	9	64
	Amikacin	>=64	>=64	27	9	64
	Ampicillin	>=32	>=32	9	18	73
	Cephalothin	>=32	>=32			100
	Cefotaxime	>=64	>=64	27	9	64
	Cefotetan	>=64	>=64	14		86
	Ceftazidime	>=32	>=32	36		64
	Ciprofloxacin	>=4	>=4	27		73
	Gentamicin	>=16	>=16	45		55
	Meropemen	2	4	100		
	Imipenem	<=0.5	1	100		
	Piperacillin	>=128	>=128	36	9	55
	Piperacillin/Tazobact.	>=128	>=128	37		63
	Trimetho/Sulfa.	>=4/76	>=4/76	27		73

Table 2 (continued)

Organism	Antimicrobial Agent	CMI 50 (µg/ml)	CMI90 (µg/ml)	S%	I%	R%
Enterobacter cloacae	Amikacin	2	2	96	4	
	Amoxi./Clavu.	>=32	>=32	4		96
	Ampicillina	>=32	>=32	3	3	94
	Cephalothin	>=32	>=64			100
	Cefotaxime	8	>=64	48	7	45
	Cefotetan	>=32	>=32	12	25	63
	Ceftazidime	2	>=32	55		45
	Ciprofloxacin	<=0.25	>=4	72	14	14
	Gentamicin	<=1	>=16	79		21
	Imipem	<=0.5	<=0.5	100		
	Meropemen	<=0.25	<=0.25	100		
	Piperacillin	16	>=128	50	9	41
	Piperacillin/Tazobact.	<=4	>=128	62	9	29
	Trimetho/Sulfa.	>=4/76	>=4/76	97		3
Escherichia colii	Amikacin	<=1	8	97	2	1
	Amoxi/Clavu.	<=2	16	80	14	6
	Ampicillin	>=8	>=32	38		62
	Cephalothin	8	>=32	46	23	31
	Cefotaxime	<=1	<=1	94		6
	Cefotetan	<=2	8	97		3
	Ceftazidime	<=1	<=1	94		6
	Ciprofloxacin	<=0.25	>=4	67	2	31
	Gentamicin	<=1	8	88	7	5
	Imipenem	<=0.5	<=0.5	100		
	Meropemen	<=0.25	<=0.5	100		
	Piperacilln	16	>=128	55	12	33
	Piperacillin/Tazobact	<=4	<=16	99	1	
	Trimetho/Sulfa	<=0.5/95	>=4/76	76		24
Citrobacter freundii	Amikacin	2	2	100		
	Amoxi/Clavu.	8	>=32	45	14	41
	Ampicillin	>=32	>=32	36	9	55
	Cephalothin	16	>=32	14	29	57
	Cefotaxime	4	16	73	27	
	Cefotetan	16	64	73		27
	Ceftazidime	<=1	16	72	14	14
	Ciprofloxacin	<=0.5	<=0.5	100		
	Gentamicin	<=0.5	2	95		5
	Meropemen	<=0.25	<=0.25	100		
	Imipenem	<=0.5	<=0.5	100		
	Piperacilln	16	>=128	57	14	29
	Piperacillin/Tazobact.	8	16	86	14	
	Trimetho/Sulfa	<=0.5/9.5	>=4/76	86		14

Table 2. (continued)

Organism	Antimicrobial Agent	CMI 50 (µg/ml)	CMI90 (µg/ml)	S%	I%	R%
Klebsiella pneumoniae	Amikacin	<=2	8	100		
	Amoxi./Clavu.	<=4	16	73	17	10
	Ampicillin	>=32	>=32	14	7	79
	Cephalothin	<=2	>=32	73		27
	Cefotaxime	<=2	64	72	7	21
	Cefotetan	2	>=32	83		17
	Ceftazidime	<=1	>=32	73		27
	Ciprofloxacin	<=0.25	2	82	9	9
	Gentamicin	<=0.5	2	100		
	Meropemen	<=0.25	<=0.25	100		
	Imipenem	<=0.5	<=0.5	100		
	Piperacillin	<=4	>=128	27	9	64
	Piperacillin/Tazobact.	<=4	8	91		9
	Trimetho/Sulfa.	4	32	65		35
Morganella morganii	Amikacin	2	>=64	89		11
	Amoxi./Clavu.	>=32	>=32			100
	Ampicillin	>=32	>=32	5		95
	Cephalothin	>=32	>=32			100
	Cefotaxime	2	8	90	5	5
	Ceftazidime	<=1	>=32	78		22
	Ciprofloxacin	<=0.25	<=0.25	100		
	Gentamicin	<=1	>=16	74	5	21
	Meropemen	<=0.25	0,5	100		
	Imipenem	<=0.5	1	100		
	Piperacillin	<=4	>=128	67	11	22
	Piperacillin/Tazobact.	<=4	32	78	11	11
	Trimetho/Sulfa.	2/38	>=4/76	89		11
Proteus mirabilis	Amikacin	4	16	100		
	Amoxi/Clavu.	4	16	83	10	7
	Ampicillin	>=32	>=32	26	74	
	Cephalothin	>=32	>=32	37		63
	Cefotaxime	2	32	68		32
	Cefotetan	2	2	100		
	Ceftazidime	<=1	8	95	5	
	Ciprofloxacin	2	>=4	42	26	32
	Gentamicin	³4	>=16	39		61
	Imipenem	4	16	80		20
	Meropemen	0,25	2	100		
	Piperacillin	64	128	37	10	53
	Piperacillin/Tazobact.	<=4	<=4	100		
	Trimetho/Sulfa.	>=4/76	>=4/76	42		58

Table 2. (continued)

Organism	Antimicrobial Agent	CMI 50 (μg/ml)	CMI90 (μg/ml)	S%	I%	R%
Staphylococcus aureus	Clindamycin	<=0.25	>=4	56		44
	Gentamicin	8	>=16	45	1	54
	Ofloxacin	4	>=4	48		52
	Penicillin	>=0.5	>=0.5	10		90
	Rifampin	0,5	4	66	4	34
	Teicoplanin	<=1	<=1	100		
	Trimetho/Sulfa.	0.5/9.5	1/18	94		6
	Vancomycin	<=1	<=1	100		
	Oxacillin	2	>=4	50		50
Staphylococcus epidermidis	Clindamycin	0,25	>=4	76	2	22
	Clarithromycin	>=8	>=8	41		69
	Gentamicin	>=16	>=16	25	3	73
	Ofloxacin	0,5	8	60		40
	Penicillin	>=0.25	>=0.25		2	98
	Rifampin	<=0.5	>=4	68	3	29
	Teicoplanin	2	4	100		
	Trimetho/Sulfa.	<=0.5/9.5	>=4/76	75		25
	Vancomycin	<=1	2	100		
	Oxacillin	>=0.5	>=0.5	12		88
Staphylococcus haemolyticus	Clindamycin	0,25	>=4	50		50
	Gentamicin	>=16	>=16	10		90
	Ofloxacin	>=8	>=8	9	9	82
	Penicillin	>=0.25	>=0.25			100
	Teicoplanin	4	32	82	9	9
	Trimetho/Sulfa	>=4/76	>=4/76	27		73
	Vancomycin	2	4	100		
	Oxacillin	>=0.5	>=0.5			100
Enterococcus faecalis	Ampicillin	<=0.5	2	99		1
	Penicillin	2	4	94		6
	Teicoplanin	<=1	1	100		
	Vancomycin	<=1	4	99		1
Enterococcus faecium	Ampicillin	16	>=16	39		61
	Penicillin	4	>=16	24		76
	Teicoplanin	<=1	1	96	2	2
	Vancomycin	<=1	4	93	2	5

REFERENCES

1. De Lalla F. Antimicrobial chemotherapy in the control of surgical infectious complications. *J Chemother* 1999; 11(6): 440-5.
2. Farthmann EH, Shoffel U. Epidemiology and pathophysiology of intaabdominal infections (IAI). *Infection* 1998; Sep-Oct, 26(5) : 329-34.
3. Nakamura T, Uchida S, Heijyo H, Masuda M, Takahashi H,Komatsu M, Aihara M, Shibata N, Yagi T, Arakawa Y. A SHV – derived extended spectrum beta-lactamase (SHV – 12) produced by an Escherichia coli recovered from wound abscess in post operative case with rectal carcinoma. *Kanseshogaku Zasshi* 2000 Feb; 74(2): 112-19.
4. Mc Gowan Jr JE. The impact of changing pathogens of serious infections in hospitalised patients. *Clinical Infectious diseases* 2000; 31 (Suppl 4) : S124-30.
5. Nathens AB, Rotstein OD. Antimicrobial therapy for intaabdominal infection. *Am J Surg* 1996 Dec; 172(6A): 1S-6S.
6. Kollef MH. Inadequate antimicrobial treatment: an important detrminant of outcome for hospitalized patients. *Clinical Infectious Diseases* 2000; 31(Suppl 4): S131-38.
7. Palucha A, Mikiewicz B, Hryniewicz W, Gniadkowski M. Concurrent outbreaks of extended-spectrum beta-lactamase-producing organisms of the family Enterobacteriaceae in a Warsaw hospital. *J Antimicrob Chemother* 1999 Oct; 44(4): 489-99.

CHAPTER 2

INFECTED NECROSIS AND PANCREATIC ABSCESS

Domenico Marrano, Vincenzo Maria Greco, Andrea Conti, Nicola Marrano
Department of Surgery and Anesthesiology, 1st Surgical Clinic, University of Bologna, Bologna, Italy

Abstract
Infected necrosis (IN) and pancreatic abscess (PA) are septic complications of acute pancreatitis (AP), and are characterised by a severe prognosis and high mortality rates (20-40%). The overall incidence is 3-8% and can reach 60% in cases of acute necrotizing pancreatitis. In our experience, the overall incidence was 7,1% for IN and 6,7% for AP, with mortality rates of 30 and 14,8%, respectively. Bacterial superinfection is generally caused by enteric Gram-negative germs that reach the pancreas by translocation through the gut and the colon. These conditions produce a very bad prognosis, and require both adequate medical and intensive care as well as surgical treatment, which must be provided as early as possible. In AP, the treatment is based on surgical or, in selected cases, radiological drainage of pus. For IN, the surgical treatment is based on necrosectomy, debridement and removal of infected tissue, by using either a closed procedure and continuous postoperative lavage, or by means of laparostomy (open treatment). In this paper, we shall consider the complex diagnostic tests required in these conditions, as well as the advantages and disadvantages of different surgical procedures. Our series of 29 surgical cases of infected acute pancreatitis will also be presented.

INTRODUCTION

Infected Necrosis (IN) and Pancreatic Abscess (PA) are rare and devastating complications of Acute Pancreatitis (AP), with an overall incidence of 1-5% and 2-8% [1-5], respectively. Incidence rates are much higher (40-60%) in necrotic hemorragic conditions [6, 7]. In our experience, incidence was 7,1% for IN and 6,7% for PA, i.e. 15 and 14 cases, respectively, of a total 210 cases of acute pancreatitis observed during the last ten years [8].

These conditions present different anatomic, pathological and clinical features with different prognostic implications; they therefore require different

A.M. *Farinon (ed.), Advances in Abdominal Surgery 2002*, 13-35.

treatments. IN is an early septic complication of acute necrotizing pancreatitis, where infection tends to spread to the pancreas, peripancreatic tissues, retroperitoneum and occasionally to the peritoneal cavity. Severe and rapid deterioration of the clinical condition may lead to septic shock and multiorgan failure with a mortality of 20-40% [3-5]. With IN, infection occurs under extremely severe clinical conditions, on account of the systemic impact of the ongoing severe acute pancreatitis. Bacterial contamination of necrotic tissue generally occurs within 2 weeks of onset of the acute episode, and the risk of superinfection is proportional to the extent of necrosis. The risk is minimal if necrosis is present in less than 30% of the gland, high if between 30 and 50%, and maximal when the necrosis affects over 50% of the pancreatic surface [9-10]. Morphological features of IN are similar to those observed in sterile necrosis, the only difference being the presence of secondary bacterial superinfection, that causes pus formation in the necrotic tissue, but without any real circumscribed pus collection [4].

Morphologically, PA is characterised by a circumscribed collection of pus, either in a capsulated form or embedded in the pancreas and the adjacent organs [1-4, 11]. The bacterial load is high, with frequent multimicrobial associations and abundant necrotic tissue. Unlike infected necrosis, it is a late complication of AP (4-5 weeks from onset) and infection occurs with no active AP. Bacteria and toxins are gradually incorporated into the blood stream through the capsular vessels causing intermittent fever and sepsis, but no multiorgan failure as in IN, and prognosis is better (average mortality 20%) [1-4, 11].

If capsular rupture occurs, sudden and dramatic toxemia and bacteremia may develop, leading to fulminant generalised sepsis with shock and multiorgan failure, and mortality rates increasing two fold [3].

As reported in the literature, our experience showed that mortality rates were high in IN (30%), due to the generalized infection and the presence of a number of organ-failure related conditions (renal failure, respiratory failure, cardiovascular failure, etc.) [8].

By contrast, mortality rates were considerably lower in PA cases (14,3%), due to its later onset, when active pancreatitis is no longer present [8].

IN and PA are two different anatomic and clinical entities whose common feature is the absolute indication for surgery, with debridement of necrotic tissue and removal of pus by means of multiple and effective drainage. From a nosographic point of view, both conditions are included in the AP classification developed at the Atlanta International Symposium (1992) [12], which is aimed at complying both with morphological and developmental criteria, as well as with clinical findings (Tab. 1).

Table 1. Morphological and clinical classification of A.P.

ACUTE OEDEMATOUS P. (MILD):	inflammatory periacinous oedema with no parenchymal destruction; favourable clinical course.
ACUTE NECROTISING P. (SEVERE):	isolated and diffuse destruction of pancreatic and peripancreatic tissue (sterile necrosis); variable bleeding; severe prognosis associated with organ failure and/or local complications.
INFECTED P. NECROSIS:	secondary bacterial infection of necrotic tissue.
PANCREATIC ABSCESS:	circumscribed, peripancreatic collection of pus with little necrotic tissue and abundant bacterial flora. Late onset during severe A.P.
	1992 Atlanta International Symposium (modified)

PATHOGENESIS AND PATHOPHYSIOLOGY

Bacterial superinfection in pancreatic necrosis, either in necrotising pancreatitis or in a post-pancreatitis collection of pus, may be a cause of IN and PA [1-4, 7].

The organisms most frequently isolated in cases of bacterial contamination are Gram-negative bacteria of enteric origin (Escherichia Coli, Klebsiella Pneumoniae, Pseudomonas Aeruginosa, Enterobacter, etc.), which are observed to be present both in IN and PA. Multimicrobial infections seem to be possible in both conditions, and produce a worse prognosis than monomicrobial contaminations [9]. In our experience, the micro-organisms that are most frequently isolated in IN and PA are the ones included in Table 2; in 15% of cases there was a multimicrobial infection. Bacterial strains and their incidence are the same ones as are reported by other authors in the literature [9, 13-16].

These organisms may reach the pancreas through four possible routes: a) hematogenous spread through the systemic circulation; b) duodenal spread through the ascending canalicular route of the pancreatic duct; c) liver spread through the bile ducts or the portal system; d) transmural lymphatic migration from the colon or by contiguity (translocation). Bacterial translocation through the gastro-intestinal tract is considered the main route of infection [9, 13]. Many possible explanations have been proposed for the phenomenon of bacterial translocation [17-18].

Table 2. Most frequently isolated micro-organisms in I.N and P.A.- Observation of 29 cases of infected acute pancreatitis (personal experience)

BACTERIAL STRAINS	%
AEROBES G+	
Staphylococcus Aureus	12
Streptococcus Faecalis	7
AEROBES G-	
Escherichia Coli	22
Pseudomonas	14
Proteus	10
Klebsiella	8
Citrobacter	8
ANAEROBES	
Bacterioides	10
Clostridium	6
FUNGI	
Candida	3

Severe Acute Pancreatitis has a complex pathophysiological background which includes tissue necrosis and fat necrosis, alongside with systemic and enzyme-mediated conditions, such as hypovolemic shock, bleeding and cardiovascular failure [19-23]. These pathophysiological events cause a remarkable reduction in splanchnic blood flow, with reduced oxygen supply to enteric mucosal membranes and subsequent direct damage to enteric cells which are the cellular components with the highest regeneration turnover. This process leads to anatomic and functional damage of the mucosal membrane, which is no longer able to act as a barrier against micro-organisms [17-18, 24-25].

Splanchnic malperfusion is associated with dynamic ileus, which may enhance translocation. This situation leads to increased intraluminal bacterial load due to peristaltic stasis as well as to distended intestinal loops, with additional reduction in blood supply to the gut walls, and increased ischemic damage and mucosal barrier deficit [17-18, 24-25].

Finally, systemic immunosuppression observed in AP is an additional triggering mechanism leading to increased risk of infection alongside with local immunosuppression, with lack of clearance of translocated bacteria and increase in bacterial load (Tab. 3) [26-28].

Table 3. Main pathophysiological mechanisms of intestinal bacterial translocation

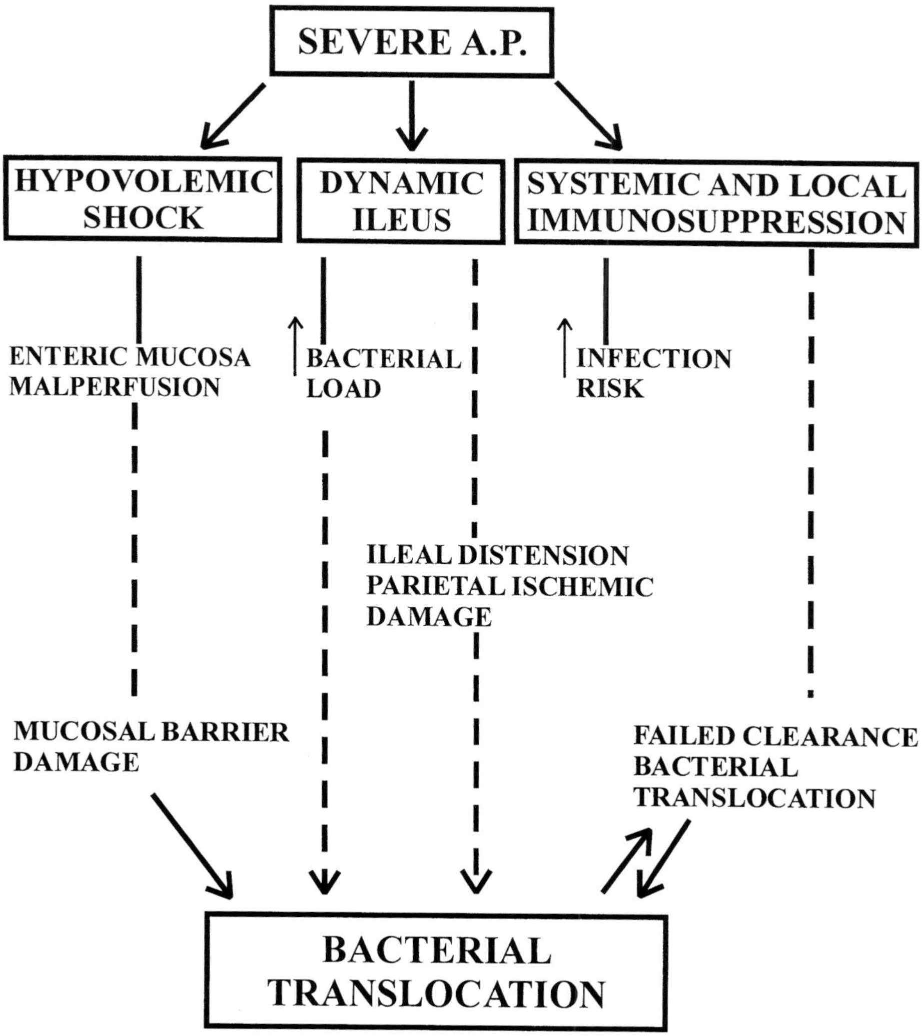

Bacteria and endotoxins then lead to the activation of monocytes, macrophages, endothelial cells, Kupfer cells and other immunocompetent cellular elements and to the release of chemical mediators (Cytokines, Interleukins, Endorphine, Histamine, etc.), that are responsible for metabolic disorders leading to septic shock, and eventually to Multi Organ Failure (MOF) [29-33].

The first and reversible metabolic alterations are cardiovascular depression and Multi Organ Dysfunction Syndrome (MODS) [34], which causes the functional deficit of individual organs and systems without inducing total failure, as observed with MOF. These pathophysiological features are observed in reversible septic shock, and can be removed by applying adequate treatment and attacking the underlying cause [35-36]. Failure to interrupt this cascade of events inevitably leads to MOF, and death of the patient due to myocardial, peripheral circulation, coagulation, lung, kidney, liver, alimentary canal and CNS failure [37-38] (Tab. 4).

DIAGNOSIS

The evolution of AP is extremely unpredictable at the time of clinical onset. It is therefore very important to be able to rely on a number of parameters that can help evaluate the severity of the condition and its prognosis, on the patient's admission to the hospital. Several prognostic markers have been proposed, based either on clinical and laboratory findings (Ranson's score, Imrie, Apache II Score, C-reactive protein, granulocytic elastase, Interleukine-2 and 6, etc.), or on radiological findings (CT-grading according to Balthazar) [39-43]. The combined use of these parameters (and particularly of C-reactive protein + CT) is extremely reliable in the differential diagnosis between mild AP and severe AP [41], but it is not very specific in the identification of septic complications of the disease. C-reactive protein is an indicator of pancreatic necrosis, but elevated levels are not predictive of infected necrosis. Similarly, when large necrotic areas are identified at CT examination, no morphological distinction is possible between sterile and infected necrosis, except for the presence of gas bubbles. PA and IN present different diagnostic problems and, therefore, a separate analysis is necessary.

PA is characterised by acute and exacerbating symptoms with intermittent fever, pain, abdominal distension, possible palpable mass and altered intestinal loops. Laboratory findings always show considerable neutrophilic leukocytosis, while amilase and lipase levels are seldom increased, since no exacerbation of pancreatitis is generally present [1-4, 7, 10-11].

Ultrasound examination shows a hypoechoic area with irregular profile and non-homogeneous content, similar to the one observed in abscesses in other or-

Table 4. Pathophysiology of septic shock in infected acute pancreatitis

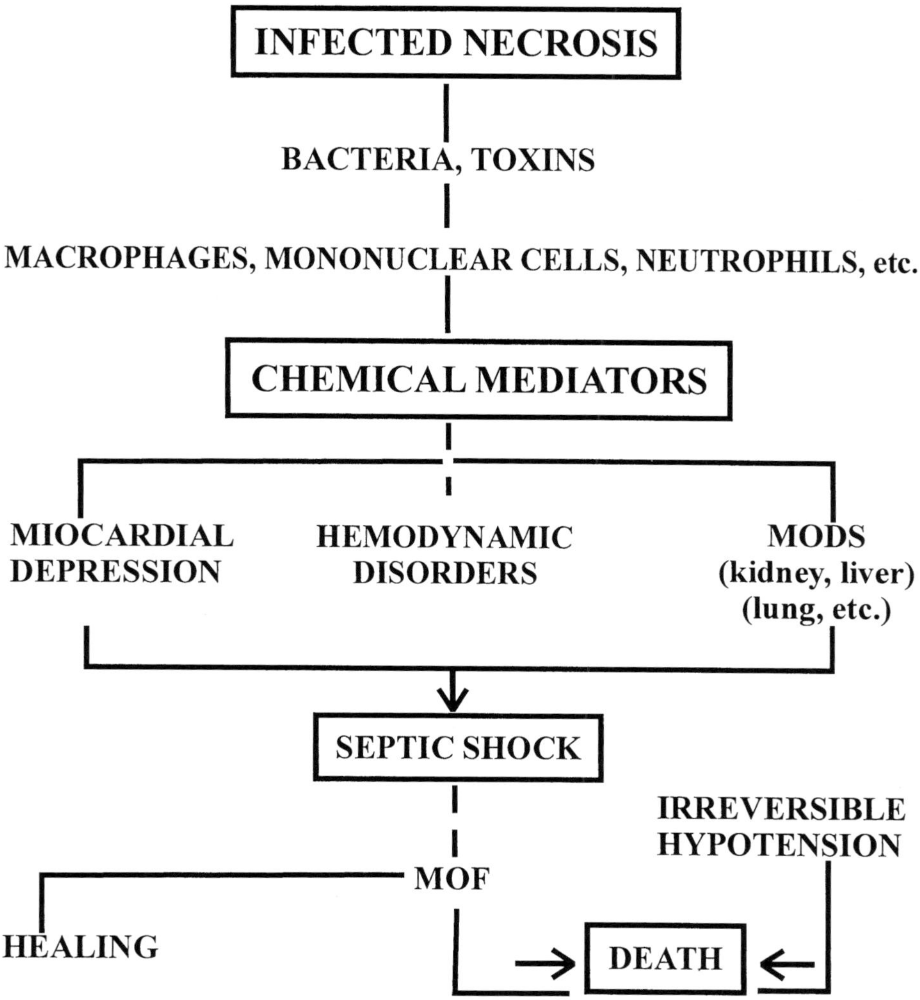

gans (Fig. 1a). In advanced cases, anechoic areas can be observed due to the

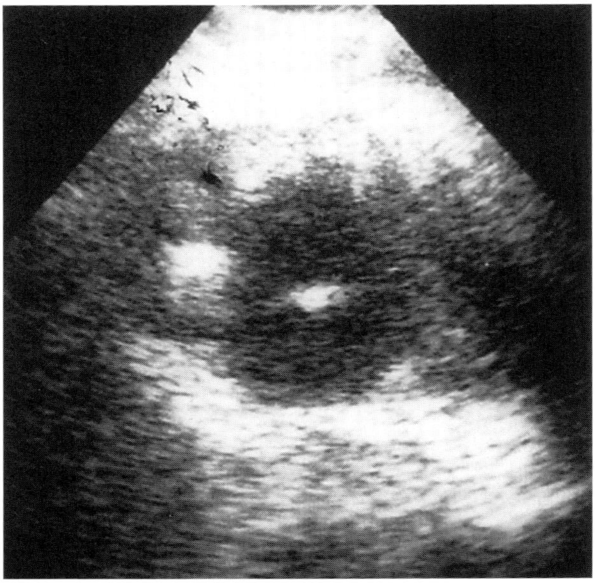

Figure 1A

Ultrasound and CT findings of a pancreatic abscess: predominantly fluid hypoechogenic area with irregular contour and non homogeneous content suggestive of a recently formed pancreatic abscess. (Personal experience)

fluid present in the upper part of the abscess, and hyperechoic areas due to the material deposited in the inferior segments (Fig. 1b) [44-45]. CT scanning is the most specific and reliable diagnostic procedure, as pancreas and abscess can be accurately examined by focusing on walls, contents and relationships with surrounding organs. CT findings in AP generally correspond to stage D

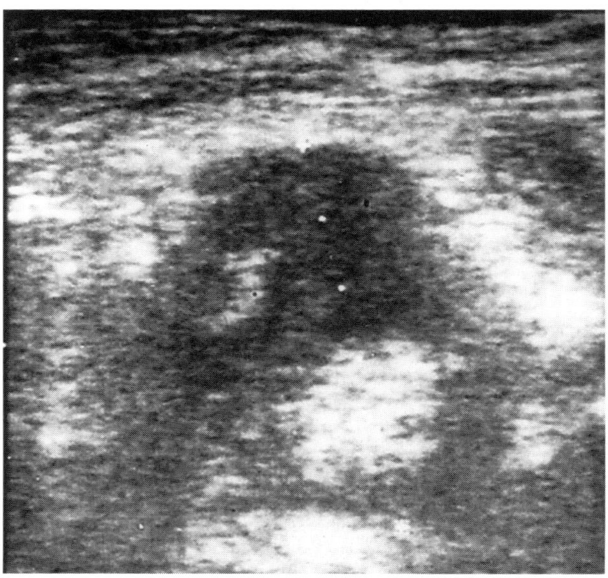

Figure 1B

Advanced abscess, with anechoic fluid component in the upper part and abundant echogenic material at the bottom. (Personal experience).

(morphological and structural alterations in the pancreas with a single and well-defined extrapancreatic collection of pus) and stage E (multiple extrapancreatic collections), in CT-guided radiological grading according to Balthazar (Fig. 1c-d) [42-47].

When AP is diagnosed on the basis of these clinical and instrumental find-

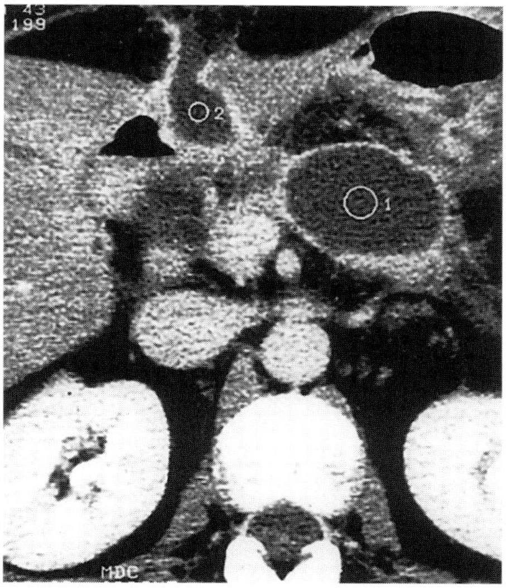

Figure 1C

Double, circumscribed and well-capsulated abscess (Stage D according to Balthazar. (Personal experience)

ings, absolute indication to surgery is to be considered. The diagnostic process in IN is much more complex and questionable, as a number of laboratory, clini-

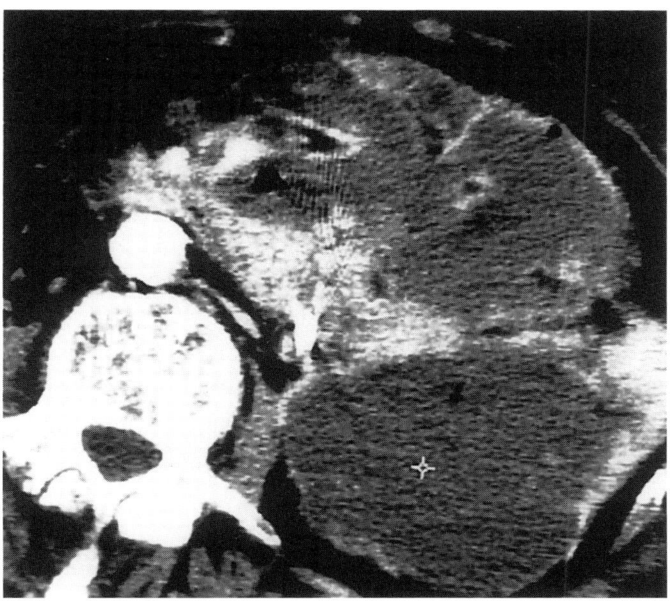

Figure 1D

Gross, multilobar and multicompartmental abscess occupying the left hemiabdomen, almost completely CT finding (Stage E according to Balthazar) (D). (Personal experience) cal and morphological data are very similar to those observed in severe necrotising (sterile) AP [1-3, 5, 7].

A clinical study carried out by Beger et al. [48] on 161 patients with pancreatic necrosis (66 IN and 95 sterile necrosis), confirmed that certain clinical and laboratory parameters are significant indicators of sepsis (temperature 38.5C, excess of bases - 4 mmol/l, Po2 60 mmHg, hematocrit 35%). The score reported by the authors indicated that the presence of three or two factors simultaneously, or of one factor only, corresponds to infection risk rates of 83%, 57-69% and 33-45%, respectively.

In our experience, we have always used Ranson's score, C-reactive protein and CT-guided staging, in the assessment of diagnosis and prognosis of AP cases [20, 40, 46-47]. In our 15 IN cases, we observed that the sepsis indicators proposed by Beger were always present, and concluded that they could effectively be used as possible IN markers versus sterile necrosis, even if they are not sufficient and must be supplemented by a careful evaluation of the clinical and radiological evolution of the disease. We believe that diagnosis must always be confirmed by CT investigation, which, in infected necrosis, can help identify stages D and E according to Balthazar, as well as stage C patients (impaired pancreas and peripancreatic fat tissue with no collection of fluid) [42-43, 46-47]. These findings may be similar to those obtained in non-infected necrotic AP. The presence of gas bubbles produced by bacterial activity (the so-called soap bubbles appearance), which is the only specific radiological indicator of infection, is unfortunately detected only in 20% of cases (Fig. 2).

In extremely doubtful cases, CT-guided aspiration of necrotic tissue, with bacteriological examination and culture of collected material, can be very useful [49-50].

Banks and co-workers [51] proposed a rationale for CT-guided aspiration in the differential diagnosis of infected and severe sterile AP. While surgery is essential in the former, a wait-and-see approach can be adopted in the latter. According to the authors, this rationale depends on the degree of systemic impairment (Systemic Toxicity), and therefore aspiration is indicated whenever persistent or ingravescent impairment is observed, while it is of no use if there is severe general impairment, when an improvement is observed, or in irreversible clinical cases.

We believe that the assessment of the patient must be based on multiple parameters [20, 40, 44-47]: i.e. clinical, laboratory and radiological findings. Indications to surgery must be considered in the case of systemic impairment, fever, positive laboratory findings for sepsis and stages C, D, E according to Balthazar.

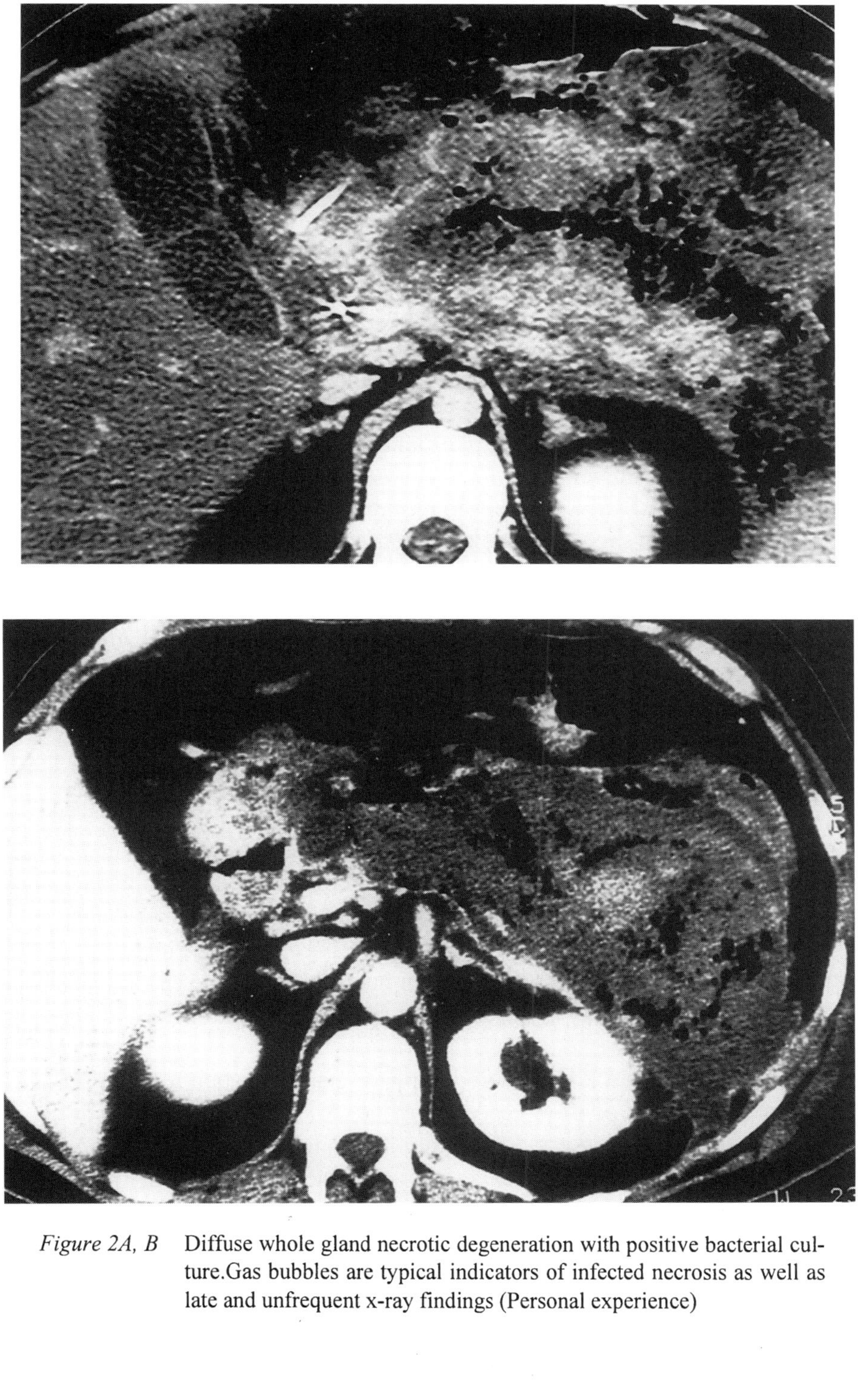

Figure 2A, B Diffuse whole gland necrotic degeneration with positive bacterial culture.Gas bubbles are typical indicators of infected necrosis as well as late and unfrequent x-ray findings (Personal experience)

MEDICAL TREATMENT

Patients with IN and PA require adequate medical and intensive care, and especially correct surgical management. Early treatment leads to longer survival and to a lower incidence of complications.

Medical treatment is essential in any form of AP. It must be started immediately and in infected pancreatitis cases it supplements surgical management, which is absolutely fundamental [20, 44, 52-55].

Medical care in infected AP is similar to that for severe AP and is based on a number of essential steps to be followed in order of priority [20, 44]:

a) symptomatic and support medical care, aimed at maintaining circulation and volemia, at restoring the electrolytic balance, achieving pain relief, correcting hyperglicemia, providing antibiotic treatment and adequate nutritional support;

b) "specific" medical treatment, in order to put gland function at rest and inhibit pancreatic enzymes;

c) intensive medical care, in order to monitor vital functions, ensure prevention and treatment of shock and systemic complications, such as cardiovascular and renal failure.

As far as medical care is concerned, antibiotic treatment and nutritional support deserve special attention, with respect to infected AP, i.e. IN and PA.

ANTIBIOTIC TREATMENT

The issue of antibiotic treatment in AP has long been debated. Based on clinical and experimental observations, as well as on the results of several controlled trials, antibiotic treatment is currently considered useless in mild and edematous AP, while it is essential whenever necrosis is present [56-58].

Results have shown that there is no risk of bacterial superinfection in the natural history of edematous AP, while in necrotic forms the risk of infection may range from 20 to 70%, and is proportional to the extension of necrosis [6-7, 9-10].

Antibiotic treatment is considered as playing an important role both in prevention and treatment of infected AP.

Wallace and co-workers [59] have demonstrated the presence of a "blood-pancreas barrier", which performs a function similar to that of the blood-brain barrier, and is believed to be responsible for selective transit of antibiotics and other substances into the pancreas.

This barrier seems to have greater affinity with and therefore greater permeability for fat soluble compounds, compared to water soluble ones.

Bradley III and co-workers [57] have shown that when antibiotics are present in the pancreatic juices, they are to be found also in the gland parenchyma and vice versa, i.e. the lack of antibiotics in pancreatic juice means that they have failed to cross the blood-pancreas barrier and to reach the parenchyma.

Antibiotic concentration in pancreatic juice has been found to be proportional to serum concentration [56-57]. The main data on antibiotic penetration into the pancreas were obtained from studies on pancreatic fistulae, or cannulation of the main pancreatic duct during ERCP. Pharmacokinetic analysis on a large number of systemically administered antibiotics showed that semisynthetic penicillins, third generation cephalosporins, quinolones, imipenem and metronidazole were present at therapeutic levels in pancreatic juice (Tab. 5) [56-60].

Table 5 Appearance of antibiotics at therapeutic levels in human pancreatic juice.

	ANTIBIOTICS	HOW OBTAINED
*	**ACYLUREIDOPENICILLINS**	
	MEZLOCILLIN	* ERCP - PF **
	PIPERACILLIN	PF
*	**3rd GENERATION CEPHALOSPORIN**	
	CEFTAZIDIME	PF
	CEFOTAXIME	PF
*	**CHINOLONS**	
	CIPROFLOXACIN	PF
	OFLOXACIN	PF
*	**IMIPENEM**	PF
*	**METRONIDAZOLE**	IERCP - PF

* ERCP - SECRETION STIMULATION
** PANCREATIC FISTULA

Mc Clelland et al. [61] have proved the bactericidal properties of quinolones and Imipenem against the Gram-negative bacterial strains that are most frequently isolated in IN, whilst metronidazole was exclusively used in the treatment of anaerobic infections. Finally, an Italian multi-center trial [57], looking at the prophylactic use of Imipenem (3 x 0.5 g/day) in acute necrotizing pancreatitis, showed that infection was less frequent in the Imipenem-treated group compared to the control group (12 vs 30%). However, this antibiotic prophylaxis did not lead to statistically significant results in terms of mortality in both groups [57]. We have always performed bacteriological examination of intra-operative specimens, or CT-guided aspiration in two cases of PA after percutaneous drainage, and we always applied a targeted antibiotic treatment. If blind antibiotic treatment had to be applied pre-operatively, the drug of choice was always Imipenem [8, 39].

NUTRITIONAL SUPPORT

Nutritional support in severe AP can contribute to “putting the pancreas at rest”, as well as providing adequate calorie and energy intake to the patient [20, 44, 62-63].

In edematous AP with a more favourable prognosis, nutritional support is not necessary. On the contrary, in severe or infected cases, nutritional support is absolutely necessary, since the patient is going through prolonged fasting, and has a high energy expenditure due to the disease, with rapid deterioration of the nutritional status. Total Parenteral Nutrition (TPN) has so far been considered as the nutritional gold standard in severe AP [62-64]. Recent clinical studies were aimed at comparing TPN with enteral nutrition (EN) showing that the latter can provide a good alternative [65]. In particular, the disadvantages of TPN are a risk of infection of the central venous catheter, hyperglycemia, which may be difficult to control, high costs and especially the risk of increasing intestinal permeability, and interfering with the function of the enteric mucosal barrier against intraluminal germs [66]. Experimental studies in the rat (Alverdy et al.) [67] claimed to have shown that TPN reduces Intestinal Secretory Immunoglobulin A (S-IgA), a secretion whose production is, on the contrary, stimulated by intestinal transit in oral feeding. Since S-IgA represents a defence mechanism for the enteric mucosa, against the direct damage of toxins and intestinal bacteria, TPN was found to favour bacterial translocation, by producing a state of intestinal immunosuppression. The same favourable conclusions for EN were reached by a clinical trial carried out by Kalfarentos et al. [68] on two groups of patients with severe AP, one treated with TPN and the other with EN. According to the authors, the main advantage offered by early EN lies in the fact that it can maintain the anatomical and functional integrity of the intestinal mucosal barrier, with reduced risk of bacterial translocation and of infection of the necrosis. EN must be administered after placing a nasojejunal tube or, postoperatively, by means of a jejunostomy. In fact, gastric or duodenal EN can induce a major pancreatic secretory response. Nutritional support must contain semi-elementary components, and must have a low fat content and a neutral pH, in order to avoid pancreatic stimulation.

Based on these findings, we believe that EN is to be preferred to TPN in severe AP, in order to reduce the risk of bacterial translocation, and use a more physiological route of artificial nutrition [68-69].

Our nutritional protocol in severe AP is adjusted according to the three different stages of the disease:

1) stage of circulatory instability (initial 2-3 days), with a condition of severe shock, which is treated by supplying hemodynamic and respiratory support and restoring the electrolytic balance. In this stage, no nutritional support is necessary.

2) stage of full-blown disease (4-15 days) when total nutritional support is necessary, due to prolonged fasting and the hypercatabolic condition, which induce a state of malnutrition and cause more dangerous complications.

3) stage of complications (over 15 days), during which adequate nutritional support is required, depending on the conditions observed (septic complications, pancreatic fistulae, etc.).

In the past, according to this protocol, we always used TPN, which is now limited to the initial stage in order to guarantee fast calorie intake. We then prefer to switch to early EN through a naso-jejunal tube, or a jejunostomy if the patient has been operated on.

SURGICAL TREATMENT

The distinction between IN and PA is important not only in terms of prognosis, since IN mortality rate is twice that of PA, but also because surgical treatment may differ considerably in the two conditions [1-4, 11].

In PA, treatment is based on early and effective surgical drainage of the collection of pus [3-4, 70-71] and, as an alternative, on radiologically guided percutaneous drainage in selected cases [72, 73]. In expert hands, both surgical and radiologically guided drainage are easily performed, and are not controversial.

The problem of surgical treatment in IN is much more complex, since it requires necrosectomy, debridement and removal of infected necrotic areas [74-75]. This treatment is currently performed according to two different procedures, both entailing advantages and disadvantages. Choice of treatment is based on the surgeon's personal experience, or is a team decision. These procedures include necrosectomy, drainage and continuous postoperative lavage according to Beger's method [76-79], and necrosectomy with open laparostomy according to Bradley's method [80-81].

Open treatment offers the advantage of guaranteeing better debridement of IN, since it renders possible the performance of dressing manoeuvres on an open abdomen. The procedure starts with necrosectomy and debridement of the pancreatic lodge. The pancreatic region can be explored every 24-48 hours through a laparostomy, for pus drainage and removal of necrotic tissue remnants. Complications include pancreatic fistulae (7%), bleeding (7%) and laparocele (32%), as reported by Bradley [80-83]. The main disadvantage of the procedure is discomfort caused to the patient by repeated anaesthesia, which is necessary for correct exploration of the open cavity.

Closed treatment, with continuous postoperative lavage, requires accurate inflow and outflow drainage, in order to guarantee optimal access for postoperative lavage [76-79]. Lavage is performed with 8-10 litres of saline containing antibiotics and protease inhibitors, whenever necessary. Postoperative drainage care requires special attention; inflowing and outflowing fluid balance must be accurately checked [76]. This method entails high risk of bleeding complications (30%), due to the possible erosion of the inferior mesenteric vein and/or its branches caused by drains pressure [84]. Revision surgery is more frequently performed than the open technique, due to the occurrence of secondary sepsis (23-27% according to Beger) [76-78].

In our opinion, the most complex problems caused by IN treatments are not due to the surgical procedure performed (closed vs open treatment), but to incorrect surgical timing. Whenever surgery is necessary, in fact, the ultimate goal of any procedure is to remove and drain infectious necrotic tissue and/or pus, and the most reliable technique is certainly the one that the surgeon is most familiar with [44-45, 85-86].

Intra-operative ultrasound is extremely useful during the first stage of surgical exploration [87-88]. Direct contact of the ultrasound probe with the surfaces to be explored, and the use of high-frequency, high-definition and easy to handle probes, make it possible to perform an instrumental exploration of great diagnostic value. The conditions of the pancreas can be thoroughly assessed before undertaking dangerous surgical dissection manoeuvres, and the gland can be explored through the gastric wall. Intraparenchymal necrotic and degenerative tissues can be identified as hypo-anaechoic focal areas. (Fig. 3 A-B). Similarly, by means of the ultrasound probe, exploration can be extended to the areas surrounding the gland, the retroperitoneum, the parietocolonic fold, the mesenteric root, etc, in order to detect collections of pus. Ultrasound examination can help undermine necrotic and degenerative tissue, remove collections of pus and then correctly position drainage tubes (Fig. 3 C-D) [87-88].

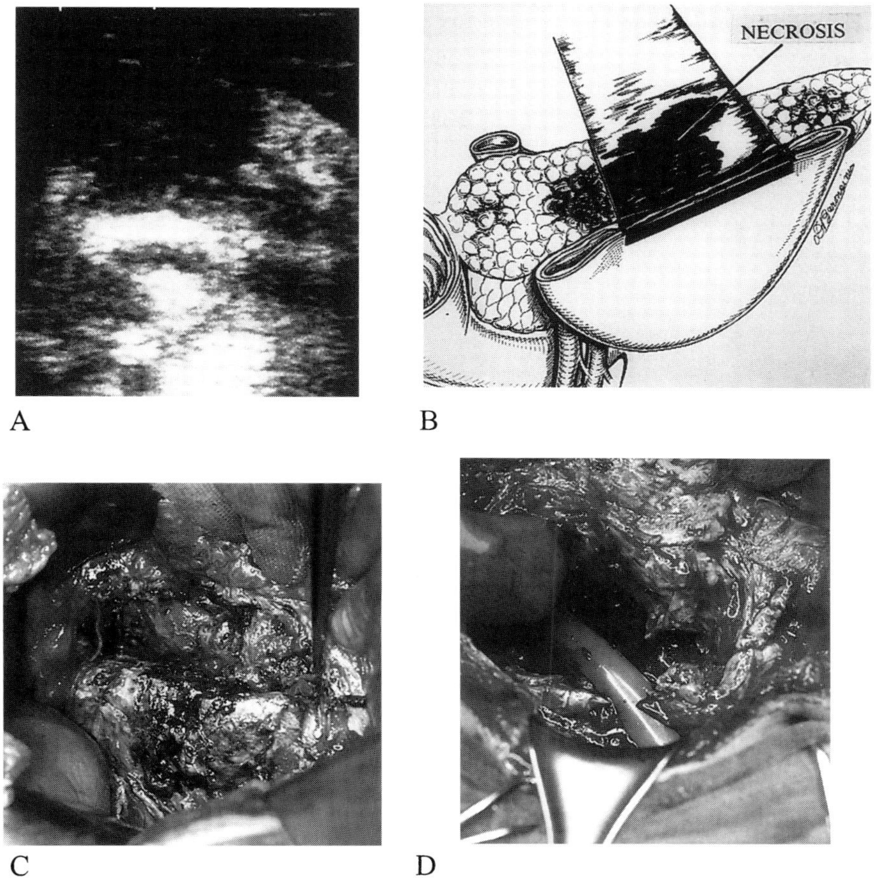

Figures 3 Intraoperative transgastric ultrasound exploration showing a large echogenic area indicating the presence of necrotic tissue (A - B)
Ultrasound findings are confirmed by targeted surgical exploration (C) followed by drainage positioning (D) (Personal experience) *See color plates.*

We operated on 29 cases of infected AP with severe general clinical conditions. IN was detected intraoperatively in 15 patients (50,1%) and PA in 14 patients (49,9%) (Tab. 6). The surgical procedure included necrosectomy, debridement, multiple drainage and postoperative lavage in all IN cases (Fig. 4 A-B-C-D). Results were characterised by high mortality rates (30% or 5 cases); death was caused by MOF, secondary to sepsis in 4 cases, and hemoperitoneum in 1 case. Morbidity rate was 30% (5 cases) with 2 cases of pleural effusion, 1 case of ARDS and 2 cases of pancreatic fistula. In PA, surgical treatment depended on intraoperative findings and abscess features: debridement and drainage of abscess were the most frequently performed procedures, with removal of necrotic remnants and multiple drainage (10 cases, i.e. 71.4%); in 2 cases (14.2%) left pancreatectomy with splenectomy was performed, due to a large and poorly degenerated abscess affecting both the body and tail of the pancreas.

Table 6 Clinical and x-ray findings in 29 operated cases of infected A.P. (personal series)

DIFFERENTIAL DIAGNOSIS between I.N. and P.A.		
CLINICAL DATA	**I.N.**	**P.A.**
Onset	early	late
Severity	+++	++
Temperature	+++	+++
Sepsis markers	+++	+
Leucocytosis	+++	++
Palpable mass	+ -	+ -
COMPLEMENTARY TESTS		
Ultrasound	irregular echoes	transonic aspect
CT	localized or diffuse necrosis; gas bubbles	localized collection; gas bubbles

In both cases there was also a pancreatic-pleural fistula infiltrating the diaphragm, and a left pleural effusion that had to be sutured intraoperatively. Finally, in 2 recent cases (14.2%) CT-guided drainage of the abscess was performed (double in one of the two cases). Both patients had previously undergone necrosectomy and drainage; relapsing sepsis at 12 and 16 days from the first operation, respectively, was observed. Results showed that surgical treatment was effective (mortality rate 14.8%, i.e. 2 cases), since localised infection and lack of severe AP were favourable prognostic factors. However, higher morbidity rates (57%, i.e. 8 cases) were due to respiratory complications (4 cases or 28.5%) and pancreatic fistulae (6 cases or 42.8%).

As regards the debate on CT-guided percutaneous drainage of abscesses, we believe that it is not in conflict with surgical indications (surgical drainage vs CT-guided drainage). CT-guided drainage should never be considered as a first procedure, and should instead be applied in adequately selected cases: in critical patients at very high surgical risk, and in previously operated patients with recurrent abscesses, for whom revision surgery is more risky due to the presence of firm adhesions and local degeneration. It should be undoubtedly used whenever ultrasound and CT examinations show a liquid collection of pus, since a mixture of necrotic tissue and pus may not be effectively removed by means of a thin CT-guided drainage tube (generally 14-20 F) [89-90].

In conclusion, we believe that the progress of medical and intensive care has lead to a reduction of mortality due to systemic complications in the initial phases of severe AP. However, local septic complications have increased

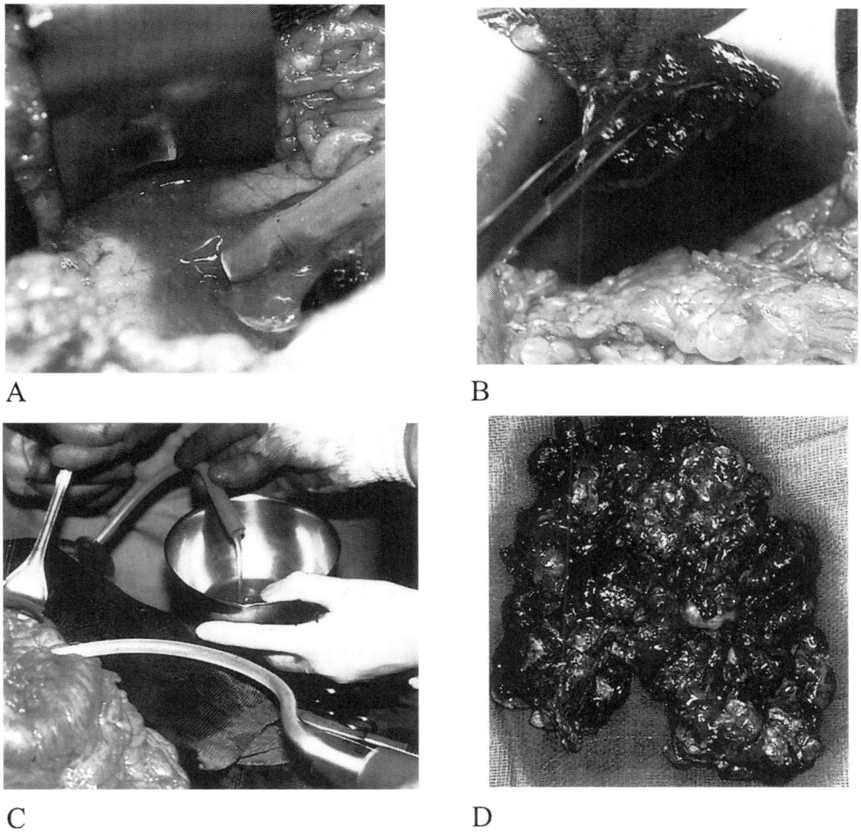

Figures 4 Intraoperative sequence of surgical treatment of infected pancreatic necrosis: the abdomen is opened and an abundant amount of purulent material is removed (A); then necrosectomy is performed (B) and tubes are positioned for postoperative drainage (C). Detail of removed I.N. (D) (Personal experience). *See color plates.*

(20-70%), as a consequence of longer patient survival, and these complications are the first cause of death in advanced cases. Moreover, we believe that early diagnosis of pancreatic sepsis and correct surgical timing are essential, in order to improve the prognosis in these patients.

REFERENCES

1. Lumsden A, Bradley III EL. Secondary pancreatic infections. *Surg Gynecol Obstet* 1990; 170: 459-67.
2. Howard TJ, Wiebke EA, Mogavero G, Kopecky K, Baer JC, Sherman S, Hawes RH, Lehman GA, Goulet RJ, Madura JA. Classification and treatment of local septic complications in acute pancreatitis. *Am J Surg* 1995; 170: 44-50.

3. Bittner R. Clinical significance and management of pancreatic abscess and infected necrosis complicating acute pancreatitis. *Ann Ital Chir* 1995; 2: 217-22.
4. Bittner R, Block S, Büchler M, Beger HG. Pancreatic abscess and infected pancreatic necrosis. Different local septic complications in acute pancreatitis. *Dig Dis Sci* 1987; 32 (10): 1082-7.
5. Banks PA. Infected necrosis: morbidity and therapeutic consequences. *Hepato-Gastroenterol* 1991; 38: 116-9.
6. Beger HG, Block S, Bittner R. The significance of bacterial infection in acute pancreatitis. In: Beger HG, Büchler M Eds. Acute pancreatitis. Berlin - Heidelberg: Springer-Verlag, 1987: 79-86.
7. Widdison AL, Karanjia ND. Pancreatic infection complicating acute pancreatitis. *Br J Surg* 1993; 80: 148-54.
8. Greco VM, Conti A, Barberio G, Casadei R, Taffurelli M, Minni F, Marrano N, la Donna M, Marrano D. Physiopatological aspects of infected acute pancreatitis (AP). *Hepato-Gastroenterol* 1998; 45 (1): XXXVII.
9. Uhl W, Schrag HJ, Wheatley AM, Büchler MW. The role of infection in acute pancreatitis. *Dig Surg* 1994; 11: 214-9.
10. Frey CF, Bradley III EL, Beger HG. Progress in acute pancreatitis. *Surg Gynecol Obstet* 1988; 167: 282-6.
11. Glazer G. Epidemiology and pathology of pancreatic abscess. In: Bradley III EL Ed. Acute pancreatitis: diagnosis and therapy. New York: Raven Press, 1994: 153-9.
12. Bradley III EL. The necessity for a clinical classification of acute pancreatitis: the Atlanta system. In: Bradley III EL Ed. Acute pancreatitis: diagnosis and therapy. New York: Raven Press, 1994: 27-32.
13. Hancke E, Marklein G. Bacterial contamination of the pancreas with intestinal germs: a cause of acute suppurative pancreatitis? In: Beger HG, Büchler M Eds. Acute pancreatitis. Berlin - Heidelberg: Springer-Verlag, 1987: 87-9.
14. Beger HG, Bittner R, Block S, Büchler M. Bacterial contamination of pancreatic necrosis. A prospective clinical study. *Gastroenterology* 1986; 91: 433-8.
15. Banks PA, Gerzof SG, Chong FK, Worthington MG, Doos WG, Sullivan JG, Johnson WC. Bacteriologic status of necrotic tissue in necrotizing pancreatitis. *Pancreas* 1990; 5(3): 330-3.
16. Medich DS, Lee TK, Melhem MF, Rowe MI, Schraut WH, Lee KK. Pathogenesis of pancreatic sepsis. *Am J Surg* 1993; 165: 46-52.
17. Gianotti L, Munda R, Alexander JW, Tchervenkov JI, Babcock GF. Bacterial translocation: a potential source for infection in acute pancreatitis. Pancreas 1993; 8(5): 551-8.
18. Wells CL, Maddaus MA, Simmons RL. Role of the macrophage in the translocation of intestinal bacteria. *Arch Surg* 1987; 122: 48-53.
19. Banks PA. Practice guidelines in acute pancreatitis. *Am J Gastroenterol* 1997; 92(3): 377-86.
20. Marrano D, Campione O, Greco VM. Pancreatite acuta. In: Ceccarelli G Eds. *Manuale di Patologia Chirurgica*. Padova: Piccin, 1996: 2635-61.
21. Campione O, Greco VM, Marrano D. Fisiopatologia della pancreatite acuta. Atti VIII Congresso Nazionale S.I.Fi.Pa.C. - S. Pellegrino Terme 15-17 maggio 1994: 355-65.
22. Steer ML. Pathophysiology and pathogenesis of acute pancreatitis. In: Bradley III EL Ed. Acute pancreatitis: diagnosis and therapy. New York: Raven Press, 1994: 3-11.
23. Glasbrenner B, Adler A. Pathophysiology of acute pancreatitis. *Hepato-Gastroenterol* 1993; 40: 517-21.
24. Alexander JW, Boyce ST, Babcock GF. The process of microbial traslocation. *Ann Surg* 1990; 212: 496-512.
25. Wells CL, Rotstein OD, Pruett TL, Simmons RL. Intestinal bacteria traslocate into experimental intra-abdominal abscesses. *Arch Surg* 1986; 121: 102-7.

26. Runkel NSF, Moody FG, Smith GS, Rodriguez LF, La Rocco MT, Miller TA. The role of the gut in the development of sepsis in acute pancreatitis. *J Surg Res* 1991; 51: 18-23.
27. Wang X, Andersson R, Soltesz V, Leveau P, Ihse I. Gut origin sepsis, macrophage function, and oxygen extraction associated with acute pancreatitis in the rat. *World J Surg* 1996; 20: 299-308.
28. Runkel NSF, Rodriguez LF, Moody FG. Mechanisms of sepsis in acute pancreatitis in opossums. *Am J Surg* 1995; 169: 227-32.
29. Baxter F. Septic shock.. *Can J Anaesth* 1997; 44(1): 59-72.
30. Parrillo JE, Parker MM, Natanson C, Suffredini AF, Danner RL, Cunnion RE, Ognibene FP. Septic shock in humans. Advances in the understanging of pathogenesis, cardiovascular dysfunction, and therapy. *Ann Intern Med* 1990; 113(3): 227-42.
31. Parrillo JE. Pathogenetic mechanisms of septic shock.. *N Engl J Med* 1993; 328(20): 1471-7.
32. Glauser MP, Zanetti G, Baumgartner JD, Cohen J. Septic shock: pathogenesis. *Lancet* 1991; 338: 732-6.
33. Giroir BP. Mediators of septic shock: new approaches for interrupting the endogenous inflammatory cascade. Crit Care Med 1993; 21(3): 780-9. 34. Nathens AB, Marshall JC. Sepsis, SIRS, and MODS: what's in a name? *World J Surg* 1996; 20: 386-91.
35. Rackow EC, Astiz ME. Pathophysiology and treatment of septic shock. *JAMA* 1991; 266: 548-54.
36. Vincent JL. New therapies in sepsis. *Chest* 1997; 112: 330S-8S.
37. Sriskandan S, Cohen J. The pathogenesis of septic shock. *J Infect* 1995; 30: 201-6.
38. Dugernier Th, Starkel P, Laterre PF, Reynaert MS. Severe acute pancreatitis: pathophysiologic mechanisms underlying pancreatic necrosis and remote organ damage. *Acta Gastroenterol Belg* 1996; LIX: 178-85.
39. Damman HG, Dreyer M, Walter TA, Gebhard J, Grabbe E. Prognostic indicators in acute pancreatitis: clinical experience and limitations. In: Beger HG, Büchler M Eds. Acute pancreatitis. Berlin - Heidelberg: Springer-Verlag, 1987: 181-97.
40. Marrano D. Fattori prognostici nella pancreatite acuta. Atti VIII Congresso Nazionale S.I.Fi.Pa.C. - S. Pellegrino Terme 15-17 maggio 1994: 331-53.
41. Uomo G, Rabitti PG, Laccetti M, Manes G, Carraturo I, Esposito P, Visconti M. Évaluation prédictive de la pancréatite aiguë nécrosante: résultats d'une étude prospective. *Presse Med* 1995; 24: 263-6.
42. Balthazar EJ, Ranson JHC, Naidic DP. Acute pancreatitis: prognostic value of CT. *Radiology* 1985; 156: 767-72.
43. Balthazar EJ, Robinson DL, Megibow AJ, Ranson JHC. Acute pancreatitis: value of CT in establishing prognosis. *Radiology* 1990; 174: 331-6.
44. Marrano D, Campione O, Greco VM. Pancreas. In: Mazzeo F, Mozzillo N Eds. Chirurgia delle infezioni - prevenzione, clinica e terapia. Milano: Masson, 1991: 658-75.
45. Marrano D, Campione O, GrecoVM, Casadei R. Complicanze e sequele delle pancreatiti. In: Ceccarelli G Ed. *Manuale di Patologia Chirurgica.* Padova: Piccin, 1996: 2689-702.
46. Greco VM, Golfieri R, Campione O, Ceccarini A, Giampalma E, Casadei R, Negri L, Lalli A, Gavelli G, Marrano D. Significato prognostico del grading TC secondo Balthazar nella pancreatite acuta. Atti XXII Congresso Società Italiana Chirurgia d'Urgenza - Giardini Naxos (CT) 7-9 novembre 1993: 120.
47. Golfieri R, Tetta C, Fadda E, Sbrozzi F, D'Arienzo P, Lalli A, Casadei R, Greco V, Marrano D, Gavelli G. Stadiazione della pancreatitie acuta mediante indagine TC. Valutazione di un nuovo grading e suo significato prognostico. *Gli Ospedali della Vita* 1997; 3: 33-40.
48. Block S, Büchler M, Bittner R, Beger HG. Sepsis indicators in acute pancreatitis. *Pancreas* 1987; 2(5): 499-505.

49. VanSonnenberg E, Wittich G, Casola G, Stauffer AE, Polansky AD, Coons HG, Cabrera OA, Gerver PS. Complicated pancreatic inflammatory disease: diagnostic and therapeutic role of interventional radiology. *Radiology* 1985; 155: 335-40.

50. Gerzof SG, Banks PA, Robbins AH, Johnson WC, Spechler SJ, Wetzner SM, Snider JM, Langevin RE, Jay ME. Early diagnosis of pancreatic infection by computed tomography-guided aspiration. *Gastroenterology* 1987; 93: 1315-20.

51. Banks PA. The role of needle-aspiration bacteriology in the management of necrotizing pancreatitis. In: Bradley III EL Ed. Acute pancreatitis: diagnosis and therapy. New York: Raven Press, 1994: 99-103.

52. Goebell H, Singer MV. Acute pancreatitis: standards of conservative treatment. In: Beger HG, Büchler M Eds. Acute pancreatitis. Berlin - Heidelberg: Springer-Verlag, 1987: 259-65.

53. Folsch VR. Principles of intensive care of patients with acute pancreatitis. In. Beger HG, Büchler M Eds. Acute pancreatitis. Berlin - Heidelberg: Springer-Verlag, 1987: 289-92.

54. Stenberg W, Tenner S. Medical progress: acute pancreatitis. *N Engl J Med* 1994; 330: 1198-210.

55. Uomo G, Visconti M, Manes G, Calise F, Laccetti M, Rabitti G. Nonsurgical treatment of acute necrotizing pancreatitis. *Pancreas* 1996; 12(2): 142-8.

56. Bradley III EL. Antibiotics in acute pancreatitis. Current status and future directions. *Am J Surg* 1989; 158: 472-8.

57. Pederzoli P, Bassi C, Vesentini S, Campedelli A. A randomized multicenter clinical trial of antibiotic prophylaxis of septic complications in acute necrotizing pancreatitis with imipenem. *Surg Gynecol Obstet* 1993; 176: 480-3.

58. Bassi C, Pederzoli P. Antibiotics in necrotizing pancreatitis. In: Bradley III EL Ed. Acute pancreatitis: diagnosis and therapy. New York: Raven Press, 1994: 93-8.

59. Wallace JR, Cushing RD, Bawdon RE, Sugawa C, Lucas CE, Ledgerwood AM. Assessment of antimicrobial penetrance into the pancreatic juice in humans. *Surg Gynecol Obstet* 1986; 162: 313-6.

60. Tyden G, Malmborg AS. Penetration of antibiotics into pancreatic juice. *Lancet* 1985; 1046.

61. McClelland P, Murray A, Yaqoob M, Van Saene HKF, Bone JM, Mostafa SM. Prevention of bacterial infection and sepsis in acute severe pancreatitis. *Ann R Coll Surg Engl* 1992; 74: 329-34.

62. Durr GHK. Enteral and parenteral nutrition in acute pancreatitis. In: Beger HG, Büchler M. Acute pancreatitis. Berlin - Heidelberg: Springer-Verlag, 1987: 285-8.

63. Latifi R, McIntosh JK, Dudrick SJ. Nutritional management of acute and chronic pancreatitis. *Surg Clin North Am* 1991; 71(3): 579-95.

64. Goodgame JT, Fischer JE. Parenteral nutrition in the treatment of acute pancreatitis: effect on complications and mortality. *Ann Surg* 1977; 186: 651-8.

65. Sigurdsson G. Enteral or parenteral nutrition? Pro-enteral. *Acta Anaesthesiol Scand* 1997; 143-7.

66. Sax HC, Wamer BW, Talamini MA, Hamilton FN, Bell RH, Fischer JE, Bower RH. Early total parenteral nutrition in acute pancreatitis: lack of beneficial effects. *Am J Surg* 1987; 153: 117-24.

67. Alverdy JC, Aoys E, Moss GS. Total parenteral nutrition promotes bacterial translocation from the gut. *Surgery* 1988; 186: 185-90.

68. Kalfarentzos F, Kehagias J, Mead N, Kokkinis K, Gogos CA. Enteral nutrition is superior to parenteral nutrition in severe acute pancreatitis: results of a randomized prospective trial. *Br J Surg* 1997; 84: 1665-9.

69. Karamitsios N, Saltzman JR. Enteral nutrition in acute pancreatitis. *Nutr Rev* 1998; 55(7): 279-82.

70. Katsohis CD, Jardinoglou E, Basdanis G, Aletras HA. Pancreatic abscess following acute pancreatitis. *Am Surg* 1989; 55: 427-34.

71. Warshaw AL, Jin G. Improved survival in 45 patients with pancreatic abscess. *Ann Surg* 1985; 202(4): 408-17.
72. Mithöfer K, Mueller PR, Warshaw AL. Interventional and surgical treatment of pancreatic abscess. *World J Surg* 1997; 21: 162-8.
73. Steiner E, Mueller PR, Hahn PF, Saini S, Simeone JF, Wittenberg J, Warshaw AL, Ferrucci JT. Complicated pancreatic abscesses: problems in interventional management. *Radiology* 1988; 167: 443-6.
74. Ranson JHC. The role of surgery in the management of acute pancreatitis. *Ann Surg* 1990; 211(4): 382-93.
75. D'Egidio A, Schein M. Surgical strategies in the treatment of pancreatic necrosis and infection. *Br J Surg* 1991; 78: 133-7.
76. Beger HG, Rau B. Necrosectomy and postoperative local lavage in necrotizing pancreatitis. *Ann Ital Chir* 1995; LXVI(2): 209-15.
77. Beger HG, Büchler M, Bittner R, Rosher R. Necrosectomy and postoperative local lavage in necrotizing pancreatitis. *Br J Surg* 1988; 75: 207-12.
78. Beger HG, Krautzberger W, Bittner R, Block S, Büchler M. Results of surgical treatment of necrotizing pancreatitis. *World J Surg* 1985; 9: 972-9.
79. Ranson JHC, Berman RS. Long peritoneal lavage decreases pancreatic sepsis in acute pancreatitis. *Ann Surg* 1990; 211(6): 708-18.
80. Bradley III EL. Management of infected pancreatic necrosis by open drainage. *Ann Surg* 1987; 206(4): 542-50.
81. Bradley III EL. A fifteen year experience with open drainage for infected pancreatic necrosis. *Surg Gynecol Obstet* 1993; 177: 215-22.
82. Bradley III EL, Fulenwider JT. Open treatment of pancreatic abscess. *Surg Gynecol Obstet* 1984; 159: 509-13.
83. Davidson ED, Bradley III EL. Marsupializzation in the treatment of pancreatic abscess. *Surgery* 1981; 89: 252-6.
84. Pederzoli P, Bassi C, Falconi M, De Santis L, Bonora A, Salvia R, Caldiron E, Sartori N, Butturini G. La necrosectomia ed il drenaggio a perfusione continua nella necrosi acuta pancreatica grave. Atti S.I.C. 1996; 3: 186-73.
85. Marrano D, Campione O, Greco VM. La chirurgia delle complicanze e sequele della pancreatite acuta.. 8th International Congress of Emergency Surgery - Milano 21-24 giugno 1987: 783-94.
86. Marrano D, Campione O. Chirurgia delle complicanze e sequele delle pancreatiti acute. *Argomenti di Chirurgia* 1982; III: 401-8.
87. Marrano D. Ecografia intraoperatoria. Valori e limiti in chirurgia generale. Atti 88 Congresso S.I.C. - Roma 12-16 ottobre 1986: 497-576.
88. Marrano D, Barbara L, Campione O, Monti F, Roversi CA, Pasqualini E, Festi D, Frabboni R. Imaging in pancreatic surgery. An atlas of intra-operative echography. *International University Press* 1992; 25-33.
89. Rotman N, Mathieu D, Anglade MC, Fagniez PL. Failure of percutaneous drainage of pancreatic abscesses complicating severe acute pancreatitis. *Surg Gynecol Obstet* 1992; 174: 141-4.
90. Baron TH, Morgan DE. The diagnosis and management of fluid collections associated with pancreatitis. *Am J Med* 1997; 102: 555-63.

CHAPTER 3

EFFECTS OF IL-2 IMMUNOMODULATION ON INFECTIOUS COMPLICATIONS IN COLORECTAL SURGERY

Nespoli A, Brivio F, Fattori L, Valerio M, Nespoli L, Arsena V, Corso V, Totis M.
3rd Department of Surgery, S. Gerardo Hospital Monza, University of Milan, Bicocca, Italy

INTRODUCTION AND BACKGROUND

Immunosuppression and starvation are the most important risk factors for sepsis after major abdominal surgery; both of them are present in advanced cancer disease, and infective complications are frequent in such patients.

The relationship between malnutrition and the impairment of immune response is a well-documented phenomenon, and is always observed during cachexia.

Surgical trauma itself is followed by a period of severe immunosuppression, and catabolism in the first three post-operative days cannot be reversed with any nutritional support.

Immune events after surgical trauma

The main immune events after surgical trauma are two: first lymphocytopenia and the impairment of cellular mediate immunity, second the increase of mononuclear cells with secretion of pro-inflammatory cytokines such as IL-1 IL-6 and TNF.

Pro-inflammatory cytokines increase is related to the severity of septic complication and to morbidity and mortality after major surgery [1]. The cascade of cytokine caused by severe disease or injury, is characterised by the law of "all or nothing".

The immune response is the same in sepsis and in neoplastic cachexia as in injury: the only difference is quantitative.

Neutrophilia and lymphocytopenia are both present in infections and advanced malignancies. Particularly lymphocytopenia seems related to prognosis.

A.*M. Farinon (ed.), Advances in Abdominal Surgery 2002*, 37-51.

We can recognise two main systems of activation on lymphocytes function: one function related to macrophage activity, and the second system of suppression related to Th2 lymphocyte activation.

Aspecific lymphocyte activation IL-2 related or T helper 1 system

T Helper type 1 lymphocytes are the main source of IL-2 secretion. This cytokine, called also T cells growth factor, has been long considered the main factor in promoting anti-tumoral immunity. The fundamental role of IL-2 is to induce lymphokine-activated killer cells' (LAK) generation from Natural Killers [2]. LAK cells are able to kill a fresh line of tumour cells regardless of their antigenicity. IL-2 triggers a typical cascade of cytokines activation, inducing IL-5 and interferon gamma secretion.

IL-2 stimulates also: the growth of all T lymphocytes subsets and macrophages, inducing their inflammatory cytokine production.

Nowadays, IL-2 is the only cytokine available for clinical use, and has been demonstrated as counteracting malignant cells' growth in solid malignancy, particularly renal cells carcinoma and melanoma.

Specific antigen related cytotoxic system

The specific antigen related cytotoxic system has as effector-cells CD 8 cytotoxic lymphocytes, and needs an antigen-presenting cell (APC) to carry out this function.

The most important APC are dendritic cells (DC), which are the main sources of IL-12 secretion. IL-12 is an autocrine growth-factor for dendritic cells, and promotes the differentiation from CD 34+ progenitors cells, and their subsequent maturation.

Human blood contains two subsets of dendritic cells: one immunologically immature, identified as CD 123+, and the other mature one identified as CD 11c+ [3]. The number of circulating mature DC and high levels of IL-12 correlate with an anticancer immunoactivity.

During IL-2 immunotherapy in renal cells carcinoma, responder patients are those who increase IL-12 serum levels and the number of DC [4].

Macrophage activation

Macrophages are cells derived from monocytes and cannot be found in blood; their maturation and activity occurs in tissues and they play a fundamental role in phagocytosis of bacteria and toxic debris. The granulocyte macrophage colony-stimulating factor (GM-CSF) is the main activator and

growth factor for macrophages. Secretion of inflammatory cytokine (IL-1, IL-6, and TNFα) follows the activation of macrophages with important metabolic effects:
1) fever (mainly due to IL-1),
2) catabolism of protein from muscle,
3) acute phase protein production (mainly mediated by IL-6),
4) increased clotting activity with endothelial toxic effect (mainly due to TNF),
5) IL-6 particularly has an important immunosuppressive function in lymphocytes replication [5], and differentiation of DC [6].

T helper 2 lymphocytes function

The growth of these cells depends on IL-2, and their function is to produce mainly IL-4 and IL-10. While IL-4 is a growth factor for β-lymphocytes, promoting the transformation into plasmacells and antibody production, IL-10 have an important suppressive effect against IL-2, with a mechanism of negative feedback. Probably IL-10 represents a mechanism of self-regulation of immune activation, with the aim of modulating the cytokine cascade upregulation.

Effects of major surgical trauma on immunity

Surgical trauma is followed by a period of severe immunosuppression of cellular-mediated immunity [7, 8], in both aspecific Th-1 related system [8, 9, 10, 11, 12], and specific dendritic cells cytotoxic lymphocytes function [13].

In Th-1 system the most evident phenomenon is the lack of total lymphocytes, natural killers and T-Helper lymphocytes.

It has been reported that after major surgery there is an impaired production of IL-2 [9], and so we can suppose that the antitumor response due to this cytokine activity is reduced [10].

Another effect of surgery is the increase of serum levels of soluble IL-2 receptor [11], that binds IL-2 so impairing its activity [12].

Lymphocytopenia occurs early in the post-operative period, and may be detected after a few hours; and after only seven days the lymphocytes count reaches the baseline levels.

Lymphocytes migration in damaged tissue is fundamental for wound-healing. Unfortunately this migration reduces the blood-immune reactivity against infections and cancer.

Dendritic cells peripheral count follows the same tendency as lymphocytes, and the most important decline affects mature DC (CD11c).

Cytotoxic lymphocytes are significantly reduced in the blood and IL-12 concentration generally falls to the minimum (according our evaluation) on the third post-operative day.

It is still difficult to understand whether the lack of DC is a dependent phenomenon due to the IL-12 impairment, or vice versa. Nevertheless, this results in a complete abrogation of antigens-related cellular immunity.

The increase of pro-inflammatory cytokine IL-6 [14] in the post-operative period is the hallmark of inflammation, and the increase of its blood-levels correlate with the severity of septic complications [15].

IL-6 causes important metabolic effects, and has a suppressive function on immunity [5], inhibiting Lymphocytes replication and DC maturation [16].

Inflammatory cytokines are the response to macrophage activation and replication.

Macrophages presence is mandatory to fight bacterial invasions, and the preservation of macrophages' function is vital to surviving an infection.

A fall of monocyte HLA-DR antigen expression in patients undergoing major abdominal surgery has been reported, due to an increase of IL-10 and IL-10 mRNA expression, detected in the first post-operative days.

Monocyte HLA-DR expression remains low during all the first operative week. This may explain the immunosuppression associated with surgical injury [16].

For a surgeon, this reported onservation might be considered as fundamental: "The impairment of the immune system due to surgical trauma is a constant phenomenon, and promotes a vulnerable post-operative period, both for the spreading of neoplastic cells [10, 17], and infectious complications, particularly in major abdominal surgery" [15-16].

Perioperative blood transfusion and postoperative infections in patients undergoing colorectal surgery

Several factors have been identified as risk factors predisposing to infective complications in colorectal surgery, such as hypovolemia, operative blood loss, length of operation, drains, malnutrition and last but not least, that the colon is opened on the surgical field.

Since Opelz and Coll. [18] reported an association between the length of survival of renal allograft and blood transfusion, it has been supposed that blood transfusion may induce immunosuppresion in recipients. The possible relationship between transfusion and infective complication in surgery was also investigated.

Adequate animal models clearly demonstrated a relationship between transfusion and risk of infective complications. The mechanisms that may explain this immunosuppressive effect are not fully understood. However, in transfused animals several immunological alterations were observed. In particular, interesting changes were found in the recipient's mononuclear cells function, such as decreased NK cell activity, decreased macrophages migration in the peritoneal cavity, and antigen presentation, decreased helper/suppressor T-cell ratio, impaired response to skin test for delayed-type hypersensitivity. [19, 20, 21, 22]

All these changes may be related to the reduction in IL-2 production (up-regulation of immune system) and the increase in PGE-2 production (powerful immunosuppressive signal 20-22)

It was also assessed that white blood cells are the blood component responsible for increased susceptibility to infections, as observed in animal models and in clinical trials [23, 24].

The role of homologous blood transfusion as a risk-factor for infective complications in colorectal surgery is still a matter of debate.

In the last ten years several clinical trials reported an association between homologous blood transfusion and infections [25, 26, 27, 28]; others did not [29]. Different factors can explain this controversy: the large number of retrospective studies, lack of adequate controls, the choice of control groups and other risk-factors that have an influence on patients who need a blood transfusion.

Anyway, it cannot be ignored that prospective, well-designed, clinical trials reported that homologous blood transfusion may effect the outcome in surgical patients, so increasing infective complications, probably through a dose-dependent mechanism; it has also been assessed that even a single unit of allogenic blood may have adverse effects [30].

Then, it is reasonable to point out a correct perioperative transfusion policy, avoiding unnecessary transfusions and single-unit blood transfusion (that is also inadequate to correct anaemia); the use of autologous blood or leukocyte-depleted blood should be considered if blood transfusion is required.

Rationale and possibility to modulate the immune system in surgery

The statements reported above are the cultural background of a modern approach to cancer surgery, and high infection-risk surgery; it appears clear that we need immunomodulation, to improve the surgical prognosis both in malignant disease and in septic patients.

In order to perform immunotherapy we have to find the way to manipulate the most important parameter (or parameters) to improve prognosis.

It is well-known that lymphocyte count in peripheral blood represents an independent factor related to survival in advanced cancer [31, 32, 33], and a high T-lymphocytes count in the post-operative period is an index related to a good prognosis [31, 34].

As far as infections are concerned, the attention of physicians is focused on mononuclear cells, and particularly on macrophages and their related cytokines.

Nevertheless, when an infection occurs the fall of lymphocyte-count and neutrophilia are constant phenomena.

Recently it has been experimentally demonstrated that in sepsis lymphocytes apoptosis is related to a poor prognosis.

The impairment of the immune system and growth of malignancy was reported in 1979, when an immunorestorative drug was suggested as an adjuvant to surgery [35].

At the present time, the discovery of cytokines makes immune activation possible. Nevertheless, the clinical use of cytokines is followed by severe side-effects, which explain the delay in affirming the safety of this therapeutic approach.

IL-2 is able to induce the cytokines cascade. It is commercially easy to find, and its clinical use has achieved sufficient experience to avoid important toxicity.

Biological effects of IL-2 immunotherapy are well-known, and surely may improve the lymphocytes peripheral count; this is one of the most important goals to be considered in order to improve prognosis in surgical cancer patients.

Experimental models on animals suggested that IL-2 therapy may reduce tumour growth after a standard surgical trauma [36] and is able to mediate protection against abscess-formation in an experimental model of sepsis [37].

The rationale of a therapeutic use of IL-2 in surgical patients, with the aim of improving both cancer prognosis and septic complications, is an interesting perspective.

The application of therapy requires the answers to three questions:

1) What is the right timing for immunotherapy?

2) How long should immunotherapy be administered?

3) What is the appropriate dose, to obtain lymphocytosis without important side-effects?

The experience of IL-2 immunotherapy for metastatic renal cancer may give an answer to all these questions:

1) During IL-2 immunotherapy lymphocytes migrate from the blood to the interstitium where they actively reproduce themselves. The peripheral lymphocytosis begins 36 hours after the last administration, and this is the right timing for operation.

2) To induce long-lasting lyphocytosis we need almost three days of therapy.

3) The proper dosage is 12.000.000 UI/day, better if split into two sub-cutaneous administrations.

Clinical experience with pre-operative IL-2 immunotherapy

In 1990, a clinical trial with pre-operative IL-2 [38] began in our department.

We demonstrated that a short three-days' course of IL-2 immunomodulation is able to induce a statistically-significant increase of post-operative total lymphocytes, T-lymphocytes and Natural Killer Cells [38-39]; these data are confirmed by other authors [40-41]. Moreover, immunomodulation may modify histological findings, by inducing important lymphocyte and eosinophilic cells-infiltration in tumour tissues [42].

The purpose of pre-operative immunomodulation is to counteract malignant cells' proliferation in the post-operative period, and to treat the minimal residual disease, with a possible improvement of prognosis [43-44]. Therefore, by improving the immune response, immunomodulation may also enhance wound-healing and reduce septic complications.

The aim of this study is to evaluate the post-operative course of patients treated with pre-operative IL-2 immunomodulation in order to detect a possible reduction of infectious complications in comparison with patients operated on without immunomodulation.

MATERIAL AND METHODS

This clinical study was carried out in Third Department of Surgery in Monza Teaching Hospital. We have evaluated the post-operative course of 41 patients who underwent colorectal surgery for cancer and were treated pre-operatively with IL-2 immunotherapy, in comparison to 73 patients operated on in the same period, without immunotherapy.

All patients received a bowel preparation, and a short-term antibiotic prophylaxis.

Inclusion criteria	histologically-documented adenocarcinoma of the colon or rectum,
	age-range 20-80 years,
	elective surgery,
	informed consent of patients.
Exclusion criteria	emergency surgery,
	Dukes A stage,
	history of previous neoplasm,
	presence of second tumour,
	steroid therapy or other immunosuppressive treatment,
	liver failure,
	cardiovascular failure,
	renal dysfunction.
Characteristics of patients	The characteristics of patients of both groups are reported in Table 1.

Table 1. Characteristics of patients

Table 1	IL-2 group	control group
Number	41	73
Mean age	60.3	65.5
Range of ages	36-80	36-80
Dukes B	11 (26.8%)	35 (47.9%)
Dukes C	9 (21.9%)	18 (24.6%)
Dukes D	21 (51.2%)	20 (27.4%)

IL-2 immunomodulation

The immunomodulation started four days before surgery with 6.000.000 UI of IL-2 administered subcutaneously twice a day for three consecutive days, followed by a day of rest, and surgery 36 hours after the last injection, according to the biological effect of IL-2 treatment.

IL-2-related toxicity was mainly fever recorded in 40/41 patients; in 32 of them fever was recorded as over 39°C.

Medication with paracetamol every 8 hours is recommended to control fever after the first day of therapy. One patient refused therapy on the third day because of cutaneous rash; one patient presented cutaneous exfoliation in the post-operative period.

No important side-effects such as hypotension, oliguria or capillary leak syndrome were reported, and no patient interrupted the treatment for toxicity.

Biological and clinical evaluation

Subset lymphocytes count CD3, CD4, and NK (CD16) were detected preoperatively in control-patients, and before immunotherapy in treated patients.

The same analyses were performed on the third and seventh post-operative days.

Subset lymphocytes-counts were obtained with colour cytofluorometry, using monoclonal antibodies (Becton-Dikinson California).

Recently, in 14 patients of IL-2 group and in 14 controls, we tested IL-6 serum concentration by RIA (normal value 30 pg/ml) preoperatively, and on 3rd and 7th post-operative days, with the aim of obtaining a biological target of inflammation.

In the post-operative period, white blood cells and total lymphocytes were evaluated daily until the seventh post-operative day.

Infective events were evaluated clinically, recording white blood cells, fever, respiratory rate, heart rate and blood acidosis.

The infective events are reported as minor infection (wound infections), anastomotic leakage, and intra-abdominal sepsis.

Because of the well-known relationship between transfusions and infections, patients who required homologous transfusions in both groups were stratified, with the purpose of showing an eventual positive effect of immunomodulation on the well-known risk of infection related to transfusions.

RESULTS

Lymphocytes count

As shown by table A1, baseline total lymphocytes were minimally lower in the IL-2 group before the beginning of treatment (1995 ± 127 treated vs 2122 ± 114 untreated), such differences were observed also in lymphocytes subsets (T lymphocytes 1314 ± 104 vs 1378 ± 76 NK 205 ± 30 vs 394 ± 44, T helper 731 ± 65 vs 836 ± 51).

Table A1. Lymphocytes count before starting IL-2 treatment

basal values at day –3	IL-2 treatment group	control group
Total lymphocytes	1995 ± 127	2122 ± 114
T lymphocytes	1314 ± 104	1378 ± 76
NK	205 ± 30	394 ± 44
T helper	731 ± 65	836 ± 51

All data are reported as average U/ml ± SE

Despite lower basal levels, IL-2 is able to induce a significant postoperative increase in peripheral lymphocytes counts. At postoperative day 3, a very significant difference could be observed in total lymphocytes (2137 ± 143 vs 1667 ± 149 p=0.002). As expected T lymphocytes population showed a similar pattern (1538 ± 93 vs 1030 ± 84 p.0001). Natural Killer population did not show any difference. We were also able to detect a significant increase in T-helper population (948 ± 68 vs 621 ± 51 p.0001). Blood cells count at day 3 are resumed in Table A2.

Table A2 Lymphocytes at 3rd postoperative day

day + 3	IL-2 treatment group	control group	significance
Total lymphocytes	2137 ± 143	1667 ± 149	p=0.002
T lymphocytes	1538 ± 93	1030 ± 84	p<0001
T helper	948 ± 68	621 ± 51	p<0001

All data are reported as average U/ml ± SE

As explained, blood samples were drawn at postoperative day 7: lab results demonstrated a significant increase in total lymphocytes counts in the treatment group (2378 ± 134 vs 1742 ± 138 p.0001), significant increase in T-lymphocytes (1703 ± 95 vs 1106 ± 81 p.0001) and significant increase in T-helper subsets (1067 ± 67 vs 699 ± 61 p.0001). Seven days after operation also NK population was significantly increased in treated patients (346 ± 48 vs 239 ± 32 p=0.03). See Table A3.

Table A3 Lymphocytes at 3rd postoperative day

day + 7	IL-2 treatment group	control group	significance
Total lymphocytes	2378 ± 134	1742 ± 138	p<0001
T lymphocytes	1703 ± 95	1106 ± 81	p<0001
NK	346 ± 48	239 ± 32	p=0.03
T helper	1067 ± 67	699 ± 61	p<0001

All data are reported as average U/ml ± SE

In the 14 treated patients IL-6 serum concentration was tested: the pre-operative data showed no difference between controls and treatment group (20.7 ± 5 pg/ml vs 20.8 ± SE 4.8 pg/ml). But in the control group we observed an important increase in IL-6, while in IL-2 treated patients this increase was less evident (110.8 ± 17.5 vs 35.0 ± 5.1 p.003). See Table A4.

Table A4 IL-6 figures

IL-6	IL-2 treatment group	control group	significance
Preoperative	20.7 ± 5	20.8 ± 4.8	n.s.
Day +3	35.0 ± 5.1	110.8 ± 17.5	p<003

All data are reported as average pg/ml ± SE

Lymphocytes count after blood transfusions

As often occurs after major surgery, some patients required blood transfusions; 41.4% of IL-2 treated patients and 36.9% of control patients received one or more blood units (Tab. B1).

Table B1 Transfusion request

transfusion request	IL-2 treatment group	control group
Number	17/41	27/73
Percentage	41.4%	36.9%

After transfusion IL-2 treated patients had more total lymphocytes in periferial blood than transfused controls. (2171 ± 201 vs 1600 ± 196 p.001). T-lymphocytes and T-helpers counts were also increased in IL-2 treated and transfused, rather than in control transfused patients (T Lymphocytes 1542 ± 217 vs 960 ± 224, T helper 917 ± 254 vs 606 ± 243 p.001). See Table B2.

Table B2 Lymphocyte counts derangement in transfused patients at postoperative day 3

	IL-2 treated	**controls**	**significance**
Total Lymphocytes	2171 ± 201	1600 ± 196	p<001
T Lymphocytes	1542 ± 217	960 ± 224	p<001
T helper Lymphocytes	917 ± 254	606 ± 243	p<001

All data are reported as average U/ml ± SE

Infectious complication

The rate of major septic complication was 2.5% (1/41) in IL-2 treated patients, while in the control group it was 5.8% (5/73) p.003.

The wound-infection rate was significantly lower in treated patients (2.5% vs 16.4% p=0.032). To assess anastomotic leakage, we routinely performed a water soluble contrast enema: both groups had an incidence of 2.5% of anastomotic leakage, relaparotomy was never requested (Tab. C1). No significant difference was observed in pneumonia and urinary tract infection rate.

As reported in Table C2, despite the same request of blood transfusions in the two study groups, the rate of wound infection in transfused patients was significantly lower among IL-2 treated patients. Only 1 out of the 17 transfused and treated patients developed wound infection (5.8%); on the other hand 8 out of 27 transfused controls had wound infection (33.3%) p=0.002. No statistical difference between the 2 groups was observed in the postoperative pneumonia incidence (11.6% vs 11.1%).

Table C1 Clinical complications

	IL-2 treatment group	**control group**	**significance**
SEPSIS	1/41	5/73	n.s.
	2.5%	6.8%	
Wound	1/41	12/73	p=0.032
Infection	2.5%	16.4%	
Anastomotic	1/41	2/73	n.s.
Leakage	2.5%	2.7%	

Table C2 wound infection and transfusion

	IL-2 treatment group	control group	significance
Wound infection	1/17	9/27	p=0.002
	5.8%	33.3%	
Pneumonia	2/17	3/27	n.s.
	11.6%	11.1%	

CONCLUSIONS

Immunostimulation with IL-2 induces a cascade of immune events, which includes either antitumoral response or macrophages stimulation and humoral immunity.

Although the original aim of immunomodulation by IL-2 was the activation of antitumoral response, in order to improve long-term outcome in cancer patients [43], immunostimulation is effective also against infectious complications, and improves wound-healing by the induction of a lymphocytes infiltration of tissues necessary for repair processes.

This study evaluates postoperative infectious complications after high-risk surgery such as colorectal surgery; it shows a significant reduction of septic complications among patients treated with immunomodulation. We would like to stress that the same surgical team operated on the patients of both groups. Therefore, differences between the two groups are not due to operators.

The increase of immune response, well-documented by the increase of lymphocytes counts and subset counts in the postoperative period, is able to prevent failure of the wound-healing process and infectious complications in patients transfused with homologous blood, usually more affected by infections. The reduction of inflammatory events is confirmed by a minimal increase of IL-6 that is, without any doubt, the most important marker of inflammation.

We believe that preoperative immunomodulation is a well-tolerated treatment, necessary to control malignant cell-spreading during the postoperative period, but it is likely to be even more useful in preventing septic complications after major surgery. The side-effects related to therapy are limited to fever, easily controlled by paracetamol, and the cost of immunomodulation is similar to antibiotic prophylaxis. Wide experience in our department can provide assurance of this procedure, excluding interactions with anaesthesia and the early post-operative course. Even if, at the present time, the main indication for IL-2 immunotherapy in surgical praxis is still oncological surgery, this study may open up new prospects for patients with high risk of sepsis, and surely may be considered a good prophylactic approach for septic complication in colorectal surgery.

REFERENCES

1. Menetrier-Caux C, Montmain G, Dieu MC, et al. Inhibition of the differentiation of dendritic cells from CD 34+ progenitors by tumour cells: role of interleukin 6 and macrophage colony-stimulating factors. *Blood* 1998; 92: 4778-4791
2. Grimm EA, Mazumder A, Zhang HZ, Rosenberg SA. Lymphokine-activated killer cell phenomenon. *J Exp Med* 1982; 155: 1823-41
3. Doherty U, Peng M, Gezelter S, et al. Human blood contains two subsets of dendritic cells, one immunologically mature and the other immature. *Immunology* 1994; 82: 487-493
4. Bonfanti A, Lissoni P, Bucocev R, Rovelli F, Brivio F, Fumagalli L. Change in circulating Dendritic cells and IL-12 in relation to the angiogenic factor VEGF during IL-2 immunotherapy of metastatic renal cell carcinoma. *Int J Biol Markers* 2000; (15) 2: 161-164
5. Zhou D, Munster AM, Winchurch RA. Inhibitory effects of interleukin-6 on immunity. *Arch Surg* 1992 ; 127: 65-69
6. Fong Y, Moldawer LL, Dhires GY, Lowry SF. The biologic characteristics of cytokines and Their implication in surgical injury. *Surg Gynecol Obstet* 1990; 49: 215
7. Roth JA, Golub SH, Grimm FR, Morton DL. Effect of operation on immune response in cancer patients: sequential evaluation of in vitro lymphocyte function. *Surgery* 1976; 79: 46-51
8. Park SK, Brady JJ, Wallance HA, Blakemore WS. Immunosuppressive effect of surgery. *Lancet* 1971; 1: 53
9. Akiyoshi T, Koba F, Arinaga S, Miyazaki S, Wada T, Tsuji H. Impaired production of IL-2 after surgery.Clin. *Exp Immunol* 1985; 59: 45-49
10. Eggermont AMM, Steller EP, Sugarbaker PH. Laparotomy enhances intraperitoneal tumour growth and abrogates the antitumor effects of Interleukin-2 and lymphokine-activated-killer cells. *Surgery* 1987; 102:71-78
11. Brivio F, Lissoni P, Mancini D, Tisi E, Tancini G, Barni S, Nociti V. Effect of antitumor surgery on soluble Interleukin-2 Receptor serum levels. *Am J Surg* 1991; 161: 466-469
12. Rubin LA, Jay G, Nelson DL. The released interleukin-2 receptor binds interleukin-2 efficiently. *J Immunol* 1986; 137 : 3841-3844
13. Brivio F, Gilardi R, Bucocev R, Ferrando R, Rescaldni R, et al. Surgery induced decline in circulating dendritic cells in operable cancer patients: a possible explanation of post-operative immunosuppression. *Hepatogastroent* 2000 in press
14. Shenkin A, Fraser WD, Seris J. The serum interleukin-6 responses to elective surgery. *Lymphokine res.* 1989; 8: 123-127
15. Damas P, Leduox D, Nys M, Vrindts Y, De Groote D, Franchimont P, Lamy M. Cytokine serum level during severe sepsis in human. IL-6 as a marker of severity. *Ann Surg* 1992; 215 (4): 356-361
16. Klava A, Windsor AC, Farmery SM, Woodhouse LF, Reynolds JV et al. Interleukin-10. A role in the development of post-operative immunosuppression. *Arch Surg* 1997 Apr; 132(4) 425-429
18. Opelz G, Sengar DPS, Mickey MR, Terasaki PI. Effect of blood transfusion on subsequent kidney transplants. *Transplant proc* 1973; 5:253-9
19. Gianotti L, Pyles T, Alexander JW et al. Impact of blood transfusion and burn injury on microbial translocation and bacterial survival. *Transfusion* 1992; 32:312-7
20. Waymack JP, Gallon L, Barcelli U, Trocki O, Alexander JW. Effect of blood transfusion on immune function. Alterations in macrophage arachidonic acid metabolism. *Ann Surg* 1987; 122:56-60
21. Kaplan J, Sarnaik S, Gitlin J, Lusher J. Diminished helper/suppressor lymphocyte ratios and natural killer activity in recipients of repeated blood transfusion. *Blood* 1984; 64:308-10
22. Stephan RN, Kisala JM, Dean RE, Geha AS, Chaudry IH. Effect of blood transfusion on antigen presentation function and on IL-2 generation. *Arch Surg* 1988; 123:235-40

23. Gianotti L, Pyles T, Alexander JW, Fukushima R, Babcock GF. Identification of the blood component responsible for increased susceptibility to gut-derived infection. *Transfusion* 1993; 33:458-465
24. Jensen LS, Kissmeyer-Nielsen P, Wolff B, Qvist N. Randomised comparison of leucocyte-depleted versus buffy-coat poor blood transfusion and complications after colorectal surgery. *Lancet* 1996; 348:841-5
25. Tartter PI, Quintero S, Barron DM. Perioperative blood transfusion associated with infectious complications after colorectal cancer operations. *Ann Surg* 1986; 152:479-482
26. Tartter PI. Blood transfusion and infections in colorectal cancer surgery. *Br J Surg* 1988; 75: 789-792
27. Braga M, Vignali A, Radaelli G, Gianotti L, Di Carlo V. Association between perioperative blood transfusion and postoperative infections in patients having elective operations for gastrointestinal cancer. *Eur J Surg* 1992; 158:531-536
28. Ota D, Alvarez L, Lichtiger B et al. Perioperative blood transfusion in patients with colon carcinoma. *Transfusion* 1985; 25: 392-394
29. Mc Alister FA, Clark HD, Wells PS, Laupacis A. Perioperative allogenic blood transfusion does not cause adverse sequelae in patients with cancer: a meta-analysis of unconfounded studies. *Br J Surg* 1998; 85:171-178
30. Vignali A, Braga M, Gianotti L et al. A single unit of transfused allogenic blood increases postoperative infections. *Vox Sang* 1996; 71:170-175
31. Kim U, Papatestas A, Aufses AH. Prognostic significance of pheripheral lymphocyte counts and carcynoembryogenic antigens in colorectal carcinoma. J Surg Onc 1976; 8 : 257-262
32. Riesco A. Five year cancer cure: relation to total amount of peripheral lymphocytes and neutrophils. *Cancer* 1970 ; 25: 135-140
33. Maltoni M, Pirovano M, Nanni O, Marinari M, Indelli M, Gramazio A, Terzoli E, Luzzani M, De Marinis F, Caraceni A, Labianca R. Biological indices predictive of survival in 519 italian termilnally ill cancer patients. *J Pain Symptom Manage* 1997; 13: 1-9
34. Yamaguchi K, Maeda S, Kitamura K. Prognostic factors in colorectal carcinoma: significance of peripheral T lymphocytes. *Int Surg* 1989; 74: 232-239
35. Lundy J, Lovett EJ, Wolinsky S. Immune impairment and metastatic tumour growth: the need for an immunorestorative drug as an adjuvant to surgery. *Cancer* 1979; 43: 945-951
36. Weese JL, Emoto SE, Sondel E. Reduced incidence of hepatic metastases by peri-operative treatment with rIL-2. *Dis Colon Rectum* 1987; 30: 503-507
37. Colacchio TA, Yeager MP, Hildebrandt LW. Perioperative immunomodulation in cancer surgery. *Am J Surg* 1994; 167: 174-179
38. Brivio F, Lissoni P, Tisi E, Erba L, Barni S, Tancini G, Rescaldani R, Alderi G, Nociti V. Effects of a pre-operative therapy with interleukin-2 on surgery-induced lymphocytopenia in cancer patients. *Oncology* 1992; 49 (3): 215-218
39. Brivio F, Lissoni P, Barni S, Tancini G, Ardizzoia A, Erba L, Alderi G, NocitiV. Effect of a pre-operative course of interleukin-2 on surgical and immunobiological variables in patients with colorectal cancer: a phase II study. *Eur J Surg* 1993; 159: 43-47
40. Nichols PH, Ramsden CW, Ward U, Sedman PC, Primrose JN. Perioperative immunotherapy with recombinant interleukin-2 in patients undergoing surgery for colorectal cancer. *Cancer Res* 1992 15; 52 (20): 5765-5769
41. Deehan DJ, Heys SD, Ashby J, Eremin O. Interleukin-2 (IL-2) augments host cellular immune reactivity in the perioperative period in patients with malignant disease. *Eur J Oncol* 1995; 21: 16-22
42. Bovo G, Brivio F, Brenna A, Fumagalli L, Perego P, Brivio O, Uggeri F, Lavorato F, Bratina G. Pre-operative Interleukin-2 immunotherapy induces eosinophilic infilltration in colorectal neoplastic stroma. *Pathologica* 1995; 87: 135-138

43. Brivio F, Lissoni P, Ffumagalli L, Girlando M, Marsili MT, Nespoli A, Uggeri F. Pre-operative IL-2 immunoprophilaxis of cancer recurrence: long term clinical results of a phase II study in radically operable colorectal cancer. *Oncol Report* 1999, 6: 1205-1207

44. Tzianabos Ao, Russel PR, Onderdonk AB, Gibson FC et al. IL-2 mediates protection Against abscess formation in an experimental model of sepsis. *Jour of Immun* 1999, 163: 893-897

SECTION II

HEPATO-BILIARY AND PANCREATIC SURGERY

CHAPTER 4

EVALUATION OF RENAL TUBULAR DAMAGE IN RATS WITH BILIARY OBSTRUCTION

Attilio Maria Farinon, Francesco Rulli, Michele Grande, Marco Gallinella Muzi, Paolo De Sole*, Mauro Piantelli**, Mario Bosco***, Antonio Villani***

*Department of Surgery, University of Rome "Tor Vergata", and Institutes of *Physiology, **Pathology and ***Anesthesiology, Catholic University of the Sacred Heart, Rome, Italy*

Abstract

Background. It is widely believed that liver disease predisposes towards acute tubular necrosis. The present study evaluates the reliability of urinary enzymes (AGL, AAP) assay in jaundiced rats, its relationship with biochemical data of renal function and pathologic findings of kidney damage.

Methods. Acute cholestatic liver disease was induced by ligation of the common bile duct (40 CBDL rats). These animals, as well as the 20 sham operated (SO), were randomly chosen to be sacrificed under anesthesia, on the 5th , 10th, 20th and 30th postoperative day. Renal injury was assessed by blood urea nitrogen, plasma creatinine, urine creatinine, creatinine clearance, urinary sodium, urinary potassium, α-glucosidase (AGL), alanineaminopeptidase (AAP) concentrations, plasma and urine osmolality, and renal histology.

Results. A significant variation of creatinine clearance (p.0001) and diuresis (p-01) was recorded in CBDL rats sacrificed on the 10th postoperative day. A progressive decrease in sodium urinary excretion was observed in CBDL rats sacrificed on the 20th postoperative day. A significant decrease from 5th to the 30th day was observed in urinary osmolality, in CBDL rats with a minimum peak in the 30th postoperative day. In CBDL rats a significant correlation was also found between the severity of tubular lesions and the fractional excretion of urinary enzymes (Ufr AGL/24h: r=0.77, p.001; Ufr AAP/24h: r=0.69, p.01).

Conclusions. Our study shows that common bile duct ligation in rats, is responsible for a complex functional response of the kidney, and that renal function is variously threatened by jaundice. The diagnostic role of urinary enzymes remains confined to the detection of acute renal failure which, in our experimental settings, is only one aspect of the impairment of renal function in bile duct ligated animals.

A.M. *Farinon (ed.), Advances in Abdominal Surgery 2002*, 55-66.

INTRODUCTION

Impairment of renal function represents a known consequence in a setting in which the kidney is exposed to ischemic or nephrotoxic insults, and such insults are considered to be more likely to instigate acute tubular necrosis, when liver function is concomitantly and significantly impaired by hepatocellular or cholestatic lesions [1-2].

Bile and its constituents are normally excreted via the biliary and gastrointestinal tracts, and, whenever this route is obstructed the kidney becomes the main excretory organ, and the jaundiced animals survival is critically dependent upon its function. For this reason, as stated by Better [3], bile duct ligation represents indeed a valid model for the study of kidney dysfunction due to liver disease. In this field, the alteration of proximal tubules represents the most striking lesion induced by obstructive jaundice [4].

Under normal conditions, most enzymes derived from renal parenchyma are excreted in urine, as a result of normal turnover rate and permeability of tubular cells. However, the increased excretion of these enzymes (parenchymatous enzymuria) is related to their leak from the damaged tubular cells, and accounts for the presence of an anatomic lesion [5-6].

Among these latter enzymes, a-glucosidase (AGL), a lysosomal enzyme of tubular cells [7], and alanineaminopeptidase (AAP), a protease widely represented in the brush border of the renal tubular cells [8], may be considered as highly specific indicators of proximal tubular damage.

This study was then undertaken to evaluate the reliability of urinary enzymes (AGL, AAP) assay in jaundiced rats and to assess its relationship with biochemical data of renal function and pathologic findings of kidney damage.

MATERIAL AND METHODS

Seventy-five male Sprague-Dawley rats, weighing between 180 and 250 g, were employed. Ligation of the common bile duct or sham operation was performed under anesthesia with intraperitoneal diazepam (1 mg/100 g body weight) and intramuscular ketamine hydrochloride (2 mg/100 g body weight).

In forty rats, following an upper midline abdominal incision, the bile duct was isolated, and double ligated. Sham-operated rats underwent laparotomy and mobilization of the gut, without manipulation or ligation of the bile duct. Both groups of rats had free access to tap water and standard rat chow (Altromin-R, Rieper, Vandoies,Italy) prior to and after surgery.

The rats were therefore individually housed in metabolic cages, and the animal states of consciousness and diuresis were checked daily.

0ut of the 40 common bile duct ligated (CBDL) rats 21 survived, and they were considered for the study. These animals, as well as the 20 sham operated (SO) rats, were randomly chosen to be sacrificed on the 5th (group A: 6 CBDL, 6 SO), 10th (group B: 4 CBDL, 5 SO), 20th (group C: 8 CBDL, 6 SO), and 30th (group D: 3 CBDL, 3 SO) postoperative day.

The day before sacrifice, 24-hour urine samples were collected and assayed for sodium, potassium, creatinine, protein, and urine osmolality, as well as 2-hour fresh urine samples which were assayed for enzymuria.

In the fresh urine, centrifuged at 2,500 rpm for ten minutes, the activities of AGL and AAP were measured using two commercially available kits (No. G1342 for AGL and No. 3002 for AAP) from FAR (Verona, Italy). The kinetics measurements were performed at 37°C , at 405 nm according to the instructions of the manufacturer. The values of AGL and AAP urinary excretion were divided by creatinine clearance (Ccr) to obtain fractional excretion (Ufr) of the urinary enzymes. Data were expressed in this form, considering that urinary excretion of enzymes is related to glomerular filtration rate [9].

Because there is no generally accepted view regarding a suitable reference basis for urinary enzymes [10], ten rats were poisoned by subcutaneous injection (0.1 mg/100 g body weight) of solution of mercury bichloride (HgCl2), a well-known nefrotoxic agent, which produces tubular necrosis with renal insufficiency [11]. In these animals urine samples were collected before and 24 hours after mercury poisoning, and assayed for enzymuria (AGL, AAP) according to the method previously described (Ufr AGL/24h: basal = 1.1 + 0.6, after poisonning = 2.5 + 1.3; Ufr AAP/24h: basal = 64 + 50, after poisonning = 205 + 53).

On the appropriate day, the rats were sacrificed under anesthesia and blood samples were collected from the left cardiac ventricule, to be assayed for bilirubin, urea nitrogen, creatinine, sodium, potassium, and plasma osmolality.

Urea nitrogen, creatinine, total bilirubin, sodium and potassium were measured by the ASTRA-8 automatic analyzer (Beckman Instr.,Brea, CA-USA).

Plasma and urine osmolality were determined by means of DIC osmotic pressure analyzer AUTO-STATOM 6010 (DIC, Kioto, Japan).

Proteinuria was determined by the sulfosalicylic turbidity method, according to Bradley et al.[12].

Basal values of all parameters were recorded from 5 untreated male rats (mean weight: 308 + 12 g), housed in metabolic cages for 10 days and sacrificed by exsanguination (cardiac puncture) under light ether anesthesia. Plasma and urine samples were assayed for baseline determination of plasma bilirubin (n.v.: 0.2 + 0.0 mg/dl), plasma urea nitrogen (n.v.: 13.7 + 0.9 mg/dl), plasma and urine creatinine-(n.v.: 0.6 + 0.1 mg/dl and 9.6 + 4.4 mg/dl/24h, respectively), urinary sodium and potassium excretion (n.v.: 1.4 + 0.2 mEq/l/24h and 1.3 + 1.2 mEq/l/24h, respectively), and plasma and urine osmolality (n.v.: 320

+ 19 mOsm/Kg and 1899 + 270 mOsm/Kg, respectively). The mean values of diuresis and creatinine clearance were 10.2 + 7.4 ml/24h and 0.1 + 0.1 ml/24h respectively. Glomerular filtration rate accounted for 0.8 + 0.1 ml/min.

At sacrifice, liver and kidneys were removed for histopathological assessment. Tissues were fixed in 10% formalin and embedded in paraffin. Sections of liver and kidneys were stained with hematoxylin and eosin; silver metenamine PAS stain was also employed for the assessment of glomerular membrane thickening. Renal histologic findings were classified according to the score proposed by Amodio et al. [4], concerning interstitial, tubular, and glomerular cells lesion. Parameters considered, with a lesion score from 0 to 4, were: the extent of cellular degeneration; the amount of bile deposits in the cells; the number of biliary thrombi; the degree of interstitial fibrosis and phlogosis; the extent of tubular degeneration; the presence of glomerular proliferation or glomerular membrane thickening.

Statistical analysis

Results are expressed as mean ± standard deviation (SD), and are considered statistically significant for p.05.

For comparison between unpaired groups, the Student t test and Bonferroni Student – Newman Keuls test were employed as appropriate. Comparison of histologic findings between groups was performed, using Mann-Withney's test for non-parametric data.

RESULTS

All rats submitted to common bile duct ligation developed obstructive jaundice, with a peak of mean plasma bilirubin values (9.2 + 1.7 mg/dl) in group A CBDL animals (Tab. 1). On the contrary, no variation in the plasma bilirubin levels was found in the group D. At gross necroscopy, this observation was explained as the consequence of spontaneous recanalization of common bile duct. This was found in 2 CBDL rats of group B, in 1 CBDL rat of group C, and in all 3 rats of group D which survived until the 30th postoperative day.

As expected, no variation of plasma bilirubin levels was recorded in SO rats.

In Table 1, mean values of biochemical indices of renal function are reported, as well as fractional excretion (U fr) of assayed urinary enzymes (AGL, AAP). Diuresis, after a first unclear trend, showed a statistically significant rise in group B CBDL rats, when compared with urine volume of SO rats of the same group (37.0 + 12.6 vs 9.6 + 1.7; p 0.01). A polyuric trend was reported in Figure 1.

Table 1. Laboratory indices in CBDL and SO rats at time of sacrifice

	Group A		Group B		Group C		Group D	
	CBDL n = 6	**SO** n = 6	**CBDL** n = 4	**SO** n = 5	**CBDL** n = 8	**SO** n = 6	**CBDL** n = 3	**SO** n = 3
Plasma bilirubin (mg/dl)	9.2 ± 1.7**	0.1 ± 0.0	8.4 ± 2.5**	0.1 ± 0.0	7.3 ± 1.3**	0.2 ± 0.0	0.1 ± 0.0	0.1 ± 0.0
Diuresis (ml/day)	17.3 ± 5.2	18.7 ± 12.7	37.0 ± 12.6**	9.6± 1.7	24.8 ± 22.1	33.0 ± 17.9	66.7 ± 24.4	25.3 ± 17.7
Blood urea nitrogen (mg/dl)	18.5 ± 5.9	18.6 ± 2.5	13.3 ± 6.7	25.0 ± 9.3	43.3 ± 29.4	29.0 ± 13.6	11.7 ± 6.4	26.0 ± 7.8
Plasma creatinine (mg/dl)	0.5 ± 0.1	0.5 ± 0.1	0.3 ± 0.1	0.5 ± 0.1	0.5 ± 0.1	0.5 ± 0.1	0.6 ± 0.1	0.5 ± 0.1
Urine creatinine (mg/dl/24h)	2.7 ± 0.9	1.9 ± 0.8	15.0 ± 6.0	2.6± 1.3	4.2 ± 1.0	6.1 ± 2.1	7.4 ± 1.8**	0.8 ± 0.5
Creatinine clearance (ml/min)	0.4 ±0.1	0.3 ± 0.1	3.1 ± 0.6‡	0.4 ± 0.2	0.6 ± 0.2	0.9 ±0.4	0.8 ± 0.2‡	0.1 ± 0.0
Urinary sodium (mEq/l/24h)	0.8 ± 0.1	0.3 ± 0.1	0.7 ± 0.5	0.4 ± 0.2	0.2 ± 0.1†	0.7 ± 0.4	0.4 ± 0.2	0.6 ± 0.3
Urinary potassium (mEq/l/24h)	3.0 ± 0.9	0.6 ± 0.2	3.0 ± 0.9**	1.4 ± 0.8	1.4 ± 0.7	1.7 ± 1.0	1.7 ± 0.2	1.4 ± 0.7
Plasma osmolality mOsm/kg)	313 ± 30*	270 ± 18	323 ± 20	307 ± 15	332 ± 29	329 ± 68	327 ± 26	284 ± 34
Urine osmolality (mOsm/kg)	1154 ± 99**	490 ± 120	721 ± 436	1144 ± 451	641 ± 103	516 ± 270	152± 94*	900 ± 451
Ufr AGL / 24h	19.6 ± 10.3	17.9 ± 9.3	4.7 ± 1.7	7.0 ± 2.1	17.2 ± 8.3	18.3 ± 7.8	2.4± 0.37	6.6± 2.1
Ufr AAP / 24h	275 ± 100	394 ± 180	85 ± 20	90 ± 42	148 ± 90	153 ± 78	87 ± 20	102 ± 16

CBDL vs SO: *=p<0.05; **p<0.01; †=p<0.005; ‡=p<0.0001

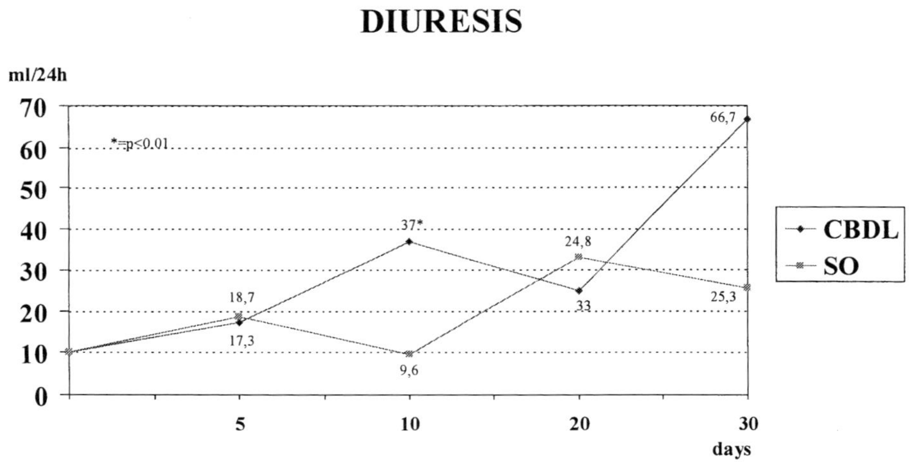

Figure 1. Comparison of mean 24 hour urinary volume between CBDL and SO rats sacrificed on the 5th, 10th, 20th and 30th day following surgery

However, no change in blood urea nitrogen and plasma creatinine was observed in CBDL rats. A significant variation of creatinine clearance (p.0001) was recorded in CBDL rats of group B and, in a less marked way, in group D (p.004) (Fig. 2).

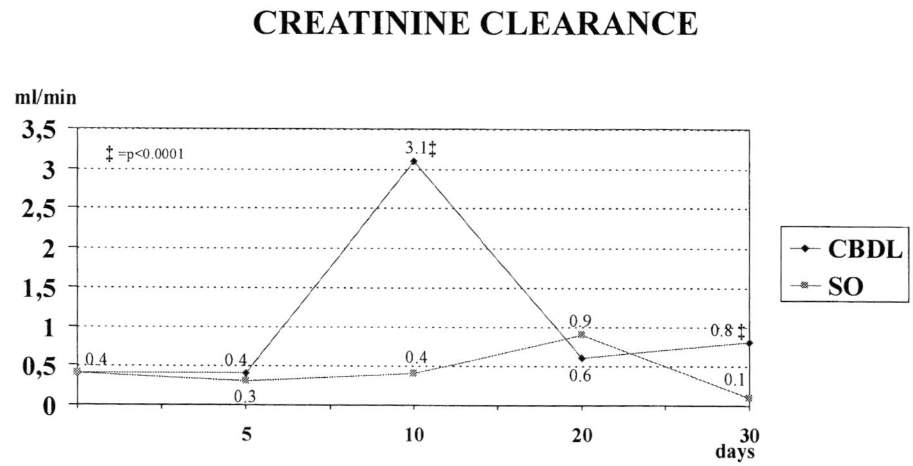

Figure 2. Comparison of urinary creatinine excretion and creatinine clearance mean values between CBDL and SO rats sacrificed on the 5th, 10th, 20th and 30th day following surgery

A progressive decrease in sodium urinary excretion was observed in CBDL rats, with a minimum peak (0,20 ± 0,1 mEq/l; p.005 vs SO) in the group C sacrificed on the 20th postoperatively day. On the contrary, concenring the urinary potassium, as well as serum sodium and potassium concentration, significant variations were not notified in the CBDL rats with respect to the SO rats.

A significant decrease from 5th to the 30th day was observed in urinary osmolality in CBDL rats, with a minimum peak in the 30th postoperatively day (152 ± 133 mOsm/kg) (Fig. 3). No remarkable variation between CBDL and SO rats was observed in plasma osmolality.

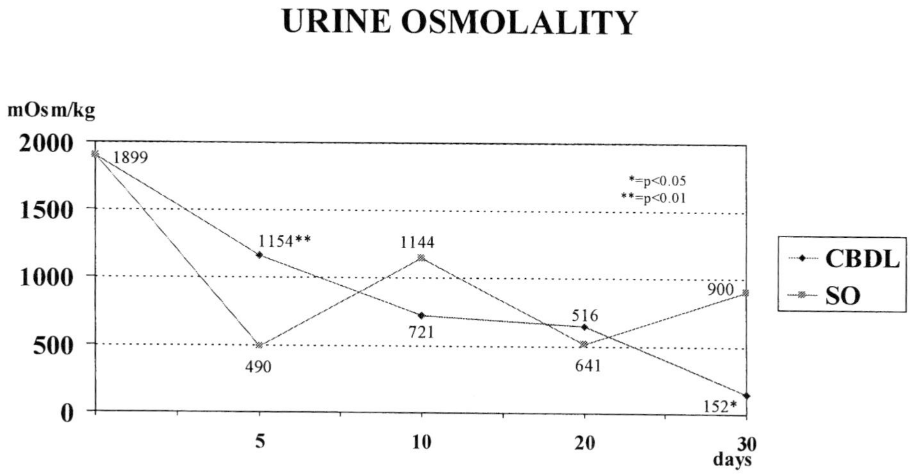

Figure 3. Comparison of urine osmolality mean values between CBDL and SO rats sacrificed on the 5th, 10th, 20th and 30th day following surgery

Glomerular filtration rate resulted as being slightly decreased (0.4 ± 0.3 ml/min) in group A CBDL rats, whereas it was considerably increased (4.9 ± 4.5 ml/min) in group B CBDL rats.

No variations were observed in urine protein levels that were not indicative of renal damage.

Light microscopic examination of kidney specimens revealed prevalently tubular cells degeneration, as well as the presence of biliary thrombi and bile deposits in cells; glomerular lesions were not observed (Tab.2).

Table 2. Kidney damage histological score in CBDL rats

Parameters	group A n=6	group B n=4	group C n=8	group D n=3
Cellular degeneration	12	5	14	6
Bile deposits in cells	9	6	20	6
Biliary thrombi	3	3	16	6
Interstitial fibrosis	0	0	0	0
Interstitial phlogosis	0	0	2	0
Tubular degeneration	15	6	14	4
Glomerular proliferation	0	0	0	0
Glomerular membrane thickening	0	0	0	0
Total score	39	20	66	22
Mean score	6.5	5.0	8.3	7.3

Group A vs B mean score: $p<0.05$; Group A and B vs C and D: $p<0.05$

The degenerative appearances were more prominent in group C CBDL rats, as was confirmed by statistically significant differences between mean lesion score of various groups (B vs C: p 0.05; A and B vs C and D: p 0.05). Large amounts of bile deposits in cells, as well as a high number of biliary thrombi, were more frequently detectable in group C CBDL rats (total score: 66; mean score: 8.3). Concerning SO rats, kidney histology showed minimal vacuolar lesions of tubular cells only in group A.

Significant correlations were obtained by comparing laboratory parameters to kidney damage score (urinary osmolality vs score: r=0.59, p.05; urinary sodium vs score: r=0.53, p.05; urinary potassium vs score: r=0.62, p.05).

In CBDL rats, a significant correlation was also found between the severity of tubular lesions and the fractional excretion of urinary enzymes (Ufr AGL/24h: r = 0.77, p.001; Ufr AAP/24h: r = 0.69, p.01). In spite of a lack of statistical significance of fractional excretion mean values (Tab.1), significant differences were found when comparing enzymes activity in urine from two animal groups with different score of tubular lesions (Tab.3).

Table 3. Correlation between fractional excretion of urinary enzymes and severity of tubular lesions

	tubular score = 2	tubular score > 2	Significance
Ufr AGL/24h	5.7 ± 2.6	25.0 ± 13.4	p<0.01
Ufr AAP/24h	131 ± 96	397 ± 136	p<0.01

DISCUSSION

Biliary obstruction acutely induced by common duct ligation produces hyperbilirubinemia with a mean peak value after 5 days. Levels of bilirubin, even in the presence of a progressive slight decrease, remain elevated until the 20th postoperative day, thereafter showing a sharp drop in values in surviving animals. The explanation for this latter phenomenon does not appear univocal: hepatic insufficiency increased renal excretion of bilirubin [13], recanalization after bile duct ligation [14], or even development of an internal bilio-digestive fistula [15-16] have all been repeatedly advocated. High mortality associated with bile duct ligation could then be related to liver failure, whereas survival of CBDL rats could be envisaged as being at least partly dependent upon spontaneous internal biliary drainage. As a consequence, bile duct ligation may be considered as a reversible model of biliary obstruction in some animals, even though it is not designed to be such in an experiment. This aspect appears of interest, in view of the fact that no animal model of reversible obstructive jaundice is simple, reproducible, and suitable for long-term longitudinal studies warranted for metabolic investigation [17].

Renal dysfunction due to impaired biliary outflow is mainly related to lesions of the proximal tubules. The correlation of these lesions to renal function parameters demonstrates that the kidney may express a protective response in critical condition induced by jaundice. Notwithstanding hypovolemia and a high level of antidiuretic hormone [18-20], generally reported after acute cholestasis in the rat, an increased diuresis was surprisingly observed. This increase appears to be dependent on the reduced urinary concentrating capacity substantiated by a decrease in urinary osmolality, more than likely due to changes in intrarenal blood flow [21-22], with concomitant reduction in outer cortical perfusion [19]. The enhancement of medullary flow with decreased medullary tonicity [23] would then be responsible for the reduced concentration ability of the kidney in jaundice [4].

Glomerular filtration rate resulted as being notably enhanced in our study, although others [4] failed to evidentiate relevant changes.

No proteinuria was found, in spite of tubular proteinuria related to impairment of proximal tubules, and glomerular proteinuria advocated by others [4] but not substantiated in our experience by the relief of alteration in any glomerular membrane morphology.

In our study, we found an increase, even if not significant, in the excretion of urinary sodium in the CBDL rats sacrificed on the 5th and 10th day postoperatively, while the minimum value (0.2 + 0.7 mEq/l/24h; p.005 vs SO) was found in group C CBDL in respect to SO rats. We believe that changes in the renal sodium excretion are due to the progressive proximal tubular damage responsible of loss of sodium.

The change in renal function following bile duct ligation has been primarily attributed to reduction in cortical perfusion [24]. The reduction in cortical perfusion may be due to increased activity of the renal α-adrenergic receptors, which are important determinants of renovascular tone [25]. This reduction in renal perfusion can explain the fall in urine osmolality after bile duct ligation, as has been underlined in our and in other studies [22]. The mechanism underlying these phenomena remains unclear, but the development of renal ischemic injury may play a role in the clinical evolution of postoperative acute renal failure in jaundiced rats.

Spontaneous internal biliary drainage significantly reduced renal impairment, the urinary sodium levels increased moderately, even though remaining lower than basal values, whereas creatinine clearance, urinary creatinine and glomerular filtration rate were in the normal range. Differently from Heidenreich et al [26] we have not found changes in plasma sodium concentration. The marked diuresis and decrease in urinary osmolality observed in group B and C CBDL rats suggested the presence of tubular refractoriness to antidiuretic hormones to be attributed to the progression of the cellular damage. In fact, the microscopic study of renal tissue from CBDL rats showed biliary thrombus and, in most samples, signs of tubular degeneration due to the presence of bile deposits in cells.

In jaundiced rats a highly significant relation between laboratory parameters and kidney damage score was found; moreover, the severity of tubular lesions presents a significant correlation with fractional excretion of urinary enzymes.

The interpretation of this data is multifaceted because it is difficult to separate the physiological response to surgical trauma from the effects related to the jaundice. On the other hand, renal function may be influenced by several factors such as rough handling of the animals during experiments [4], and changes in fluid and food intake [3-4].

Recently Leung et al. [27], outlined a novel form of acquired resistance to renal injury and speculated that such potentially cytoprotective alteration may safeguard the kidney against irreversible functional and structural injury, in the hepatorenal syndrome.

In conclusion, our study shows that common bile duct ligation in rats, is responsible for a complex functional response of the kidney, and renal function is variously challenged by the jaundice. Impaired renal function in the epatorenal syndrome can, in fact, lead to recovery when liver function is restored, as indicated by the amelioration of normal renal function, after spontaneous recanalization of the common bile duct, as observed by us and others [14].

So far, we have also found a correlation between tubular lesions and the fractional excretion of urinary enzymes. Anyway, the diagnostic role of urinary enzymes remains confined to the detection of acute renal failure which, in our experimental settings, is only one aspect of the impairment of renal function in bile duct ligated animals. In fact, the detection of enzymuria, even if not statistically significant, was observed in the rats of the C group, with unrecovered hepatic function.

In summary, our studies demonstrate that the animal model introduced by Trams and Symenoidis [14] can be employed to study both functional (i.e. hepato-renal) and organic (i.e. acute renal failure) renal impairment, and confirm that the detection of enzymuria is diagnostic only in the case of acute renal failure.

REFERENCES

1. Epstein M: Hepatorenal syndrome: emerging perspectives of pathophysiology and therapy. *J Am Soc Nephrol* 1994; 4:1735-1753.
2. Woolfson RG, Hillman K: Causes of acute renal failure, in *Comprehensive Clinical Nephrology*, edited by Johnson RJ, Feehally J, New York, Mosby, 2000, pp 16.1-16.16.
3. Better O S: Bile duct ligation: an experimental model of renal dysfunction secondary to liver disease. In: Epstein M (ed): *The kidney in liver disease*, New York, Elsevier, 1983, pp 289-301.
4. Amodio P, Rigotti P, Bazzerla G, Pagnini-Arslan C, Bonvicini P, Milani L, Ancona E, Gatta A: Are urinary enzymes useful markers of kidney damage in obstructive jaundice? *Nephron* 1985; 39: 377-381.
5. Burchard U, Haschen RJ, Krosch H: Clinical usefulness of enzyme determinations in urine; in Dubach, Schidt (ed): *Diagnostic significance of enzyme and proteins in urine*. Bern, Huber, 1979, pp 106.
6. Bonini PA, Guarnieri GF, De Nadai-Frank A, et al: Significato fisiopatologico e applicazioni cliniche degli enzimi urinari. *Quad Sclavo Diagn.* 1973; 9(1):419-441.
7. Ceriotti G, Bonini PA: Specificita dell'α-glucosidasi urinaria nelle lesioni citolitiche del tubulo renale. *Minerva Nefrol* 1971; 18:126.
8. Peters JE, Mampel E, Schneider I, Burchardt U, Fukala E, Ahrens I, Haschen RJ: Alanine aminopeptidase in urine in renal diseases. *Clin Chim Acta* 1972; 37:213-224.
9. Ceriotti G, Guarnieri GF: Physiological background for a possible utilisation of urinary enzymes in clinical diagnosis. *Proc 6th Int Symp Clin Enzymol.* Venice, 1974, p.255.
10. Yung K, Scholz D: An optymized assay of alanine aminopeptidase activity in urine. *Clin Chem* 1980; 26: 1251-1254.
11. Schreiner GE, Maher JF: Toxic nephropathy. *Am J Med* 1965; 38: 409-439.
12. Bradley M, Schumann GB, Ward PCJ: Examination of urine. In: Henry JB (ed.): *Clinical diagnosis and management by laboratory methods*-Todd Sanford. Philadelphia, Saunders, 1979, pp 559-634.
13. Stein TA, Burns GP, Wise L: Diagnostic value of liver function tests in bile duct obstruction. *J Surg Res* 1989; 46:226-229.
14. Trams GE, Symeonidis A: Morphologic and Functional changes in the liver of rats after ligation or excision of common bile duct. *Am J Path* 1957; 33:13-25.
15. Van Vleet JF, Alberts JO. Evaluation of liver function tests and liver biopsy in experimental carbon tetrachloride intoxication and extrahepatic bile duct obstruction in the dog. *Am J Vet Res* 1968; 29:2119.
16. Kirshner R, Hartung H, Trendelenburg C: Experimentelle Untersuchimgen bei kurtkistigen und dauerhaftem gallengsverschluss. *Leber Magen Darm* 1980; 220-225.

17. Posner MC, Burt ME, Stone MD, Lihan B, Narren RS, vydelingum NA, Brennan MF: A model of reversible obstructive jaundice in the rat. *J Surg Res* 1980; 48: 204-210.
18. Aarseth P, Aarseth S, Bergan A: Blood volume partition after acute cholestasis in the rat. *Eur Surg Res* 1976; 8:61-70.
19. Yarger WE: Intrarenal mechanisms of sat retention after bile duct ligation in rats. *J Clin Invest* 1976; 57: 408-410.
20. Better OS, Massry SG: Effect of chronic bile duct obstruction on renal handline of salt and water. *J Clin Invest* 1972; 51:402-411.
21. Better OS, Aisenbrey GA, Berl T: Role of antidiuretic hormone in impaired urinary dilution associated with chronic bile duct ligation. *Clin Sci* 1980; 58:493-500.
22. Allison MEM, Moss NG, Fraser MM: Renal function in chronic obstructive jaundice: a micropuncture study in rats. *Clin Sci Mol Med* 1978; 54:649-659.
23. Massry SG, Klein KL: Effects of bile duct ligation on renal function. In: Epstein M. (ed): *The kidney in liver disease*. New York, elsevier, 1978; pp 151-162.
24. Better OS, Bomzon A: Effects of jaundice on the renal and cardiovascular systems. In: Epstein M (ed.): *The kidney in liver disease*. Baltimore, Williams & Wilkins 1988;pp 508-534.
25. Bomzon A, Better OS, Blendis LM: Renal alpha-1-adrenoreceptors in rats with obstructive jaundice. *Nephron* 1986; 42: 258-261.
26. Hidenreich S, Brinkema E, Martin A, Dusing R, Kipnowski J, Kramer HJ : The kidney and cardiovascular system in obstructive jaundice: functional and metabolic studies in conscious rat. *Clin Sci* 1987; 73: 593-599.
27. Leung N, Croatt AJ, Haggard JJ, Grande JP, Nath KA. Acute cholestatic liver disease protects against glycerol-induced acute renal failure in the rat. Kidney Int 2001; 60:1047-157.

CHAPTER 5

THE EVOLUTIONARY PATTERN OF PRIMARY SCLEROSING CHOLANGITIS: FROM A BENIGN TO SEVERE DISEASE

Sara D'Innocenzo, Francesca Russo, Lucia Miglioresi, Marco Bacosi, Giovanni L. Ricci
Liver Pathophysiology Laboratory, Department of Clinical Sciences, University of Rome "La Sapienza", Rome, Italy

Acknowledgements
This work is largely based on reports presented at the Single Topic Conference on Primary Sclerosing Cholangitis organised by the American Association for the Study of Liver Disease at Emory University, Atlanta GA, in September 2000.

DIFFERENT CLINICAL VARIETIES OF PSC.

The natural history of primary sclerosing cholangitis (PSC) is, to say the least, puzzling in its variability, in terms of age of onset, symptoms and prognosis.[1-2] As a matter of fact there are several, unfortunately independent areas of observation: the Doctor following a patient with Ulcerative Colitis (UC) or Crohn's Disease (CD), who sees quite a benign increase of serum alkaline phosphatase (sALP) and is not worried about it, the Hepatologist who is quite happy to have found a rare disease, or the Endoscopist willing to perform exploration and diagnosis, but little interested in the radiologic aspect.

With this procedure, there is no possibility of measuring the progression of disease of the single patient. The prognostic models are only descriptive, and there is no true way of predicting the onset of liver failure, which is the reason to transplant, or identify a prodromic stage of PSC where inflammation can still be counteracted.

A.M. *Farinon (ed.), Advances in Abdominal Surgery 2002*, 67-84.

Asymptomatic versus symptomatic

Originally, many patients who were recognized as having this disease presented features of advanced liver disease. Now, increasingly, it appears that more cases are being discovered incidentally, often during evaluation for abnormal liver tests, seen in association with inflammatory bowel disease. During the time span in which the PSC progresses, more than a third of patients will eventually develop one or more symptoms. Over an average period of 10-15 years, patients often progress to the end-stages of liver disease, and suffer the consequences of a failing liver or require liver transplantation..

Although this course can be highly variable with some patients surviving 25 years or more, with nearly asymptomatic PSC, other patients develop end-stage disease within a year of diagnosis. Symptoms that can occur in these patients include fatigue most commonly, pruritus, jaundice, weight loss or gastrointestinal bleeding [1, 3-4]. Patients may have intermittent symptoms of fever, chills, and pain in the right upper quadrant consistent with cholangitis in about 10% of patients.

The clinical course can follow a number of paths. Perhaps the most common is that of halting progression towards the development of signs and symptoms of advanced liver disease, with portal hypertension, eventual symptoms of liver failure, and need for liver transplantation. A smaller number of patients experience intermittent episodes of cholangitis.

Patients with primary sclerosing cholangitis may also develop portal hypertension. There are no good medical history studies regarding the frequency or cause of the portal hypertension that occurs in these patients. They can develop gastroesophageal varices and suffer from variceal hemorrhage. A unique complication of portal hypertension in patients with primary sclerosing cholangitis, after a colectomy and ileostomy, is the development of peristomal varices[5]. If these peristomal varices bleed, they can be difficult to control and may require either placement of TIPSS, portocaval shunt surgery, or liver transplantation.

The estimated average survival from the time of diagnosis to death, for liver transplantation, is within the range of 10-15 years [6, 7]. Both variceal bleeding and cholangiocarcinoma can complicate the course of the disease. Patients presenting symptoms seem to have a shorter estimated survival, although asymptomatic patients frequently become symptomatic during the course of the disease and seem to follow a parallel course which is only slightly longer but is otherwise comparable [8].

The cholangiographic distribution of abnormalities, either extra- or intra-hepatic versus both intra- and extra-hepatic, does not seem to influence the course of the disease.

Several models have been developed to describe the course of disease and to better asses the difference in survival between asymptomatic and symptomatic patients [6-7, 9-10]. A recent report, still in abstract form, has pointed out two variables identifying bad prognosis and the timing for transplantation [11], i.e. when consistently high serum cholesterol and raising sALP slow down their increase and start to drop.

Age of onset

The age of onset is present as a variable in many models of survival (Tab.1): it is not clear what its real meaning is. In Scandinavian experience, the range of onset is between 8 and 88 years [13-14]: this casts a doubt as to whether the observed disease is the same. The consideration is that a fibrotic stenosis of bile ducts of different magnitude, resulting in a rise of SALP, appears as it is, a fibrotic stenosis more or less concentric around remnants of the original duct, and with different degrees of cellularity: the preceding damage and inflammation probably started with different pathogenetic mechanisms.

In children the disease resembles an auto-immune hepatitis, with a whole array of auto-antibodies and normal sALP [15-18] This could still be a sampling error, as in children a liver biopsy is more feasible than an ERCP; at the same time it could be a prodromal lesion. If this is the case, it is still unsettled as to whether the inflammatory cells are activated by peptides of unknown origin (biliary, viral, intestinal through the spaces of Disse and then in the linphatic peribiliary plexus) co-expressed with specific HLA-II [19-23], or whether the damage is aspecific, the inflammation being elicited by other mechanisms. In the latter case, the inflammation could simply produce ischemic, mechanical damage to the biliary epithelial cells, with a mechanism reproduced in similar settings [24].

Table 1. Models of medical history for Primary Sclerosing Cholangitis: some of them include the results of liver biopsy, i.e. not only intrahepatic localization of PSC but also the consequences of extrahepatic strictures. The age is both age at onset and age at time of evaluation: in general a young age of onset is associated with very rapid deterioration and bad prognosis.

Institution	**King's College (n=126) (15>**	**Swedish (n=305) (16)**	**Mayo (n=174) (20)**	**Multicenter (n=426) (21)**
Variables	Age	Age	Age	Age
		Hepatomegaly		
	Bilirubin	Bilirubin	Bilirubin	
	Histological	Histological	Histological	Histological
	Stage	Stage	Stage	Stage
	Splenomegaly		Hemoglobin	Splenomegaly
	Alkaline Phosph.			Inf. Bowel Disease

Time of diagnosis

Mathematical prognostic models are a useful tool in the stratification of disease both in clinical decisions and in conducting clinical trials; the variable "age" appears again with a different meaning. An advanced age with absence of bilirubin must probably be considered as being associated to a good prognosis: the disease existed a long time before producing clinically evident cholestasis, and will probably take time before becoming life-threatening.

These survival scores can be useful in helping to optimize timing for liver transplantation, although with increasingly long waiting lists, and current policies which assign livers to patients with the longest time on the waiting list, or to the most critically ill, providing an organ at the optimal time for transplantation has become increasingly difficult.

One of the characteristics of most of these models is the requirement for histologic staging. As noted above, sampling variability renders histologic staging of somewhat limited value in patients with primary sclerosing cholangitis; this is a flaw of many of these models. A recently developed model from Mayo Clinic relies on bilirubin, AST, history of variceal bleeding, and serum albumin [9, 24] , while histologic assessment is not required. The model has shown good correlation between estimated and actual survival. Other models that have been used include the Child-Pugh score: in comparison the Mayo Risk Score seems more apt to this specific disease [24, 26]. This is particularly evident for patients early on in the course of their liver disease when the Mayo model is compared to the Child-Pugh Score which was developed for patients with much more advanced liver disease.

A clinical onset with partcularly advanced disease at a younger age is correlated to a bad prognosis: the only treatment is ortotopic liver transplantation, and there is chance of recurrence of disease. At a more advanced age PSC follows a milder, clinical course, and palliative, surgical or endoscopic treatment of dominant biliary strictures may ensure reasonable well-being.

Mean of diagnosis

ERCP. In a review from Mayo Clinic 70 episodes of suspected dominant bile duct strictures, for which patients with PSC underwent ERCP, were found during a ten-year period among 1,000 patients [27]. This suggests that the rate of developing symptomatic dominant strictures is quite low. Occasionally, patients will develop intermittent fever or vague right upper quadrant discomfort, which may or may not be due to a dominant stricture, or represent true bacterial cholangitis.

In general bacterial cholangitis is a relatively uncommon event, but the incidental finding of PSC by retrograde cholangiography reveals an advanced disease. On the other hand, biliary obstruction almost always underlies the development of bacterial cholangitis, but dominant strictures rarely occur. Even less commonly, patients develop choledocholithiasis. Fortunately, complicating cholangiocarcinoma appears infrequently: 0.5 to 1 % of patients per year, with primary scierosing cholangitis, develop cholangiocarcinoma [28].

Histologic Changes. Histologic changes have been described elsewhere and there is enormous variability. Nearly all active UC develop edema and linfo-plasmacellular inflammation centered on the bile ducts: only few of these cases will develop fibrotic stenosis, with a clinical picture dominated by the cholestasis.

Because of what appears to be a great deal of variability also in the expression of disease throughout the liver histologically, it has not been possible to determine the average rate of histologic progression in patients with primary sclerosing choiangitis, unlike the situation in primary biliary cirrhosis, where a relatively accurate prediction of the rate of histologic progression can be made [29-30].

The recently described entity of small duct PSC also seems to follow a course comparable to classic PSC. These patients show similar clinical, biochemical, and histologic features and may make up fewer than 5% of patients with a histologic diagnosis of PSC [31-32]. These patients are distinguished by normal cholangiograms in the setting of inflammatory bowel disease. Some of these patients who develop cholangiographic features of classic PSC may also develop cholangiocarcinoma, or require liver transplantation. More work is required in order to understand the medical history of this variant.

PRESENCE OF IBD AND RISK OF COLONIC CANCER

While it is well-accepted that there is no relationship between the course of PSC, and the course and presence or absence of inflammatory bowel disease (IBD), or the severity of the course, patients with inflammatory bowel disease and PSC seem uniquely predisposed to developing colon cancer.

It is well-known that patients with UC run an increased risk of developing colorectal carcinoma. The two major risk factors for this complication are the long duration of disease and extension of colitis. The cause of neoplastic change in UC remains however unexplained, and the presence of PSC has been shown to increase the risk of colorectal cancer/dysplasia [33-37].

In a study from Sweden the absolute cumulative risk of developing colorectal dysplasia/cancer in the group UC plus PSC has been calculated as 9%, 31% and 50% respectively, after 10, 20 and 25 years; in the group with UC alone the risk was 2% 5% and 10% respectively [36].

Almost identical cumulative incidence of colorectal neoplasm was found in a recent Finnish case control study, including 45 patients with UC and concomitant PSC and 45 pair-matched control patients with UC only [37]. The cumulative incidence of colorectal neoplasm was 11% at 10 years and 31% at 20 years, from onset of disease in the group with UC and PSC, and 3% at 10 years and 8% at 20 years, in the control group of UC patients without PSC ($p<0.01$).

In a population-based cohort of 125 Swedish patients with concomitant PSC and UC, the risk of developing colorectal cancer but not dysplasia was assessed [38]. The cumulative risk of colorectal cancer after diagnosis of UC was 10%, 33% and 40% after 10, 20 and 30 years, respectively. In contrast, other studies did not find an increased risk for PSC patients with UC, of developing colorectal cancer/dysplasia [39, 41]. In a study from the Mayo Clinic, 178 patients with PSC were identified and stratified by geographical area of residence, and were followed up to determine development of colorectal carcinoma [40]. Comparisons were made with a previous study, in which the risk of colorectal cancer in UC had been assessed in a large cohort of UC patients (also including patients with PSC) [42]. Among the 178 PSC patients, no increased risk of development of colorectal carcinoma was found, compared to UC patients. However, among the 178 PSC patients only 143 patients had UC. In the subgroup of PSC patients with UC, the cumulative incidence of colorectal carcinoma and dysplasia was 20% at 20 years and 67% at 30 years after diagnosis of UC, indicating that also in this study PSC patients with UC run an increased risk of developing colorectal neoplasm. The opposite findings may partly be explained by a different study design. The ideal study design to determine whether PSC is an independent risk factor for colorectal cancer in patients with concomitant UC, would be a case-control study with appropriately matched controls. Co-variables would include age at onset of UC, duration of UC and previous liver transplantation [43].

Three studies have consistently shown that PSC patients develop a more proximal colorectal cancer compared to UC patients without PSC [40, 42]. In the study by Shetty et al, 76% of patients with PSC had neoplasm secondary bile acids. Since patients with cholestasis have a higher proportion of carcinogenic secondary bile acids, and the right colon is exposed to the highest concentrations of secondary bile acids, these acids might act as a possible carcinogen. Some studies have suggested that there might be a higher incidence of colorectal cancer in the first two years after liver transplantation [47, 49]. It would be of interest to study whether colorectal cancers after liver transplantation for PSC have the same localization in the colon as for UC patients without liver disease.

It is of importance to emphasise the necessity for all patients with PSC and UC to be included in colonoscopic surveillance programs, probably at an earlier time than UC patients without PSC. Also after transplantation, an annual colonoscopy of these patients is suggested.

THE PROGRESSIVE DISEASE

The estimated average survival from the time of diagnosis to death for liver transplantation, is within the range of 10-15 years [6-7]. As noted above, variceal hemorrhage in cholangiocarcinoma can complicate the course of the disease. Patients presenting symptoms seem to have a shorter estimated survival, although asymptomatic patients frequently become symptomatic during the course of the disease, and seem to follow a parallel course which is only slightly longer, but is otherwise comparable [8].

Retrospective analysis of endoscopic treatment procedures, including stone removal, naso-bilary drainage, dilatation and stenting, revealed clinical or cholangiographic improvement in 77% of PSC patients [50]. Overall survival at 1, 3, and 5 years following endoscopic biliary dilation were 91%, 80% and 68%, respectively. Ten endoscopically treated patients (29%) underwent OLT and all remain alive to date. OLT free survival in endoscopically-treated patients, comparing non-cirrhotic versus all patients, reveals 83%, 56%, and 42% versus 76%, 55% and 36% respectively. Selected non-cirrhotic patients may benefit from biliary enteric bypass of extrahepatic strictures [52-53]. Patients with histological stage 1 or 2 PSC, predominant extrahepatic or perihilar strictures, and clinical symptomatology such as pruritus, jaundice or cholangitis are candidates for resectional therapy. There has been no demonstrated difference in survival between groups with or without previous biliary tract surgery, when undergoing subsequent OLT.

Hepatic insufficiency

Primary sclerosing cholangitis is characterised by fibrosing inflammation of the intra- and extrahepatic biliary tree, with elevation of sALP and increased prevalence of HLA-II B8, DR3 and DR4 and perinuclear antineutrophil cytoplasmic antibodies (p-ANCA) in 82% of patients.

Basically it is a disease of the biliary tract, with remarkably normal parenchima: the presence of cholestasis and bile acid retention is able to produce progressive changes and lead to hepatic insufficiency.

Various medical regimens have been used to treat PSC, including steroids, azathioprine and D-penicillamine, with varied success. Estimated median survival time, from diagnosis to either death or OLT, is 12 years. Wiesner and La Russo reported 64% of PSC patients treated without transplantation and followed longitudinally, either died or developed end-stage liver disease.

Timing for OLTx

Sclerosing cholangitis accounts for nearly 10% of all liver transplants in North America, surpassed only by post-necrotic cirrhosis, primary biliary cirrhosis and Laennec's cirrhosis [53]. Liver transplantation is recognized as the treatment of choice, once advanced disease with cirrhosis and portal hypertension are present. Patients without cirrhosis may benefit from surgical, radiological and endoscopic procedures, but these become increasingly hazardous as the liver parenchyma becomes more diseased. These patients should be referred to OLT. Improvement in surgical and anaesthetic techniques, control of coagulation disorders, the use of venous bypass and new immunosuppressives, have led to improved patient survival after liver transplantation for PSC.

The OLTx survival has been excellent in this patient population, as seen in several studies [54]. The Pittsburgh-UNOS liver transplant registry reports a one-year survival rate of 84%, which compares favourably with the 82% one-year survival for primary biliary cirrhosis [55]. At UCLA 127 patients were transplanted for primary sclerosing cholangitis and achieved 1, 2, and 5-year actuarial survivals of 90%, 86% and 85% respectively. This experience demonstrates an excellent long-term outcome for these chronically ill patients, and compares favourably with smaller group reports and the recently reported larger experience from the Mayo clinic, where review of 150 patients demonstrated survivals of 94%, 92% and 86% respectively at 1, 2, and 5 years. Some reports have associated liver transplantation after biliary surgery with longer hospital stay, and an increased rate of morbidity and mortality [56]. Recently, this same group has updated their review of 150 patients undergoing OLT, demonstrating no increase in biliary complications, or decrease in survival in those patients who previously underwent biliary procedures, or had recurrent disease [57]. In other groups, previous biliary surgery did not adversely affect long-term patient survival.

Outcome of OLTx

Until recently, the diagnosis of recurrent sclerosing cholangitis was thought to be rare, but has now been quantified at 10-20%. The Mayo series revealed twenty-four of 120 patients with evidence of recurrent disease [58]. Twenty-two out of twenty-four (91%) had cholangiographic evidence and 11 patients (46%) histopathological evidence of recurrence. Overall survival was equal to those without PSC recurrence, and no specific risk factors were found. The experience in Pittsburgh was somewhat similar: an initial review in 1991 yielded 2.5% recurrence at 1 year, but in 1996 a retrospective study of the same population for incidence of recurrent PSC increased to 25% [59, 61]. When compared to a cohort of similar patients with identical biliary reconstructions there was a 4-fold greater incidence of histologic similarities in the PSC population. Biliary strictures may be secondary to 10w-grade bacterial cholangitis, related to the Roux-en-y biliary reconstructions, required in patients with primary sclerosing cholangitis. Additionally, ischemia related to chronic rejection, preservation injury, blood group mismatches, hepatic artery thromboses and viral infections, may all play a rôle in the development of strictures. However, classical fibro-obliterative lesions and periductal fibrosis were seen almost exclusively in patients having liver transplantation performed due to primary sclerosing cholangitis [62]. This finding was reported by Harrison, after pathologic review of 51 allograft specimens, from twenty-two patients transplanted for PSC by a single pathologist were compared to a control-group of non-PSC patients who had undergone Roux- en-y reconstruction. Non-anastomotic biliary strictures were found in 11(86%) of our post-transplant patient population. The presence of these strictures had no significant effect on patient or allograft survival.

The retransplant rate for PSC is similar to the initial transplantation rate of those non-cirrhotic patients treated by resection [63]. Multicenter prospective analysis of 447 patients undergoing OLT for either PSC or PBC, revealed that 10.4% were retransplanted. Consequent increases in death risk were noted to be 3.1 fold overall, and 6.7 fold greater in the group transplanted, more than 30 following initial grafting versus those patients receiving only one graft [64].

Primary sclerosing cholangitis is associated with long standing IBD, mainly UC, which is a risk factor for colorectal carcinoma [65]; it has also been well-documented that immunosuppression after transplantation leads to the development of certain forms of cancer, and the incidence of colorectal cancer after 15 to 25 years of UC has been reported as being from 1.5% to 35%. In our series, 30 patients (23%) have undergone colectomy since the time of their liver transplant. All patients are followed with semi-annual colonoscopy, and 27 patients have been found to develop dysplasia or overt colorectal carcinoma; the remaining three had recalcitrant UC that was difficult to manage medically. In our series, the patient survival was not significantly affected by the development of dysplasia or colorectal carcinoma. We feel that all patients should undergo colonoscopy at least every six months, and that colectomy should be performed as soon as dysplasia is found.

Based on the natural history of the disease, the following criteria are offered as guidelines in listing patients for transplantation [67]:

- MAYO Risk Score >4 or Childs-Pugh Score >7, i.e. cirrhosis with poor quality of life and/or complications of portal hypertension;
- Severe recurrent bacterial cholangitis, uncontrollable with antibiotics;
- Intractable pruritus

Relative listing criteria: bile duct dysplasia with possible diagnosis of cholangiocarcinoma.

Unsuitable criteria for listing:

- elevated CA 19-9;
- inflammatory bowel disease only;
- bone disease alone.

CHOLANGIOCARCINOMA

Cholangiocarcinoma, the most-feared long term complication in PSC, was found in one study to develop more often in patients with IBD complicated by colonic dysplasia/carcinoma [30], suggesting that these patients constitute a high risk subgroup for development of cholangiocarcinoma (CCA). If this finding is confirmed by further studies, the occurrence of colonic dysplasia may reduce the threshold for referring PSC patients to liver transplantation.

Cholangiocarcinoma (CCA) occurs in 15-30% of patients with PSC. Ultrasound guided biopsy of dominant strictures revealed cholangiocarcinoma in 75% of patients with such lesions [67]. Combination of CEA and CA19-9 provides better predictive correlation for occult tumors than any single serum marker [68].

The University of Pittsburgh Medical Center found a 10.6% incidence of CCA in explanted livers: 50% of these tumors were unrecognized prior to transplantation. In patients without CCA the authors reported 1 year and 5 year survival rates of 85% and 76%, respectively. When cases with CCA were included, 5-year survival fell to 27% [70], the decrease in survival being very sharp in those patients with T2 tumors or larger [71].

At UCLA an 11% incidence of CCA was detected: patients were then stratified into two groups, patients with known pretransplant CCA, or at the time of exploratory laparotomy found to have neoplastic changes on frozen sections of the biliary tree, and a second group consisting of patients with small (<1 cm) incidental intrahepatic CCA, found at the time of explant. All patients with known CCA had recurrence of the carcinoma, and no long-term survivors are noted. In contrast, patients with incidental CCAs have similar 1,2 and 5-year survivals to non-CCA patients: the same prognosis does not hold true for the incidentally discovered CCA.

Although the pathogenesis for cancer formation and progression in this disease is unknown, several theories have been advanced to account for certain aspects of the relationship. Increased biliary epithelial cell turnover is an important initiating element of the neoplastic process. Carcinogenic constituents of bile may play a rôle in inducing irreversible DNA structural damage in cells that are undergoing heightened cell turnover. Also genetic inherited differences in repair mechanisms of DNA may play a role in influencing the risk of tumor formation and rate of cancer progression.

Although the precise relationship between IBD and PSC is unknown, the inflammatory destruction of otherwise normal-appearing cellular constituents (bile duct epithelial cells, intestinal crypt epithelium) suggests similar immunologic disturbances for both conditions. There is at present no way to predict which patients will go on to develop the other disease, and there is no histologic means to identify that subset of patients with PSC who will develop CCA. It is expected that molecular markers will provide reliable discriminating parameters to accomplish the latter objective.

The histologic picture of sclerosing cholangitis includes inflammation of larger-sized bile ducts. The inflammatory cell infiltrate insinuates directly into the biliary epithelium of the affected bile ducts, causing biliary epithelial cell death and stimulating regenerative activity of bile ducts and ductules. The inflammatory infiltrate is mainly composed of chronic inflammatory cells such as lymphocytes, histiocytes and plasma cells. Acute inflammatory cells in the form of neutrophils and eosinophils are also frequently present. A critical element in the microscopic diagnosis of sclerosing cholangitis is inflammatory destruction of the biliary epithelial lining, which must be demonstrated to establish this diagnosis.

With time, the inflammatory nature of the disease is replaced by a fibrobliterative attack on bile ducts. Concentric bands of fibrous tissue, in a characteristic whorling pattern know as onion-skinning, replace the normal bile duct at the point of injury. In this state it may be difficult to demonstrate the inflammatory nature of the lesion; however obliterative onion-skinning fibrosis may substitute for this feature and provide a basis for histopathologic diagnosis. It is important to note that the inflammatory-fibrotic reaction is discontinuous in nature, and therefore subject to significant sampling error when only limited biopsy sampling is performed. Sclerosing cholangitis is discontinuous with respect to time, as new lesions in one part of the biliary tract may alternate with advanced fibrotic lesions in other areas and CCA is a malignant proliferation of bile duct epithelial cells, that can arise at any point in the biliary tree, from microscopic portal tracts to the ampullary region. The hallmark of this condition is uncontrolled cellular proliferation, which invariably manifests invasion into the bile duct wall by neoplastic bile duct cells. While exophytic growth of biliary epithelial cells can occur, producing tumor mass obstruction of bile flow, this is not the usual pattern of tumor growth. In this uncommon pattern of tumor expansion, CCA grows exclusively as a polypoid mass, with little or no invasion of the bile duct wall. Tumor growth in this form has been associated with a relatively better prognosis, probably related to the tendency for non-invasiveness with this form of bile duct cancer. Unfortunately, this less-invasive form of bile duct cancer growth is less often seen. More commonly the direction of tumor growth is into the bile duct wall, associated with fibrotic desmoplastic reactions of supporting mesenchymal cells. Biliary obstruction in CCA in this situation is secondary to constriction of the bile duct by this desmoplastic fibrotic reaction, which very characteristically accompanies the CCA invading the structure of the bile duct.

Cholangiocarcinoma cells display a range of cellular anaplasia, with well to moderately to poorly differentiated forms of cancer. The poorly differentiated forms of this tumor are easy to recognize by their marked degree of nuclear enlargement and pleomorphism. Well and moderately differentiated forms can be difficult to recognize, as their appearance may closely resemble that of reactive non-neoplastic biliary epithelial cells, which may be seen in benign bile duct strictures or in sclerosing cholangitis unassociated with cancer formation. This consideration is relevant for the diagnosis of CCA. Analysis of biliary cytology obtained by brushing is currently the best means of detecting CCA, with the expectation that it may be identified at a stage when it is still amenable to therapy for curative intent. Due to the overlapping cellular morphology between reactive non-neoplastic bile duct hyperplasia and CCA, a definitive diagnosis is very often not achieved by cytologic analysis alone. Instead, indeterminate diagnoses of "atypical" or "suspicious" are rendered in a significant proportion of cases. This has stimulated the application of molecular methods to cytologic specimens, in an attempt to improve upon the diagnosis of CCA in this situation, and to reduce the number of samples which are diagnosed in an indeterminate fashion.

Genetic alterations in bile duct cancer

Bile duct neoplasia is characterized by the accumulation over time of somatically acquired mutations, involving many well-characterized oncogenes and tumor suppressor genes. The list of available genetic targets for mutational change in CCA is likely to increase, as our understanding of the full range of relevant human genes becomes fully comprehensive, as the human genome project nears completion.

A large number of studies have indicated that a narrow group of specific genes are more likely to be altered in bile duct cancer. While geographic differences in the rate of mutation have been shown, in general, all studies point to growth regulatory genes mutations as being critical to the formation and progression of the forms of cancer. The group includes the p53, p16 (MTS1 or CDKN2A), retinoblastoma, APC and DCC tumor suppressor genes. Gene mutation and allelic bSS have been demonstrated for each of these important genes, not only in fully developed cancers, but also in early precursor lesions including biliary epithelial hyperplasia and dysplasia. The finding of this limited yet diverse spectrum of tumor suppressor gene alterations, supports the involvement of multiple different pathways for growth deregulation in the formation of bile duct cancer. The frequency of mutational change for these genes varies from 30% to over 80%, with mutation in multiple genes being the rule. Currently, no specific clinical or pathologic pattern of tumor growth or behavior can be attributed to any particular single or group of gene alterations, although several studies have suggested that localization of tumors within the biliary tract may be associated with certain forms of acquired mutational damage.

The most common oncogene alterations in bile duct cancer is point mutation of the k-ras-2 oncogene [9-10,12,14]. K-ras-2 mutation occurs in approximately 30% of tumors, and has been identified in cytologic specimens, including bile duct brushing and fluid aspirations. Point mutation is a convenient target for molecular detection, since the presence of a single mutated cell among many normal cells can be achieved by using highly sensitive polymerase chain reaction-based detection approaches. As with tumor suppressor gene mutation, it is important to note that k-ras-2 mutation can occur early in bile duct neoplasia, preceding overt cancer formation. Hence the presence of k-ras-2 mutation, as with any other single gene alteration, should not be interpreted as definitive for the presence of cancer.

The entire biliary tract epithelium often shows evidence of diffuse oncogenic changes, although the finding of CCA is in general localized to a single site. This is made manifest by the presence of biliary dysplasia, which is often encountered adjacent to the site of cancer formation in a given subject. In common with other premalignant conditions for cancer formation involving the gastrointestinal tract, biliary dysplasia points to the existence of a multistep process of acquired genetic damage, that provides a framework for progressive clonal expansion of neoplastic cells. Detection and characterisation of this precursor field of genetic-altered cells offers the best target for early detection and potential prevention of bile duct cancer.

While histologic and cytologic methods provide the most convenient means to evaluate the biliary epithelium, most common forms of mutational change cannot be effectively assessed by microscopic staining approaches alone. Ploidy analysis can be performed in this fashion, and studies have supported the relationship between the presence of aneuploidy and increased tumor biologic aggressiveness. However, the results of ploidy analysis have not been universal, and are less effective in the analysis of premalignant biliary tract abnormalities.

An alternative approach is tissue microdissection. Microdissection-based genotyping is a two-step process, that can be carried out on all types of clinical specimens, after routine tissue fixation and thorough microscopic analysis. The first step consists of removal of individual cells from four-micron-thick histologic sections, by manual or automated means. Tissue is removed according to cellular characteristics, and collected in a highly purified state free from normal supporting cells contamination. The second step consists of PCR followed by mutational analysis, to easily detect mutational change of multiple different cancer genes, in an objective and quantitative manner.

Using microdissection-based genotyping, it has been shown that the dysplastic field, such as occurs in the biliary tract in a subject with CCA, is made up of multiple clones of epithelial cells, each manifesting a unique constellation of acquired mutational change. Different segments of the biliary tract will have different genotypic patterns of damage, reflecting the diverse accumulation of mutation occurring throughout the affected organ. Not uncommonly, a patient with CCA will have two concurrent primary tumors in different regions of the biliary tract. The genotype pattern of damage of the two tumors has been shown to be different. The material required for analysis has been microdissected off the glass slide, and collected for multiple gene analysis, and a small but highly informative panel of 10-20 cancer associated genes has been identified. This approach is readily available at this time, and can be carried out in a timely and cost-effective manner: in particular, it is suitable for diagnostic evaluation of biliary tract dysplasia, enabling an objective assessment to be made of accumulated gene damage of clusters of cells otherwise characterized as atypical or suspicious for malignancy. It should be possible in the near future to predict in the individual patient with PSC, the likelihood of progression to CCA.

REFERENCES

1. Wiesner RH, LaRusso NF. Clinicopathologic features of the syndrome of primary sclerosing cholangitis. *Gastroenterology* 1980; 79:200-6.
2. Chapman RW, et al. Primary sclerosing cholangitis: a review of its clinical features, cholangiography, and hepatic histology. *Gut* 1980; 21:870-7.
3. LaRusso NF, et al. Current concepts. Primary sclerosing cholangitis. *New England Journal of Medicine* 1984; 310:899-903.
4 Lee YM, Kaplan MM.. Primary sclerosing cholangitis. *New England Journal of Medicine* 1995; 332:924-33.
5. Wiesner RH, et al. Peristomal varices after proctocolectomy in patients with primary sclerosing cholangitis. *Gastroenterology* 1986; 90(2):3 16-22.
6. Farrant JM, et al. Natural history and prognostic variables in primary sclerosing cholangitis. *Gastroenterology* 1991; 100(6):1 710-7.
7. Broome U, et al. Natural history and prognostic factors in 305 Swedish patients with primary sclerosing cholangitis. *Gut* 1996; 38:610-5.
8. Porayko MK, et al. Patients with asymptomatic primary sclerosing cholangitis frequently have progressive disease [see comments]. *Gastroenterology* 1990; 98(6):1594-602.
9. Wiesner RH, Grambsch PM, Dickson ER, et al. Primary sclerosing cholangitis: natural history, prognostic factors and survival analysis. *Hepatology* 1989; 10:430-436.
10. Dickson ER, et al. Primary sclerosing cholangitis: refinement and validation of survival models. *Gastroenterology* 1992; 103: 1893-901.

11. Bacosi M, et al. Follow up of 53 consecutive patients with PRIMARY SCLEROSING CHOLANGITIS from a single I.B.D. clinic. *Hepatology* 2000; 32: in press.
12. Okolicsanyi L, et al. Primary sclerosing cholangitis: clinical presentation, natural history and prognostic variables: an Italian multicenter study. *Eur.J.Gastroenterol. Hepatol* 1996; 8:685-691.
13. Boberg KM, et al. Natural history of primary sclerosing cholangitis. A long term follow-up study of 394 European primary sclerosing cholangitis patients. *J Hepatol* 2000; 33: in press.
14. Schrumpf E, Abdelnoor M, Fausa O, Elgio K, Jenssen E, Koimannskog F. Risk factors in primary sclerosing cholangitis. *J Hepatol* 1994; 24:1061-1066.
15. Boberg KM, Fausa O, Haaland T, et al. Features of autoimmune hepatitis in primary sclerosing cholangitis: an evaluation of 114 primary sclerosing cholangitis patients according to a scoring system for the diagnosis of autoimmune hepatitis. *Hepatology* 1996; 23:1369-1376.
16. Mieli Vergani G, Lobo Yeo A, McFarlane BM, et al. Different immune mechanisms lead to autoimmunity in primary sclerosing cholangitis and autoimmune chronic hepatitis of childhood. *Hepatology* 1989; 9:198-203.
17. Wilschamsk M, Chait P, Wade JA, et al. Primary sclerosing cholangitis in 32 children: clinical, laboratory and radiographic features, with survival analysis. *Hepatology* 1995; 22:1415-1422.
18. Chapman RW, Varzhese Z, Gaul R, et al. Anti-neutrophil antibody: a test for autoimmune primary sclerosing cholangitis in childhood. *Gut* 1993; 34:199-202.
19. Dienes HP, Lohse AW, Gerken G, et al. Bile duct epithelia as target cells in primary biliary cirrhosis and primary sclerosing cholangitis. *Virchows Arch* 1997; 431:119-124.
20. Hashimoto E, Lindor KD, Homburger HA, et al. Immunohistochemical caracterization of hepatic linphocytes in primary biliary cirrhosis in comparison with primary sclerosing cholangitis and autoimmune chronic active hepatitis. *Mayo Clin Proc* 1993; 68:1049-1055.
21. Washington K, Clavien PA, Killenberg P. Peribiliary vascular plexus in primary sclerosing cholangitis. *Histopathology* 1991; 19:321-327.
22. Sanchez Urdapzal L, Gores GJ, Ward EM, et al. Diagnostic features and clinical outcome of ischemic-type biliary complications after transplantation. *Hepatology* 1993; 17:605-609.
23. Kubota T, Thomson A, Clouston AD, et al. Clinicopathologic findings of recurrent primary sclerosing cholangitis after orthotopic liver transplantation. *J Hepatobiliary Pancreat Surg* 1999; 6:337-381.
24. Dickson ER, Murtaugh PA, Wiesner RH, et al. Primary sclerosing cholangitis: refinement and validation of survival models. *Gastroenterology* 1992; 103: 1893-1901.
25. Farrant JM, Hayìlar KM, Wilkinson ML, et al. Natural history and prognostic variables in primary sclerosing cholangitis. *Gastroenterology* 1991; 100:1710-1717.
26. Shetty K, Rybicki L, Carey WO. The Chiid-Pugh classification as a prognostic indicator for survival in primary sclerosing cholangitis. Hepatology 1997; 25: 1049-1053.
27. Dickson ER, et al. Primary sclerosing cholangitis. Refinement and validation of survival models. *Gastroenterology* 1992; 103:1893-1901.
28. Kaya M, Petersen BT, Angulo P, Lindor KD. Balloon dilatation compared to stenting of dominant strictures in primary sclerosing cholangitis. *Gastroenterology* 2000; 118: (AGA, San Diego, CA, abstract form).
29. Angulo P, et al. Time course of histological progression in primary sclerosing cholangitis. *American Journal of Gastroenterology* I999; 94(1 I):33 10-3.
30. Locke GR, 3rd, et al. Time course of histological progression In primary biliary cirrhosis. *Hepatology* 1996; 23(1):52-6.
31. Wee A, Ludwig J. Pericholangitis in chronic ulcerative colitis: primary sclerosing cholangitis of the smali bile ducts? *Annals of Internal Medicine* 1985; 102(5):581-7.
32. Angulo P, Maor-Kendler, Donunger JJ, Lindor KD. Small-duct primary sclerosing cholangitis: prevalence and natural history. (accepted for poster presentation, DDW May 2000, San Diego, CA).

33. Broome U, Lindberg G, Lòfberg R. Primary sclerosing cholangitis in ulcerative colitis: a risk factor for the development of dysplasia and DNA aneuploidy? Gastroenterology 1992; 102:1877-1880.
34. Broome U, Lofberg R, Veress B, Eriksson LS. Primary sclerosing cholangitis and ulcerative colitis: evidence for increased neoplastic potential. *Hepatology* 1995; 22:1404-1408.
35. Brentnaii TA, Haggitt RC, Rabinovitch PS, et al. Risk and natural history of colonic neoplasia in patients with primary sclerosing cholangitis and ulcerative colitis. *Gastroenterology* 1996; 110:331-338.
36. O'Haens GR, Lashner BA, Hanauer SB. Pericholangitis and sclerosing cholangitis are risk factors for dysplasia and cancer in ulcerative colitis. *Am J Gastroentero* 1993; 88:1 174-1178.
37. Leidenius MH, Farkkila MA, Karkkainen P, et al. Colorectal dysplasia and carcinoma in patients with ulcerative colitis and primary sclerosing cholangitis. *Scand J Gastroentero* 1997; 32:706-711.
38. Kornfeld O, Ekbom A, lhre T. Is there an increased risk for colorectal cancer in patients with ulcerative colitis and concomitant primary sclerosing cholangitis? A population based study. *Gut* I997; 41:522-525.
39. Gurbuz AK, Giardiello FM, Bayless TM. Colorectal neoplasia in patients with ulcerative colitis and primary sclerosing cholangitis. Dis Colon Rectum 1995; 38:37-41.
40. Loftus EV Jr, Sandborn WJ, Tremaine WJ, et al. Risk of colorectal neoplasia in patients with primary sclerosing cholangitis. *Gastroenterology* 1996; 110: 432-440.
41. Nuako KW, Ahlquist OA, Sandborn WJ, et al. Primary sclerosing cholangitis and colorectal carcinoma in patients with chronic ulcerative colitis: a case-control study. *Cancer* 1998; 82: 822-826.
42. Ekbom A, Helmick C, Zack M, Adami H. Ulcerative colitis and colorectal cancer. *N Engl J Med* 1990; 323:1228-1233.
43. Sandborn WJ, Loftus EV Jr, Ahlquist OA. Association of primary sclerosing cholangitis and colorectal cancer in patients with ulcerative colitis: is it true and does it matter? *Gastroenterology* 1998; 115: 236-237.
44. Marchesa P, Lashner BA, Lavery IC, et al. The risk of cancer and dysplasia among ulcerative colitis patients with primary sclerosing cholangitis. *Am J Gastroenterology* 1997; 92:1285-1288.
45. Shetty K, Rybicki L, Brzezinski A, Carey WO, Lashner BA. The risk for cancer or dysplasia in ulcerative colitis patients with primary sclerosing cholangitis. *Am J Gastroenterol* 1999; 94:1643-1649.
46. Lindberg B, Broomé U, Persson B. Proximal colorectal dysplasia/cancer in ulcerative colitis. The impact of primary sclerosing cholangitis and sulfasalzine: Results from a 20-year surveillance study. *Dis Colon Rectum* 2000; in press.
47. Bleday R, Lee E, Jessurun J, et al. Increased risk of early colorectal neoplasms after hepatic transplant in patients with inflammatory bowel disease. *Dis Colon Rectum* 1993; 36: 908-912.
48. Higashi H, Yanaga K, Marsh JW, et al. Development of colon cancer after liver transplantation for primary sclerosing cholangitis associated with ulcerative colitis. *Hepatology* 1990; 11:477-480.
49. Knechtle SJ, D'Alessandro AM, Harms BA, et al. Relationships between sclerosing cholangitis, inflammatory bowel disease, and cancer in patients undergoing liver transplantation. *Surgery* 1995; 118: 615-619.
50. Lee JG, Schutz SM, England RE, et al. Endoscopic therapy of sclerosing cholangitis. *Hepatology* 1995; 21:661.
51. Ahrendt SA, Pitt HA. Surgical treatment for primary sclerosing cholangitis. Journal of Hepatobiliary and Pancreatic Surgery 1999; 6:366-372.
52. Myburgh JA. Surgical biliary drainage in primary sclerosing cholangitis. The role of the Hepp-Couinaud approach. *Archives of Surgery* l994; 129: 1057-62.

53. Gordon R, Shaw B, Iwatsuki S, et.al. Indications for liver transplantation in the cyclosporine era. *Surg Clin North Am* 1986; 66:541-556.
54. Sekido H, Takeda K, Morioka D, et al. Liver transplantation for primary sclerosing cholangitis. *Journal of Hepatobiliary and Pancreatic Surgery* 1999; 6:373-376.
55. Belle S, Detre K. Report from the Pitt-UNOS liver transplant registry. *Transplant Pros* 1993; 25: 1137-1142.
56. Wiesner RH, Porayko MK, Hay JE, et al. Liver transplantation for primary sclerosing cholangitis. Impact of risk factors on out come. *Liver Transplantation and Surgery* 1996; 2:99-108.
57. Graziadei IW, Weisner RH, Marotta PJ, et al. Long-term results of patients undergoing liver transplantation for primary sclerosing cholangitis. *Hepatology* 1999; 30:1 121-27.
58. Graziadei IW, Weisner RH, Batts KP, et al. Recurrence of primary sclerosing cholangitis following liver transplantation. *Hepatology* 1999; 29: 1050-56.
59. Iwatsuki S, Starzl T, Van Thiel D, et al. Liver transplantation for sclerosing cholangitis. *Gastroenterology* 1991; 90: 1736-1742.
60. Sheng R, Campbell WL, Zajko AB, et al. Cholangiographic features of stricture after liver transplantation for primary sclerosing cholangitis: Evidence of recurrent disease. *American Journal of Roentgenology* 1996; 166:1109-1113.
61. Balan V, Abu-Elmagd K, Demtris AJ. Autoimmune liver diseases: Recurrence after liver transplantation. *Surgical Clinics of North America* 1999; 79:147-152.
62. Harrison R, Hubscher S. Sclerosing cholangitis in liver allografts: a historical perspective {Abstract}. *J Pathology* 1992; 168(suppl): 150A.
63. Ahrendt SA, Pitt HA. Surgical treatment for primary sclerosing cholangitis. *Journal of Hepatobiliary and Pancreatic Surgery* 1999; 6:366-372.
64. Kim WR, Weisner RH, Poterucha JB, et al. Hepatic retransplantation in cholestatic liver disease: Impact of the interval to retransplantation on survival and resource utilization. *Hepatology* 1999; 30:395-400.
65. LaRusso NF, Wiesner RH, Ludwig J, et al. Primary sclerosing cholangitis. *N Engl J Med* 1984; 310:899-903.
66. Wiesner R. Primarv sclerosing cholangitis: Minimal listing criteria for liver transplantation. (Abstract) ASTP Consensus Conference, Bethesda, Maryland 1997.
67. Mirza DF, Davies M, Oliff S. Preoperative diagnosis of cholangiocarcinoma in primary sclerosing cholangitis in potential liver transplant candidates. (Abstract). *Hepatology* 1994; 20:1 54A.
68. Ramage JK, Donaghy A, Farrant JM, et al. Serum tumor markers for the diagnosis of cholangiocarcinoma in primary sclerosing cholangitis. *Gastroenterology* 1995; 108(3):865-9.
69. Chalasani N, Baluyut A, Ismail A, et al. Cholangiocarcinoma in patients with primary sclerosing cholangitis: A multicenter case control study. *Hepatology* 2000; 3 1:7-11.
70. Abu-Elmagd K, Selby R, Iwatsuki S, et al. Cholangiocarcinoma and sclerosing cholangitis: clinical characteristics and effect on survival after liver transplantation. *Transplant Proc* 1993; 25: 1124-1125.
71. Nashan B, Schlitt HJ, Tusch G, et al. Biliary malignancies in primary sclerosing cholangitis: Timing of liver transplantation. *Hepatology* 1996; 23;1105-1111.
72. Mirza DF, Davies M, Oliff S. Preoperative diagnosis of cholangiocarcinoma in primary sclerosing cholangitis in potential liver transplant candidates. Hepatology 1994; 20:154(A).
73. Ramage JK, Donaghy A, Farrant JM, et al. Serum tumor markers for the diagnosis of cholangiocarcinoma in primary sclerosing cholangitis. *Gastroenterology* 1995; 108:865-869.
74. Chalasani N, Baluyut A, Ismail A, et al. Cholangiocarcinoma in patients with primary sclerosing cholangitis: A multicenter case control study. *Hepatology* 2000; 31:7-11.
75. Abu-Elmagd K, Selby R, Iwatsuki S, et al. Cholangiocaricnoma and sclerosing cholangitis: climcal characteristics and effect on survival after liver transplantation. Transplant Proc 1993; 25: 1124-1125.

76. Nashan B, Schlitt HJ, Tusch G, et al. Biliary malignancies in primary sclerosing cholangitis: Timing of liver transplantation. *Hepatology* 1996; 23:1105-1111.
77. Tannapfel A, Weinans L, Geissler F, Schutz A, Katalinic A, Kockerling F, Hauss J, Wittekind C. Mutations of p53 tumor suppressor gene, apoptosis, and proliferation in intrahepatlc cholangiocellular carcinoma of the liver. *Digestive Diseases & Sciences* 45:317-24.
78. Hidaka E, Yanagisawa A, Seki M, Takano K, Setoguchi T, Kato Y. High frequency of K-ras mutatlons in biliary duct carcinomas of cases with a ion common channel in the papilla of Vater. *Cancer Research* 2000; 60:522-4.
79. Rijken AM, Hu J, Perlman EJ, Morsberger LA, Long P, Kern SE, Hruban RH, Yeo CJ, Griffin CA. Genomic alterations in distai bile duct carcinoma by comparative genomic hybridization and karyotype analysis. *Genes, Chromosomes & Cancer* 1999; 26:185-91.
80. Itoi T, Ohyashiki K, Yahata N, Shinohara Y, Takei K, Takeda K, Nagao K, Hisatoml H, Ebihara Y, Shay JW, Salto T. Detection of telomerase activity in exfoliated cancer cells obtained from bile. *International Journal of Oncology* 1999; 15:1061-7.
81. Yokoyama Y, Hiyama E, Murakami Y, Matsuura Y, Yokoyama T. Lack of CD44 variant 6 expression in advanced extrahepatic bile ductlar ampullary carcinoma. *Cancer* 1999; 86(9):1691-9.
82. Kamikawa T, Amenomori M, Itoh T, Momoi H, Hiai H, Machinami R, Ishikawa Y, Mori T, Shimahara Y, Yamaoka Y, Fukumoto M. Analysis of genetic changes in intrahepatic cholangiocarcinoma induced by thorotrast. *Radiation Research* 1999; 152 (6 Suppl):S1 18-24.
83. Ahrendt SA, Eisenberger CF, Yip L, Rashid A, Chow JT, Pitt HA, Sidransky D. Chromosome 9p21 and p16 inactivation in primary sclerosing cholangitis-associated cholangiocarcinoma. *Journal of Surgical Research* 1999; 84(1):88-93.
84. Tannapfel A, Engeland K, Weinans L, Katalinic A, Hauss J, Mossner J, Wittekind C. Expression of p73, a novei protein related to the p53 tumour suppressor p53, and apoptosis in cholangiocellular carcinoma of the liver. *British Journal of Cancer* 1999; 80(7):1 069-74.
85. Sturm PD, Rauws EA, Hruban RH, Caspers E, Ramsoekh TB, Huibregtse K, Noorduyn LA, Offerhaus GJ. Clinical value of K-ras codon 12 analysis and endobiliary brush cytology for the diagnosis of malignant extrahepatic bile duct. *Clinical Cancer Research* 1999; 5(3):629-35.
86. Kang YK, Kim WH, Lee HW, Lee HK, Kim YI. Mutation of p53 and K-ras, and 1055 of heterozygosity of APC in intrahepatic cholangiocarcinoma. *Laboratory Investigation* 1999; 79(4):477-83.
87. Iachino C, Catsicojannis N, Dallera F. Prognostic significance of tumor DNA content in carcinoma of the hepatic duct confluence. *Journal of Experimental & Clinical Cancer Research* 1998; 17(4)425-30.
88. Ito R, Tamura K, Ashida H, Nishiwaki M, Nishioka A, Yamamoto Y, Furuyama Jl, Utsunomiya J. Usefulness of K-ras gene mutation at codon 12 in bile for diagnosing biliary strictures. *International Journal of Oncology*1998; 12(5):1 019-23.
89. Iwamoto KS, Mizuno T, Kurata A, Masuzawa M, Mori T, Seyama T. Multiple, unique, and common p53 mutations in a thorotrast recipient with four primary cancers. *Human Pathology* 1998; 29:412-6.
90. Hruban RH, Sturm PD, Slebos RJ, Wilentz RE, Musler AR, Yeo CJ, Sohn TA, van Velthuysen ML, Offerhaus GJ. Can K-ras codon 12 mutations be used to distinguish benign bile duct proliferations from metastases in the liver? A molecular analysis of 101 liver lesions from 93 patients. *American Journal of Pathology* 1997; 151:943-9.
91. Finkelstein S, Przygodzki RM, Swalsy PA. Microdissection-based P53 Genotyping: Recommendations for Molecular Testing. *Molecular Diagnosis* 2000, in press.
92. Marchesa P, et al. The risk of cancer and dysplasia among ulcerative colitis patients with primary sclerosing cholangitis. *American Journal of Gastroenterology* 1997; 92:1285-8.
93. Pasha TM, Petz J, Ludwig J, Therneau TM, Benson JT, Malinchoc M., Dickson ER, Lindor KD. Incidence of cholangiocarcinoma in patients with primary sclerosing cholangitis. *Hepatology* 1997; 26:170A.

CHAPTER 6

MULTIDISCIPLINARY MANAGEMENT OF LIVER METASTASES FROM COLORECTAL CANCER

Giuseppe Sigismondo Sica, Achille Lucio Gaspari
Department of Surgery, University of Rome "Tor Vergata", Rome, Italy

INTRODUCTION

Numerous studies of the natural history of colorectal carcinoma have shown that liver metastasis is the primary determinant of survival [1]. Up to 25% of colorectal cancer patients have synchronous hepatic metastasis2, and 50% develop metachronous metastasis [3]. Only 5-10% of these patients will have potentially resectable liver metastasis [4]. At present surgical resection, whenever possible, is the gold standard for treatment, and there are no proven efficacious therapies that prolong survival in this group of patients.

In the late seventies Foster and Berman [5] established a liver tumour registry, showing a 48% 2-year survival and 22% 5-year survival, for patients who underwent liver resection for colon and rectum metastases, thus demonstrating, the value of such resection, with an acceptable mortality of 10%.

Modern surgical techniques have yielded an operative mortality rate for major liver resections of less than 5%, and 30 to 35% 5-years' survival rate [6, 7, 8, 9].

The spontaneous prognosis for untreated patients with hepatic metastasis from colorectal cancer is poor, and most of the patients die during the first few years after discovery of the liver recurrence.

Wilson and Adson [10] compared the survival of 60 patients having resection, with that of 60 patients of matched number and extent of metastasis having a biopsy only, and found no 5 years' survivors in the biopsy-only group, but a 25% survival in the resected group. In 1991 [11] Scheele also demonstrated no 5 years' survivors who had a potentially curable but non-resected lesion, but a 38% actuarial survival for those patients who had their lesion resected.

A.M. Farinon (ed.), *Advances in Abdominal Surgery 2002*, 85-94.

Unfortunately, the majority of patients with hepatic metastasis manifest with the disease that has spread beyond surgical resection, and only about 10% of patients with hepatic metastasis from colorectal cancer are suitable for resection.

Resection seems, at the moment, to give the best chance of long term survival. Some other modalities of ablations for liver malignancies such as alcohol injection, radiofrequency and cryosurgery are extensively used whenever the lesion(s) is unresectable. Chemotherapy has also been investigated and is currently used as the only-therapy, as adjuvant therapy and as neo-adjuvant therapy (Tab. 1).

Table 1. Survival in percentage (%) from Gillams, Dis. Col. Rectum; May 2000

	No treatment	Surgery	PCT	HAI	RF
12 months	32	92	48	64	90
24 months	10	62	21	25	60
36 months	3	48	3	5	34
48 months	-	40	-	-	22
medium	7.4 - 11	33	12	17	27

CHEMOTHERAPY

Since the number of patients with unresectable colorectal liver metastases is so high, the use of a variety of therapeutic agents has been one approach that has been extensively investigated over the last three decades. A response rate of up to 30% has been reported using systemic 5-Fluorouracil [12, 13]; other authors have showed no efficacy [14, 15]. In a review of 24 institutions, Hughes et others16 have demonstrated little benefit in patients receiving adjuvant systemic chemotherapy.

To sum up, there is lack of evidence of supporting i.v. chemotherapy, but since the liver is a frequent site of recurrence after hepatic resection , a logical adjuvant therapy is intra-arterial regional infusion of the liver (HAI). Some reports have shown substantial tumour response rate. Knowledge of different catheter placement is essential to avoid complications; intra-arterial chemotherapy can be associated with infection, bleeding, cholangitis, gastritis, duodenitis, and haematological problems associated with systemic chemotherapy. For repeated administration of chemotherapeutic agents, a catheter must be used that can be inserted transcutaneally (via the subclavian artery), with coil obstruction of the gastroduodenal artery and insertion of the catheter into the common hepatic artery. A laparotomy is necessary if the catheter is placed in the proper hepatic artery. The catheter is connected to an implantable infuser port, placed in a subcutaneous pocket in the left upper chest.

Recently, Bismuth showed a series of patients whose primarily unresectable colorectal liver metastases were downstaged by crono-modulated chemotherapy and considered suitable for radical surgery. The cumulative 5 years' survival rate was 40%, but only 14% in those patients with concomitant extrahepatic disease. [17]

RESECTION

Several studies have analysed subgroups of patients undergoing hepatic resection for colorectal metastases, in order to identify factors that may indicate a better prognosis. However, considering the impossibility of getting randomised prospective data regarding resection of colorectal cancer liver metastases, it is necessary for the surgeon to individualise each situation. Assessment of operative risk and technical feasibility is often more straightforward than determining the probability of long term disease-free survival.

However, some factors seem to be important prognostic variables, such as histological grade, extent of metastatic disease of the liver, and coexistent extrahepatic disease.

The mean survival after resection of metastasis from poorly-differentiated tumours is 7.1 months, compared with 17.9 months for moderated or well-differentiated tumours; however, as few patients with poorly-differentiated tumours undergo resection of hepatic metastases, statistical significance is difficult to demonstrate. Patients with more than three intrahepatic metastases had a 5 year disease-free survival of 7%, a statistically significant difference, if compared to 25% in those patients with three or fewer metastases.[18]

The coexistence of extrahepatic disease reduces the probability of long-term patient survival, even if the extrahepatic disease is resectable.19 20 However, Scheele and associates [21] did not find a statistically significant difference in the survival and tumor-free survival of patients with extrahepatic disease, although there was a tendency for less favourable results.

The presence of metastases in the hepatic or celiac lymph nodes is also a poor prognostic factor after hepatectomy; however, again patients with positive lymph nodes should not always be excluded from liver surgery, and moreover lymph nodes dissection may help to prevent the early occurrence of obstructive jaundice.

Recurrence occurs in approximately 65-80% of patients who undergo initial hepatectomy for hepatic metastasis from colorectal carcinoma [22, 23], with the liver being the most common location. Approximately 40% to 50% of all patients with recurrence after initial hepatectomy have liver metastases, and

20-30% are liver-only metastases [24, 25, 26, 27]. Repeat hepatic resection has been shown to be a safe and effective modality for a well-selected group of patients; the procedure carries a low operative mortality rate and survival time is comparable to that of patients with initial hepatic resections. Although operative mortality is low, the recurrence rate after second hepatectomy is high, and very few patients will ultimately survive their disease. Postoperative therapy should be considered for this high-risk colorectal cancer group.

Technical aspects of hepatic resections

The segmental anatomy of the liver has recently been emphasised by Couinaud. [28] Segmental resections based on portal segmental anatomy have been popularised by Bismuth. [29, 30] Hepatic resections are designated as anatomical (Tab. 2) when a morphologically-defined portion of the hepatic parenchyma is removed, and as non-anatomical those that consist of wedge resections and enucleations.

Table 2. Formal Anatomical resections

- Right lobectomy
- Right trisegmentectomy
- Left lateral segmentectomy
- Left lobectomy
- Left trisegmentectomy

The advantage of wedge liver resections is their relative ease of performance. The use of Harmonic Scalpel is helpful; attempts to approximate the cut liver edges by deep parenchyma sutures are inappropriate, as they can lead to sepsis and postoperative biliary fistulae. Wedge resection of segment IV are hazardous and should be avoided, as well as enucleations that do not allow a uniform safe tumour margin, and they usually bleed profusely.

Table 3. Gaspari, Columbus Hospital (Hepatectomies)

• Right trisegmentectomy	7
• Left trisegmentectomy	8
• Left lobectomy	5
• Segmentectomies	24
• Wedge	33

The technique of choice for resection of secondary malignancies is anatomical resection, but a simple wedge resection may be indicated in most cases (Tab. 3).

A comprehensive understanding of intra-hepatic vascular anatomy is critical for performing segment-oriented resection.

The three main hepatic veins divide the liver parenchyma into four sectors; each sector represents hepatic parenchyma that is supplied by an independent portal pedicle and consists of one or two segments. Segment I, the caudate lobe, is a distinct anatomic segment: it receives its vessels from both the right and left portal pedicle, but it drains directly into the IVC through numerous small veins.

The anatomic right liver consists of segments V, VI, VII and VIII, each one supplied by a single branch of the right portal pedicle. The right hepatic vein divides the right liver in two sectors: the anterior consists of segments V and VIII and the posterior right sector consists of segments VI and VII.

The left liver is divided into two anatomic sectors by the left hepatic vein: the anterior sector consists of segments IV and III; the posterior consists only of segment II.

Parenchyma dissection may proceed in one of two ways: with either the trans-parenchyma approach to vascular elements (ton-That-Tung) [31], or preliminary dissection and control of the hilar elements of the lobe to be removed [32].

By identifying the portal pedicle to individual anatomic segments, it is possible to control the inflow to the segments that are intended for resection, to minimize blood-loss during transection. Intra-operative ultrasound guidance is helpful in identifying segmental pedicles and hepatic veins as well as small nodules.

Separation of hepatic parenchyma is accomplished with kelly-clamp or finger fracture technique, Harmonic Scalpel, ultrasound or hydro-dissection.

Many authors have successfully reported laparoscopic hepatectomies [33, 34, 35].

Whatever the technique of choice, metastatic liver tumour(s) must be resectable with at least a one centimetre tumour-free margin.

Adequate tumour-free surgical margin is imperative to successful surgical treatment of colorectal cancer liver metastases. This is supported by results from the Hepatic Tumour Registry, The Gastrointestinal Tumour Study Group, as well as single institution reviews [36, 37, 38]. There is no significant increase in survival-advantage in the group of patients undergoing a non-curative resection, compared to patients with unresectable disease.

When it is believed that resection could not be accomplished because the amount of liver-tissue left in place after surgery would probably be too small, two techniques can be used: portal vein embolization and two-stage hepatectomy. Portal vein embolization induces atrophy of the liver to be resected and hypertrophy of the liver to be left. Re-hepatectomy after hypertrophy of the residual liver-tissue can be used for large bilateral lesion, in which one-stage resection of all involved segments would have led to liver failure.

RADIOFREQUENCY AND OTHER INTERSTITIAL ABLATION TECHNIQUES

Interstitial ablation techniques permit the introduction of a destructive agent directly into the neoplastic tissue, saving as much as possible of the surrounding tissue. Their use is reserved to all those cases in which tumor-destruction is required to improve the expectancy or quality of life. [39, 40]

Radiofrequency (RF) electromagnetic radiation is a safe, well-tolerated and effective treatment, to achieve tumor destruction in patients with unresectable hepatic malignancies.

The RF system consists of a generator that supplies up to 100 Watts of power, a Lee Veen monopolar array needle electrode, and an indifferent dispersive electrode pad applied to the patient's skin. This generator displays the temperature of the needle-tip, and the impedance between the needle and the grounding pad. The Lee Veen needle electrode is a 15-gauge insulated cannel that contains expandable prongs which are deployed, after ultrasound-guided placement of the needle electrode into the tumor. The tissue temperature in the tumor can be controlled between 50° and 100°C by increasing the RF power and current delivery. The final size of the sphere of ablated tissue is proportional to the square of the RF current, also known as the RF power density

RF ablation procedure can be achieved by the percutaneous approach, under local anaesthesia with conscious sedation. However, in patients with large tumors (4c. in diameter), multiple tumors or tumors that abut a major intrahepatic blood-vessel, it is possible to perform the treatment during an open surgical procedure. In this last case, hepatic inflow occlusion (Pringle's manoeuvre) facilitates RF ablation of large or hypervascular tumors and tumors near blood vessels, because heat loss or cooling effect is principally dependent on blood circulation.

We actually use RF, as the procedure of choice for nonresectable liver metastases and our results show a 100% of tumor necrosis in lesions less than 3 cm. in diameter, and 90 to 100% of necrosis in metastases between 3 and 5 centimetres. (Rossi P.: Comp. Ass. Rad. & Surg. 2001). We also use RF to ablate a tumor in the opposite lobe, when performing a hepatectomy for multiple, bilobar liver metastases.

Recently RF ablation has been successfully used in combination with intra-arterial infusion chemotherapy. [41] This modality provides a new option for treatment of multiple liver metastases from colorectal cancer.

Cryosurgery has provided a new therapeutic approach for unresectable liver tumors [42, 43]. More recent studies have even suggested that cryosurgery may achieve similar results to those of resection.

With cryoablation techniques, tumor cell death is not a direct consequence of lowering tissue temperature, but is caused by ice-crystal formation during rapid freezing, with resultant destruction of normal cellular structures.

We do not have personal experience with cryosurgery. The efficacy of cryosurgery for eradication of tumors is dependent on the size of the lesion, because it is difficult to achieve the low temperature necessary for tumor-cell destruction at the periphery of tumors 5 cm. in diameter. The overall complication rate after cryosurgery is high, up to 50 % [44, 45] and includes death, haemorrhage, biliary fistulas. Furthermore, the local recurrence rate reported after cryosurgery is very high, if compared to the local recurrence rate in the tumor treated by RF. Prospective randomised trials are therefore needed to compare the two techniques.

Alcohol injection has been extensively used to obtain a palliative destruction of liver malignancies. It is a low-invasive procedure and is easily repeatable under ultrasound guidance. Ethanol is not usually suitable for colorectal hepatic metastases, because the tumor tissue is too hard and alcohol does not diffuse inside the tumor.

Laser Induced Thermotherapy is a MR-guided ablation technique currently performed in some centres, by means of an implantable percutaneous catheter system. CT is used to control the insertion of the catheter. It seems to permit good tumor control for localised liver metastases, without extra-hepatic spreading patterns.

Microwaves and **Interstitial Rx-Therapy** are, at the moment, rarely indicated.

SUMMARY

When colorectal cancers metastasise to distant organs, usually multiple sites are involved, and treatment consists primarily of systemic chemotherapy. Median survival with optimal regimes range from 10 to 15 months. Less frequently colorectal cancer metastasises only to the liver, and in a minority of these cases surgical resection can be performed and results in a median survival of 28-46 months. Five-year survival rates range from 24 to 38 %. For liver metastases that are not suitable for surgical resection, other regional therapies that can be considered are radiofrequency ablation, cryosurgery and hepatic arterial infusion chemotherapy. The median survival after interstitial treatments is of 24-30 months. Intra arterial chemotherapy may increase survival in patients with isolated liver metastases, compared to systemic chemotherapy.

All these treatments should be considered, for an optimal multidisciplinary management of metastasis from colorectal cancer.

REFERENCES

1. Steele G Jr,Osteen RT, Wilson RE, Broows DC, Mayer RJ, Zamcheck N, Ravikmar TS. Patterns of failure after cure of large liver tumors. *Am J Surg* 1984; 147 : 554.
2. Bengmark S, Halfstrom L. The natural history of primary and malignant tumors of the liver. I. The prognosis for patients with hepatic metastases from colonic and rectal carcinoma by laparotomy. *Cancer* 1970; 23: 198.
3. Bozzetti F, Bignami P, Morabito A, et al. Pattern of failure following surgical resection of colorectal cancer liver metastases. *Ann Surg* 1987; 205: 264.
Ekberg H, Tranberg KG, Andersson R, et al: Pattern of recurrence in liver resection for colorectal secondaries. World J Surg 11:541, 1987.
4. August DA, Ottow RT, Sugarbaker PH. Clinical perspective of human colorectal cancer metastases. *Cancer Metastases Rev* 1984; 3: 303-324.
5. Foster JH, Berman MM. Liver tumor survey. *In* Solid Liver Tumors. Philadelphia, WB Saunders, pp 5-8, 1977.
6. Doci R, Genwar L, Bignami P, et al. One hundred patients with hepatic metastases from colorectal cancer treated by resection: Analysis of prognostic determinants. *Br J Surg* 1991; 78: 797.
7. Gayowski TJ, Iwatsuki S, Madariaga JR, et al. Experience in hepatic rection for metastatic colorectal cancer: Analysis of clinical and pathologic risk factors. *Surgery* 1994; 116: 703.
8. Rosen CB, Nagorney DM, Taswell HF, et al. Perioperative blood transfusion and determinants of survival after liver resection for metastatic colorectal carcinoma. *Ann Surg* 1992; 216: 493.
9. Scheele AP, Stangl R, Altendolf-Hofmann A, et al. Indications of prognosis after hepatic resection for colorectal secondaries. *Surgery* 1991; 110:13.
10. Wilson SM, Adson MA. Surgical treatment of hepatic metastases from colorectal cancers. *Arch Surg* 1976; 111: 330.
11. Scheele J, Stangl R, Altendorf-Hofmann A, et al. Indications of prognosis after hepatic resection for colorectal secondaries. *Surgery* 1991; 110: 13.
12. Chang AE, Schneider PD, Sugarbaker PH, et al. A prospective randomized trial of regional versus systemic continuous 5-fluorodeoxyuridine chemotherapy in the treatment of colorectal liver metastases. *Ann Surg* 1987; 206: 685.
13. Martin JK, O'Connell MJ, Wieand HS, et al. Intra-arterial floxuridine vs systemic fluorouracil for hepatic metastases from colorectal cancer: A randomized trial. *Arch Surg* 1990; 125: 1022.
14. Butler J, Attiyet FF, Daly JM. Hepatic resection for metastases of the colon and rectum. *Surg Gynecol Obstet* 1986; 162: 109.

15. Fostner JG, Silva JS, Golbey RB, et al. Multivariate analysis of personal series of 247 consecutive patients with liver metastases from colorectal cancer. I. treatment by hepatic resection. *Ann Surg* 1984; 199: 3,7,16.
16. Hughes KS, Simon R, Songhrabodi S, et al. Resection of the liver for colorectal study of indications for resection. *Surgery* 1988; 103: 278.
17. Bismth H, Adam R, Lévi F, Farabos C, Waechter F, Castaing D, Majno P, Engerran L. Resection of nonresectable liver metastases from colorectal cancer after neoadjuvant chemotherapy. *Ann Surg* 1994; 509: 522.
18. Registry of Hepatic Metastases. Resection of the liver for colorectal carcinoma metastases: a multi-institution study of indications for resection. *Surgery* 1988; 103: 278.
19. Bengmark S, Hafstrom L. The natural history of primary and secondary malignant tumors of the liver. I. The prognosis for patients with hepatic metastases from colonic and rectal carcinoma by laparotomy. *Cancer* 1969; 23: 198.
20. Adson MA. Resection of liver metastases – when is it worth while? *World J Surg* 1987; 11: 511.
21. Scheele J, Stangl R, Altendorf-Hofmann A, Galli FP. Indications of prognosis after hepatic resection for colorectal secondaries. *Surgery* 1991; 110: 13.
22. Nordlinger B, Jaeck D, Guiguet M, Vaillant J, Balladur P, Schaal J. Surgical resection of hepatic metastases. Multicentric retrospective study by the French Association of Surgery . In Nordlinger B, Jaeck D, eds. Treatment of hepatic metastases of colorectal cancer. New York: Springer-Verlag, 129: 46, 1992.
23. Hughes KS, Simon R, Songhrabodi S, Adson MA, et al. Resection of the liver for colorectal metastases: a multi-institutional trial of the indications for resection. *Surgery*1988; 103: 278-88.
24. Wood CB, Gillis Cr, Blumgart LH. A retrospective study of natural history of patients with liver metastases from colorectal cancer. *Clin Onc*1976; 2: 285-8.
25. Hughes KS, Simon R, Songhrabodi S, Adson MA, et al. Resection of the liver for colorectal metastases: a multi-institutional trial of the indications for resection. *Surgery*1988; 103: 278-88.
26. Vaillant J, Balladur P, Nordlinger B. Repeat liver resection for recurrent colorectal metastases. *Br J Surg* 1993; 80: 340-4.
27. Stone M, Cady B, Jenkins R, McDermott W, Steele G. Surgical therapy for recurrent liver metastases from colorectal cancer. *Arch Surg* 1990; 125: 718-22.
28. Couinaud C. Le Foie. Etudes Anatomiques et Chirurgicalle. Paris: Masson 1957.
29. Bismuth H. Surgical anatomy and anatomical surgery of the liver. *World J Surg* 1982; 6: 3-9.
30. Bismuth H, Houssin D, Castaing D. Major and minor segmentectomies "regleees" in liver surgery. *World J Surg* 19826: 10-24,.
31. Ton that Tung (Ed). Les resection majeures et mineurs du foie. Masson Editeur, Paris, 1979.
32. Lortat-Jacob JL, Robert HG. Hepatectomie droite règlèe. *Presse med* 1952; 60: 549-551.
33. Ferzli G, David A, Kiel T. Laparoscopic resection of a large hepatic tumor. *Surg Endosc* 1995; 9 (6): 733-735.
34. Azagra JS, Goergen M, Jacobs D. Laparoscopic left lateral segmentectomy (left hepatic lobectomy). *Endosurgery* 1994; 1: 7-9.
35. Gagner M, Rheault M Dubuc J. Laparoscopic partial Hepatectomy for liver tumor. *Surg Endosc* 1992; 6: 99.
36. Cady B, Stone M, Mcdermott W, et al. Technical and biologic factors in disease-free survival after resection for colorectal cancer matastases. *Arch Surg* 1992; 127: 561.
37. Registry of Hepatic Metastases. Resection of the liver for colorectal carcinoma metastases: A multi-institution study of indications for resection. *Surgery* 1988; 103: 278.
38. Steele G, Bleday R, Mayer R, et al. A prospective evalutation of hepatic resection for colorectal carcinoma metastases to the liver. Gastrointestinal study group protocol 6584. *J Clin Oncol* 1991; 9: 1105.

39. Rossi S, Di Stasi M, Buscarini E, Cavanna L, Quaretti P, Squassante E, Garbagnati F, Buscarini L. Percutaneous radiofrequency interstitial ablation in the treatment of small hepatocellular carcinoma. *J Intervent Radiol* 1993; 8: 97-103.
40. Goldberg SN, Gazella GS, Solbiati L, Livraghi T, Tanabe KK, Hahn PF, Mueller PR. Ablation of the liver tumors using percutaneous RF therapy. *AJR* 1998; 170: 1023-1028.
41. Kainuma O, Asano T, Aoyama H, Takayama W, Nakagohri T, Kenmochi T, et al. Combined therapy with radiofrequency thermal ablation and intra-arterial infusion chemotherapy for hepatic metastases from colorectal cancer. *Hep Gastr* 1999; 46: 1071-1077.
42. Ravikumar TJ, Kane R, Cady B, et al. Hepatic cryosurgery with intraoperative ultrasound monitoring for metastatic colon carcinoma. *Arch Surg* 1987; 122: 403-409.
43. Ravikumar TJ, Steele GD. Hepatic cryosurgery. *Surg Clin North Am* 1989; 60:433-440.
44. Quebbeman EJ, Wallace JR. Cryosurgery for hepatic metastases. In: Cordon RE (Ed). Current technique in general surgery. New York: Mosby 1997: 1-75.
45. Gagner DJ, Roh MS. Cryosurgery for hepatic malignancies. In: Curley SA (Ed). Liver cancer. New York: Springer-Verlag 1998:173-200.

CHAPTER 7

MORBIDITY AND SURVIVAL IN LIVER RESECTION FOR COLORECTAL METASTASES.

Gennaro Nuzzo, Felice Giuliante, Maria Vellone, Ivo Giovannini
Institute of Surgical Pathology, Catholic University of the Sacred Heart, Rome, Italy

Abstract
Liver resection is the only treatment which offers the possibility of curing patients with colorectal liver metastases. Despite the increasing complexity of resections, operative mortality and morbidity rates of liver resection have been considerably reduced. During recent years, positive late results have progressively increased, and it has been shown that this depends upon several factors, which are related to characteristics of the primary cancer, of metastases and to the accuracy of surgical technique. In the period 1990-1999, one hundred hepatic resections were performed consecutively on 94 patients for metastases from colorectal cancer; 6 were re-resections. The 30-day mortality rate was 2% (2 patients); morbidity rate was 22% (22 patients). Overall actuarial survival rate was 32% after 5 years. Primary tumor stage, time of appearance of metastases, adequacy of the margin of resection and intra-operative blood transfusions, were the factors most significantly affecting long-term results. Correct surgical technique, in terms of completeness of resection and limited intra-operative bleeding, was crucial in achieving longer survival. The margin of resection on the specimen was the most important prognostic factor, relating to the surgical procedure: actuarial 5-year survival rate was 46%, in cases with a margin of resection greater than 1 cm (71 patients), and nil in cases with a margin smaller than 1 cm (23 patients). Patients who were not intra-operatively transfused had a 5-years survival rate of 54%. Results of our analysis confirm that in specialized centers the operative risk of liver resections is low, and good late survival is observed in more than one third of the resected patients. New chemotherapy regimens, portal vein embolization and thermal ablation techniques should increase, in the near future, the number of patients who can benefit from surgery.

Keywords
Liver metastases, liver resection, colorectal cancer.

A.*M. Farinon (ed.), Advances in Abdominal Surgery 2002*, 95-113.

INTRODUCTION

Liver metastases are the most frequent secondaries of colorectal cancer. Synchronous liver metastases are discovered in 15-25% of patients during pre-operative evaluation, or at laparotomy for primary cancer [1-2]. Metachronous secondaries affect another 20-30% of patients [3], and are discovered during postoperative follow-up, with a higher incidence during the first 2 years (about 90%) [1]. In both cases, liver resection represents effective and safe treatment, even if for only a limited proportion of patients (10%) [4]. As a matter of fact, in specialized centers hepatic resection carries a low operative risk, and is associated with excellent post-operative quality of life. At present the surgical mortality rate is less than 3% and post-operative non-lethal complications occur in less than 20% [5]. With regards to long-term results, liver resection is, at the moment, the only treatment that offers the chance of a cure, with an overall 5-years survival rate of more than 30% [5, 8]. Furthermore, recently published studies of sufficient size and follow-up reported 10-year survival rates of more than 20% [5, 7-8]. Recurrence of disease is the most frequent cause of late mortality, occurring in almost 65% of patients at 5 years. Recurrence occurs in the liver alone in almost 50% of patients, and 10-50% of these patients can be treated with a complete repeat hepatectomy [9-11]. Therefore the possibility of selecting patients in different classes of risk of recurrence, is crucial to directing more accurately patients with different levels of risk, towards utilizing different protocols of treatment. New anti-cancer drugs with modified therapeutic regimens (neo- adjuvant), new therapeutic techniques such as radiofrequency, and procedures such as pre-operative portal embolization, have been introduced during recent years. The possibility of associating surgery with these new modalities of treatment could considerably increase the number of patients who might be cured, by increasing the resectability rate.

In our study, the results of 100 consecutive liver resections performed on 94 patients with colorectal cancer metastases were analyzed to evaluate immediate results, and to identify features and factors which are more closely related to long-term results.

METHODS

One hundred liver resections for hepatic metastases from colorectal cancer were performed between 1990 and 1999, on 94 patients (M/F 49/45). The median age was 59 years (range 34-76); 22 patients (23.4%) were older than 70. Six re-resections were included.

Features of primary tumors are summarized in Figure 1. The most frequent location of primary tumors was the colon (71 cases, 75.5 %), and in the

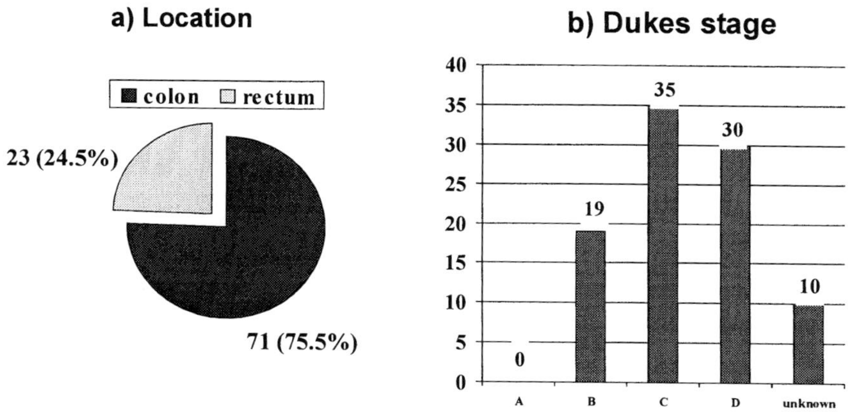

Figure 1. Features of primary tumor: a) location and b)Dukes stage

majority of cases advanced primary tumors were observed (Dukes C and D = 65%). In 10 patients who had been operated in another hospital, Dukes stage was not known.

Features of liver metastasis are summarized in Table 1.

Table 1. Features of liver metastases

	n. cases	%
TIME OF APPEARANCE		
Synchronous	26	28
Metachronous	68	72
early ≤ 12 months	24	26
late > 12 months	44	46
TUMOR DISTRIBUTION		
Unilobar	73	73
Bilobar	27	27
NUMBER OF TUMORS		
1	61	61
2 – 3	26	26
> 3	13	13
TUMOR SIZE		
< 5 cm	67	67
≥ 5 cm	33	33

Synchronous metastases were observed in 26 patients, and metachronous metastases in 68 (72.3%), with a mean disease-free interval of 22±15 months (range 3-80). In 21 cases the disease-free interval was ≤ 1 year ("early" metastases) and in 43 cases > 1 year ("late" metastases). The metastasis was single in 61 cases, and more than 5 cm in size in 33 cases (33 %).

In 4 patients an extrahepatic metastasis was present: lung metastases (2 cases), peritoneal metastasis with invasion of a jejunal loop (1 case), peritoneal metastasis with invasion of psoas muscle (1 case).

In 57 cases (57%), a major hepatectomy (resection of 3 or more segments) was performed, and in 43 cases (43%) a minor resection was carried out (Tab. 2). Sixteen out of 26 patients with synchronous metastases had a combined procedure, with simultaneous resection of the primary tumor and of the hepatic metastases. In this group, 5 major hepatectomies and 11 minor resections were performed. In the other patients with synchronous metastases, surgery was delayed by 3 months, after systemic chemotherapy.

Table 2 Extent of resection (*)

MAJOR RESECTIONS	57	
Right hepatectomy		25
Right hepatectomy + IV seg.		4
Left hepatectomy		6
Left hepatectomy + V/VIII seg.		3
Resection of 5 segments		1
Resection of 3 segments		14
Resection of 5 - 8 segments		4
MINOR RESECTIONS	43	
Resection of 2 segments		16
Resection of 1 segment		7
Limited resection		20

* according to Couinaud's classification

Extrahepatic disease was present in 4 patients. In 2 patients with lung metastases, pulmonary resection was performed 3 months after liver resection; in 2 patients with peritoneal metastases, resection of extrahepatic disease was carried out at the same time as liver resection.

Liver resection was performed in every case with the aim of obtaining a margin of resection of at least 1 cm. With this aim, intra-operative ultrasound was used in all cases to guide the resection. A margin of more than 1 cm was actually achieved in 77 liver resections. In the other 23 cases, for reasons of size, number or location of metastases, a margin smaller than 1 cm. was obtained.

Hepatic pedicle clamping (HPC) was used in 70 cases. Total vascular exclusion (TVE) of the liver was performed in 6 cases, in which the metastases were located close to the vena cava, or to the confluence of a main hepatic vein with the vena cava. In two of the latter patients, because of the small size of the future remnant liver, preoperative right portal embolization was performed, and in both patients a right hepatectomy was performed.

Six patients underwent re-resection of a recurrent hepatic metastasis at 4 to 14 months after the first resection. Features of this group of patients are summarized in Table 3.

Table 3. Features of patients who underwent re-resection

Sex	Age	1st resection	Interval (months)	N. of tumors	2nd resection	Morbidity	Follow-up (months)
1 f	52	limited resection (VII seg.)	12	1	VI segm.	-	26 (a)
2 f	64	IV-V+VIII seg.	14	1	II - III	-	52 (d)
3 f	56	Right hepatect.	9	1	IV	-	19 (d)
4 f	48	limited resection (III seg.)	4	5	II-III-V-VI-IVant + Limited resection of VIII seg.	subphrenic abscess	57 (d)
5 m	47	V seg.	13	2	IV - VI-VII	-	30 (a)
6 m	53	limited resection (III seg.)	9	2	V-VIII	-	21 (a)

[A = alive, d = dead]

Fifty-one patients received a postoperative systemic chemotherapy with 5-fluorouracil and folinic acid.

Perioperative mortality, morbidity rates and long-term results were evaluated in relation to: age of patients, ASA class, features of the primary tumor (staging and location), and of the metastases (time of appearance, number, size, lobar distribution), surgical technique (type and margin of resection, length of procedure, use of HPC, intra-operative blood transfusions), and adjuvant chemotherapy.

Values are reported as mean ± standard deviations. Statistical analysis was conducted using the chi-squared test and the Student t-test. Actuarial patient survival was calculated by the Kaplan-Meier method. Comparison of patient survival curves were made by the log-rank test. A value of $p < 0.05$ was considered to be statistically significant.

RESULTS

Operative mortality rate was 2% (2 cases). One patient was a 62 year old man with a mis-diagnosed cirrhosis, who underwent a right hepatectomy for two metastases from a sigmoid neoplasia, with continuous clamping of the pedicle for 40 minutes, and he died from liver failure on the 22nd post-operative day.

The other patient was a 60 year old man with synchronous multiple liver metastases from rectal cancer, who first underwent an anterior resection of the rectum. Then he was treated with systemic chemotherapy (12 cycles). After 14 months a reduction of the number (three in segment 4, 7 and 8) and size of liver metastases was obtained. Though they were located close to the vena cava and right hepatic vein, they were considered to be resectable with a right extended hepatectomy, but this would have left a limited, future remnant liver. Therefore he was first treated with right portal embolization. After sufficient hypertrophy of the left lobe, a right hepatectomy extended to the posterior part of segment 4 was planned. During the resection, bleeding from the confluence of the right hepatic vein to the vena cava could not be controlled; total vascular exclusion was applied, but the manoeuver was not tolerated by the patient, who died intraoperatively.

Morbidity rate was 22% (22 cases). The complications are reported in Table 4.

Table 4. Morbidity

Overall morbidity	22 (22%)
Type of complications	
Subphrenic abscess	9
Liver failure	4
Biliary fistula	2
Biliary lesion	2
Pleural effusion (thoracentesis)	5
Pulmonary embolism	2
Intestinal occlusion	2*

*2 patients required a reoperation
4 patients had more than one complication

The most common complications were abdominal fluid collection, pleural effusion and liver failure. There were no significant differences related to: age of patient, ASA class, type of resection, length of procedure and use of HPC (Tab. 5).

Table 5. Post-operative complications related to different factors

	N. CASES	MORBIDITY N. (%)	MORTALITY N. (%)	Log-rank test
OVERALL	100	22 (22%)	2 (2%)	
AGE				
≥70 aa	22	3 (13.6)	-	p=ns
< 70 aa	78	19 (24.3)	2 (2.5)	
ASA				
I	65	16 (24)	1 (1.5)	p=ns
II	7	-	-	
III	28	6 (21)	1 (3.5)	
RESECTION				
MAJOR	57	14 (24.5)	2 (3.5)	p=ns
MINOR	43	8 (18.6)	-	
LENGTH OF PROCEDURE				
≥ 300 min.	41	11 (26.8)	2 (4.8)	p=ns
< 300 min.	59	11 (18.6)	-	
SYNCHRONOUS LIVER AND COLON PROCEDURE				
YES	16	6 (37.5)	-	p=ns
NO	84	15 (17.8)	2 (2.3)	
HPC	70	16 (22.8)	2 (2.8)	p=ns
no HPC	30	6 (20)	-	
HPC ≥ 60 min.	16	8 (50)	1 (6.2)	p<0.05
HPC < 60 min.	54	16 (14.8)	1 (1.8)	
I.O. TRANSFUSIONS				
YES	35	10 (28.5)	1 (2.8)	p=ns
NO	65	12 (18.4)	1 (1.5)	

Regarding the use of HPC in patients who were clamped (70 cases), morbidity rate was significantly higher in those with ischemia time prolonged for more than 1 hour, than in those with ischemia time of less than 1 hour (50% vs. 14.8%; p< 0.05) (Tab. 5).

In patients with synchronous metastases, who underwent simultaneous hepatic and colon resection (16 cases), morbidity rate was higher, even if not statistically significant, than that of patients who underwent only liver resection (37.5% vs. 17.8%; p=ns) (Tab. 5). In this group of patients, the most frequent complication was abdominal abscess (4/6 cases, 67%); two out of 5 patients who underwent major resection developed postoperative complications (40%).

Intra-operative blood transfusions were required in 50% (15/30) of cases operated on without HPC, and in 28.5% (20/70 cases) of those in which Pringle's manoeuver was performed (p<0.01). The mean number of blood transfusions was 3.9±2.4 in non-clamped patients, and 2.6±1.1 in clamped cases ($p<0.05$) (Tab. 6).

Table 6. Number of transfused cases and of blood units per transfused case in 100 resections performed with or without hepatic pedicle clamping (HPC)

		with HPC	without HPC	p
Total resections	100	70	30	
Number of transfused cases	35 (35%)	20 (28.5%)	15 (50%)	< 0.01
Units of blood (mean±SD)	3.1±1.9	2.6±1.1	3.9±2.4	< 0.05

Morbidity rate in patients who underwent a second liver resection was 16.6% (Tab. 3).

Median postoperative stay was 17 days (range 6-78).

Overall 5-year survival rate was 32%, with a median survival of 39 months. All the analyzed criteria related to late survival are reported in Table 7.

Long-term results were significantly influenced by the stage of the primary colorectal cancer: 3-year and 5-year survival rates were better in patients without lymph node involvement (Dukes B), in comparison with those with lymph node metastases (Dukes C) (71% vs. 55%; 62% vs. 24%; p=0.01) (Fig. 2).

With regards to the time of appearance of liver metastases, synchronous metastases were associated with a less-favourable prognosis than metachronous ones; 5-year survival rate of patients with synchronous metastases was 17%, whereas patients with metachronous secondaries had a 5-year survival rate of 37% (p=0.005) (Fig. 3).

The number and size of metastases by themselves did not significantly influence long-term survival, even if there is a trend towards a significantly higher survival time in patients with single metastases than in patients with multiple metastases (36% vs. 25%), and with metastases < 5 cm in size, than in patients with metastases ≥ 5 cm in size (46% vs. 19%) (Tab. 7).

Patients with a margin of resection greater than 1 cm (71 cases) showed a 5-year survival rate of 46%; 5-year survival rate of patients with a margin of resection of less than 1 cm., or infiltrated (23 cases), was nil (p=0.0001) (Fig. 4). With regards to intraoperative blood transfusions, survival rate was higher in non-transfused patients than in transfused patients (54% vs. 9%) (p=0.0001) (Fig. 5).

Finally, the 51 patients who received postoperative adjuvant chemotherapy had a non-significantly longer survival rate, in comparison with that of untreated patients (5-year survival 33% vs. 29%) (Tab. 7).

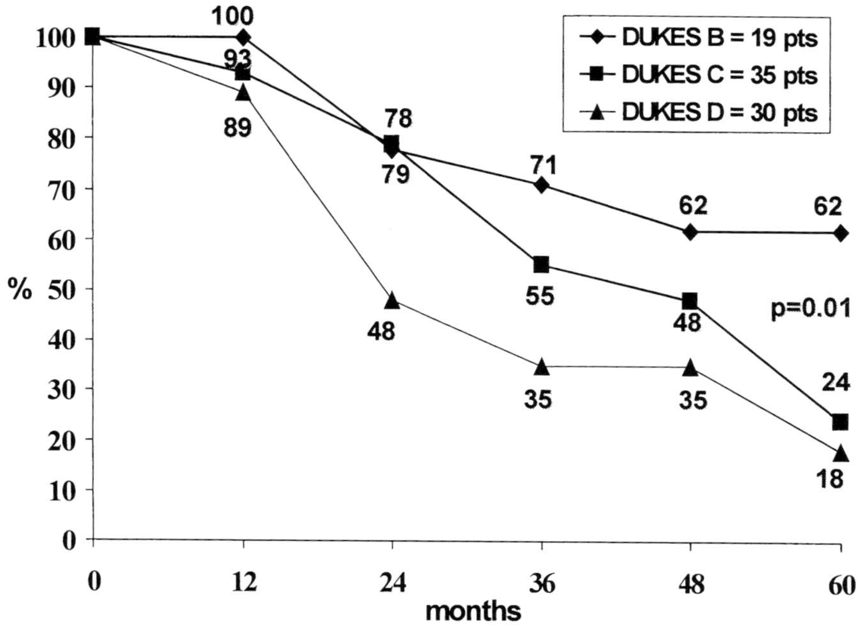

Figure 2. Actuarial survival after hepatic resection related to Dukes stage

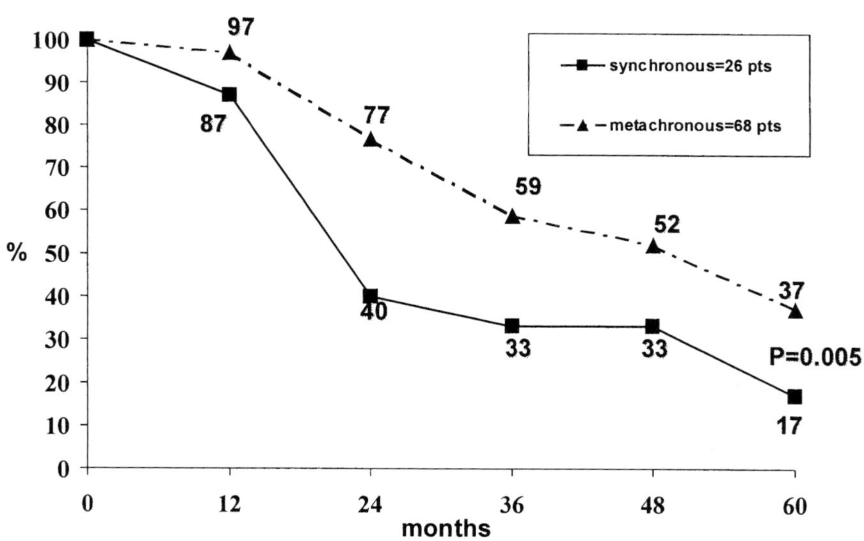

Figure 3. Actuarial survival after hepatic resection related to time of appearance of liver metastases

Table 7. Influence of various clinical and pathologic risk factors on overall survival patients

FACTOR	N.PTS	SURVIVAL 3%			Log-rank test
		1-YEAR	3-YEAR	5-YEAR	
OVERALL	94	94	52	32	
AGE (y)					
< 70	78	93	45	24	p=ns
≥ 70	16	100	82	66	
PRIMARY TUMOR					
Colon	71	95	58	39	p=ns
Rectum	23	94	33	11	
DUKES (*)					B vs C:
B	19	100	71	62	p=0.01
C	35	93	55	24	
D	30	89	35	18	
TIME OF APPEARANCE					
Synchronous	26	87	33	17	p=0.005
Metachronous	68	97	59	37	
Early (≤12m)	24	100	64	55	p=ns
Late (>12m)	44	95	57	35	
NUMBER OF TUMORS					
1	58	98	59	36	p=0.1
> 1	36	88	42	25	
SIZE					
< 5 cm	62	93	60	46	p=0.1
≥ 5 cm	32	97	42	19	
TUMOR DISTRIBUTION					
Unilobar	73	92	48	33	p=ns
Bilobar	27	100	54	27	
TYPE OF RESECTION					
Major	54	92	52	37	p=ns
Minor	40	96	51	21	
RESECTION MARGIN					
> 1 cm	71	98	65	46	p=0.0001
< 1 cm	23	82	19	0	
I.O. BLOOD TRANSFUSIONS					
Yes	33	97	26	9	p=0.0001
No	61	95	69	54	
ADJUVANT CHEMOTHERAPY					
Yes	51	98	55	33	p=ns
No	43	90	48	29	

* In 10 patients staging of the primary tumor was not known.

ns = non statistically significant

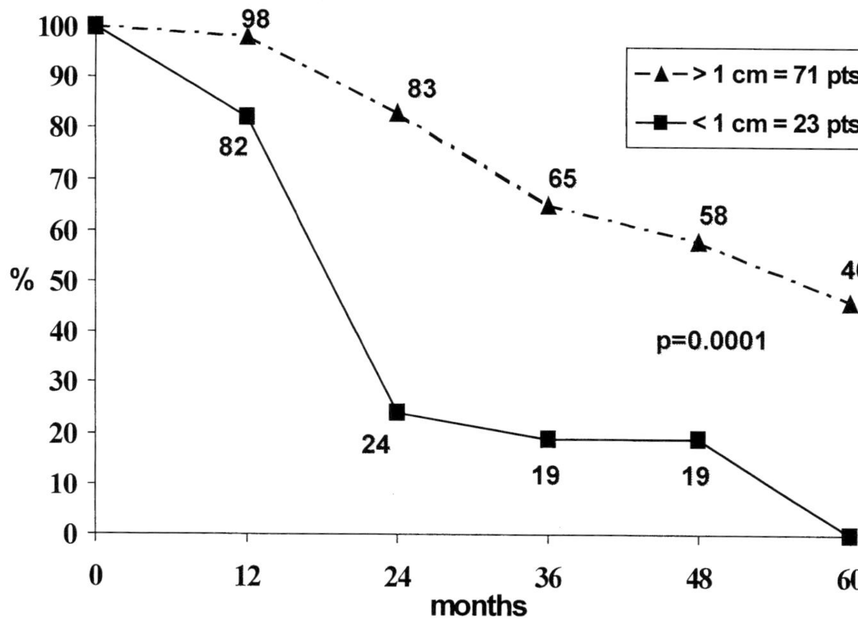

Figure 4. Actuarial survival after hepatic resection related to margin of resection

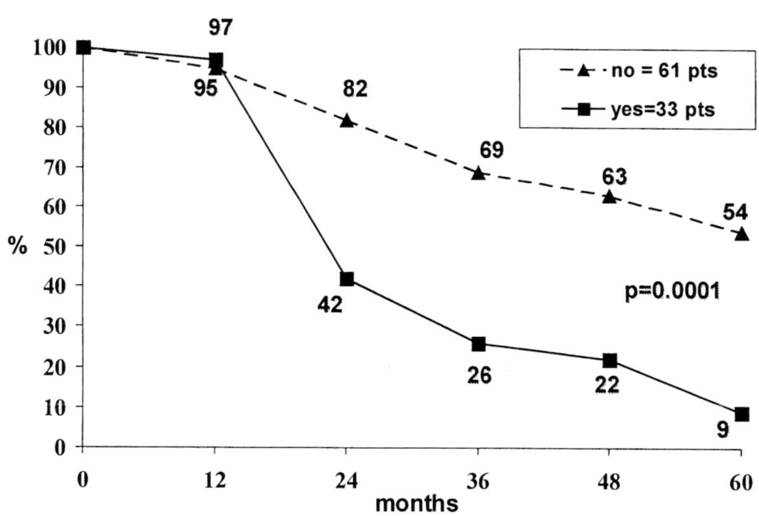

Figure 5. Actuarial survival after hepatic resection related to i.o. Blood transfusions

In patients with extrahepatic disease median survival was 31.5 months.

With regards to the re-resected patients, in three of these a median survival of 42 months [19-57] after the first liver resection was observed. The other three patients are still alive after 21, 26 and 30 months (Tab. 3).

Age of patients, location of the primary tumor (colon or rectum), lobar distribution of liver metastases and type of resection, did not influence long-term results (Tab. 7).

DISCUSSION

The good overall results of liver resection for colorectal metastases support the increasing acceptance of surgery as the preferred treatment of liver metastases. In spite of the increasing complexity of resections, surgical risk has been considerably reduced during recent decades. Several specialized centers have shown that liver resection is currently a well-controlled procedure with a mortality rate lower than 3% [5]. The results of our analysis (mortality rate 2% and morbidity rate 22%) confirm these data. With respect to operative risk regarding patients with synchronous metastases, debate still continues on the indications for performing simultaneous resection of liver metastases and of the primary colorectal tumor. At present, the most widely-accepted practice is to perform both liver and colon resection simultaneously, only in the case of low-risk procedures [12]. In our retrospective analysis a higher morbidity rate was observed in patients synchronously resected (37.5%), compared with those who were resected only on the liver (17.8%). This higher morbidity rate was probably related to the relatively high rate of major liver resections (5/16, 31%) associated with colorectal resection.

The improvements of surgical techniques have permitted the progressive increase in indications to re-resection. As a matter of fact, in spite of the greater complexity of procedures, operative risk in such re-resections is similar to that of the first resection [9-11]. The same results have been observed in our analysis: the morbidity rate of re-resections was 16%, similar to that of the overall group (22%).

With regards to the natural history of patients with liver metastases from colorectal cancer, those patients who do not undergo any treatment have a mean survival time of 8.7 months [13] and 3-year survival rate is almost nil [14]. Chemotherapy alone is capable of producing a survival of 12-18 months [14-17]. Different technical procedures of thermal ablation (cryotherapy, radiofrequency, laser-induced interstitial thermotherapy) have recently shown good results in terms of local tumor control rate, mainly in cases of small liver metastases [18-19]. However, because of the rapid evolution of such techniques, and the limited duration of available follow-up data, it is not yet possible to define the exact rôle of these treatments. Currently accepted indications for thermal ablation techniques, mainly of radiofrequency, both in intraoperative and percutaneous settings, are:

1) patients not eligible for liver resection,

2) patients not radically resected, in which these procedures can be applied associated with surgical resection. In a series of 158 liver resections for colorectal liver metastases, Elias et al. were able to conduct curative therapy in 21 cases, by combining hepatectomy and radiofrequency ablation of residual nodules in the remnant liver. The 2-year survival rate was 90% in that group of patients [20].

The only potential curative treatment currently available remains liver resection, which offers a chance of cure in more than one third of the radically resected patients; in our experience, overall 5-year survival rate was 32%. Recent publications by Fong [5] and Scheele [7] reported a 10-year survival rate of 22% and 23% respectively; results never reported for other treatment. Because no other current treatment offers the possibility of cure, hepatic resection is the treatment of choice, and serves as the standard of comparison, for treatment of metastatic disease isolated to the liver.

A large number of data confirm that long-term results are based on different parameters which include: characteristics of primary tumor, characteristics of hepatic metastases, accuracy of liver resection, and the presence of extrahepatic metastases. Based on their own experiences, several authors have proposed different prognostic scoring systems, to predict long-term results and to improve patient selection for surgery [5, 7-8, 21]. In the analysis of the experience of Memorial Sloan-Kettering Cancer Center on 1001 patients, Fong reported seven independent predictors of adverse outcome after liver resection:

1) lymph node involvement of the primary colon cancer,
2) disease-free interval less than 12 months after colorectal resection,
3) preoperative CEA levels higher 200 ng/ml,
4) number of metastases more than 1,
5) size of largest tumor more than 5 cm,
6) positive margin of liver resection,
7) presence of extrahepatic disease.

By using 5 of these criteria, a simple pre-operative clinical score was obtained, which proved highly predictive of outcome (Tab. 8) [5]. Some of the most recently published predictor factors which have been identified, are summarized in Table 9.

Several authors identify the Dukes' stage of primary tumor as a factor significantly related to long-term results [3, 5, 7, 22]. Fong reported that patients with Dukes B tumor had a 5-years survival rate, higher than those with Dukes C tumor (41% vs. 32%) [5]. Similar results were reported by Scheele, who observed a 5-year survival rate of 50% in patients with non-involved mesenteric lymph node, compared to 37% in patients with lymph node involvement [7]. Also in our study, although in 10 patients the stage of primary tumor remained unknown, 5-year survival rate was significantly influenced by the Dukes stage (B 62% vs. C 24%; $p<0.05$).

Table 8. Clinical risk score for tumor recurrence according to Memorial Sloan-Kettering Cancer Center

Score*	1 yr	3 yr	5 yr	Median (months)
0	93	72	60	74
1	91	66	44	51
2	89	60	40	47
3	86	42	20	33
4	70	38	25	20
5	71	27	14	22

- ❑ Dukes C
- ❑ Disease-free interval < 12 months
- ❑ CEA > 200 ng/ml
- ❑ Number of tumors > 1
- ❑ Size of the largest tumor > 5 cm

* Each risk factor is one point

About 20% of potential candidates for surgical procedure for colorectal cancer have synchronous liver metastases [1-2]. As already mentioned, at present it is generally accepted that a simultaneous liver and colon resection should be performed only in cases with superficial or safely resectable metastases; in cases with deeply located metastases and requiring major hepatic resection, a delay of two or three months with chemotherapy is advisable. This policy may be suggested by technical reasons (in particular the kind of surgical approach), by oncologic considerations (in particular the possibility of occult hepatic or extrahepatic lesions), and by the excessive operative risk of the two procedures in association. In our study, 26 patients had synchronous metastases, but simultaneous liver and colon resections were performed in 16 cases. In patients with synchronous metastases the 5-year survival rate was significantly lower than survival in metachronous metastases (17% vs. 37%; $p < 0.05$).

Also, for metachronous metastases the disease-free interval between colo-rectal resection and the appearance of liver metastases is often reported as an important prognostic factor. According to results reported by Fong, patients with a disease-free interval longer than 12 months have a higher 5-year survival rate than patients with a disease-free interval lower than 12 months (41% vs 30%) [5]. This difference was not observed in our experience.

Table 9. Indipendent predictors of outcome at multivariate analysis after resection of colorectal liver metastases

	Fong 1999 (5)	Iwatsuki 1999 (8)	Nordlinger 1996 (21)	Scheele 1995 (7)
Number of patients	**1001**	**305**	**1568**	**434**
Age			+	
Primary tumor stage	+		+	+
Primary tumor grade				+
Disease-free interval	+ (12 months)	+ (30 months)	+ (24 months)	+ (synchr./met achr.)
CEA level	+ (200 ng/ml)		+ (30 ng/ml)	
N. of tumors	+ (>1)	+ (> 3)	+ (> 4)	
Satellite metastases				+
Largest tumor size	+ (> 5 cm)	+ (> 8 cm)	+ (> 5 cm)	+ (>5 cm)
Tumor distribution Bilobar		+		
Type of resection				+ (anat./non-anat.)
Positive margin	+	+	+	+
Year of resection				+ (1960-70/ 1980-92)
Extrahepatic disease	+	+ (hepatic limph node involvement included)		+

With regards to the features of metastases, the number and size of lesions are relevant prognostic factors, even if different cut-off limits are used by different authors [5, 7-8, 21]. In our study, the number and size of metastases did not reach statistical significance, but a strong trend towards significance was observed in patients with single metastasis compared to those with more than one lesion (61% vs. 26%) and in patients with metastases smaller than 5 cm. in comparison to those with metastases bigger than 5 cm (46% vs. 19%).

With regards to surgical technique, the most important surgical factor is the completeness of liver resection. Scheele showed, with strong evidence, that survival of patients who underwent non-radical liver resections was very similar to that of patients who were only deliberately debulked or not resected: in these patients, 5-year survival rate was almost nil. On the contrary, in patients resected with a negative margin of resection, 5-year and 10-year survival rates of 38% and 23% respectively were reported [7]. Similar results were observed in our experience: patients with margins of resection greater than 1 cm had a 5-year survival rate of 46% and those with smaller margins had a 5-year survival rate of zero.

Also the accuracy of surgical technique, in terms of intraoperative bleeding, was a relevant factor. Intraoperative blood transfusions have an immunosuppressive effect, and have a negative impact on long-term results, in patients submitted to surgical procedures for colorectal neoplasms and liver metastases [23-24]. Rosen reported a longer 5-year survival rate in non-transfused patients, compared with transfused patients (32% vs. 21%, $p<0.03$) [23]. On the other hand, Gayowsky reported a significant difference in survival only for transfused patients receiving more than 10 units [25]. Younes confirmed that the number of blood transfusions is an important prognostic factor, but stressed that most transfused patients are also those with more advanced diseases, which probably intrinsically implies a worse prognosis [26]. In our study, we observed a higher 5-year survival rate in non-transfused patients than in transfused patients (54% vs. 9%, $p<0.05$). In order to minimize intraoperative bleeding, in our surgical technique hepatic pedicle clamping is liberally used [27], and in our experience it permitted more than a 50% reduction in the number of transfusions, and the number of transfused patients.

The presence of extrahepatic lesions is not always a contraindication to liver resection, if these can be radically resected at the same time as liver resection, or after three months of systemic chemotherapy [14, 28]. Sheele and Elias did not report any difference between survival curves in patients with or without extrahepatic lesions, if these lesions could be resected without residual disease [29-30]. In our experience, extrahepatic disease could be radically resected in 4 patients, and mean survival was 31 months.

The involvement of the hepatic pedicle lymph node was observed in 14% of patients with colorectal liver metastases [31]. Whether or not to resect liver metastases in such circumstances is still a subject of controversy. In fact, it has been shown that long-term results in these patients are definitely worse than in those without lymph node involvement [32]. However, also in this group a 5-year survival rate of 12% was reported by a multicentric French trial on 1818 patients [33]. Therefore, at present hepatic pedicle lymph node involvement should not be considered a contraindication to liver resections, but a factor of worse prognosis, which probably should direct these patients to more aggressive chemotherapy regimens.

Results of recent studies suggest that different regimens of adjuvant chemotherapy (intravenous, intra-arterial, chronomodulated) may improve survival after resection of colorectal liver metastases [34-35]. Adjuvant systemic chemotherapy with 5-FU and folinic acid after liver resection was performed, in our experience, on 51 patients, who had a non-significantly higher 5-year survival rate than untreated patients (33% vs. 29%). Although prospective trials, that clearly demonstrate the efficacy of one specific regimen of adjuvant chemotherapy after liver resection, are not yet available, the published results and the low toxicity of the new drugs seem to justify the use of postoperative chemotherapy.

In 10-20% of the resected patients with a liver recurrence, a second complete resection is technically feasible. Five-year cumulative survival rate after re-resection is 19-41% [9, 11]. Recently, Adam reported that prognostic factors in a multivariate analysis were 1) whether or not the first hepatectomy had been curative and 2) the delay between first hepatectomy and recurrence [11]. Five-year survival rate was 62% when that delay was more than 1 year and 26% when it was less. A third and a fourth hepatectomy can be performed in selected cases. In our experience, 6 patients were re-resected for recurrent liver metastases: mean survival was 42 months after the first hepatectomy, similar to that observed in the overall group (39 months). Again, even in cases with poor prognostic factors, when feasible, repeat hepatectomy can offer the best chances of prolonged survival.

With the aim of increasing the resectability rate, of patients with multiple liver unresectable metastases from colorectal cancer, the so-called "two-stage hepatectomy" has been proposed by Adam [35]. This term has been used for a first hepatectomy that permits the resection of the highest possible number of tumors, followed by a second hepatectomy performed after a period of liver regeneration, with the aim of completing the resection of the remaining metastases. Preoperative and postoperative chemotherapy is associated to surgery. By using this extremely aggressive policy, the author reported in 13 consecutive patients, a 3-year survival rate of 35%, and a median survival of 31 months, from the second hepatectomy. This limited experience needs to be confirmed by a larger number of patients, but it confirms that with close and continuous co-ordination of surgeons and oncologists, a larger number of patients might be cured.

CONCLUSIONS

This study confirms the low perioperative mortality and morbidity of the surgical treatment of liver metastases in specialized centers. It confirms that long-term results are influenced by factors and features which characterize initially the primary tumor, the patient, the liver metastases, and by the accuracy of surgical technique. Analysis of all these factors is important, in order to improve the available information on the clinical correlates of long-term survival, and the criteria for selection of surgical candidates. The data in our study provide evidence that better results are obtainable in patients without nodal involvement of the primary tumor and metachronous metastasis. Among surgical factors, we strongly confirm that the margin of resection is the most important prognostic factor, followed by the number of blood transfusions. In the near future, better results will be obtainable, by increasing the resectability rate of patients with liver metastases from colorectal cancer; this is possible in the setting of aggressive multi-treatment protocols.

REFERENCES

1. Faivre J, Rat P, Arveux P. Epidémiologie des métastases hépatiques des cancers colorectaux. In: Nordlinger B, Jaeck D. Traitement des Métastases Hépatiques des Cancers Colorectaux. Rapport du 94e Congrès de l' Association Francaise de Chirurgie. Paris, Springer-Verlag 1992; p 3-9.
2. Hunt TM, Carty N, Johnson CD. Resection of liver metastases from a colorectal carcinoma does not benefit the patient. *Ann Royal Coll Surg Engl* 1990; 72: 199-205.
3. Registry of Hepatic Metastases: Resection of the liver for colorectal carcinoma metastases: A multi-institutional study of indications for resection. *Surgery* 1988; 103: 278-288.
4. Penna C, Nordlinger B. Traitement des métastases hépatiques des cancers colorectaux : jusq'où aller ? *Gastroenterol Clin Biol* 1998 ; 22 : 1046-1047.
5. Fong Y, Fortner J, Sun R L et al. Clinical score for predicting recurrence after hepatic resection for metastatic colorectal cancer. Analysis of 1001 consecutive cases. *Ann Surg* 1999; 230(3): 309-321.
6. Ohlsson B, Stenram U, Tranberg KG. Resection of colorectal liver metastases: 25-year experience. *World J Surg* 1998; 22: 268-277.
7. Scheele J, Stang R, Altendorf-Hofmann A et al. Resection of colorectal liver metastases. *World J Surg* 1995, 19: 59-71.
8. Iwatsuki S, Dvorchik I, Madariaga J R et al. Hepatic resection for metastatic colorectal adenocarcinoma: a proposal of a prognostic scoring system. *J Am Coll Surg* 1999; 189: 291-299.
9. Muratore A, Polastri R, Bouzari H et al. Repeat hepatectomy for colorectal liver metastases: a worthwhile operation? *J Surg Oncol* 2001; 76: 127-132.
10. Nordlinger B, Vaillant J C, Guignet M et al. Survival benefit of repeat liver resections for recurrent colorectal metastases : 143 cases. Association Francaise de Chirurgie. *J Clin Oncol* 1994, 12 : 1491-1496.
11. Adam R, Bismuth H, Castaing et al. Repeat hepatectomy for colorectal liver metastases. *Ann Surg* 1997, 225: 51-60.
12. Jaeck D, Bachellier P. Quel tratement chirurgical propser dans les cancers du colon avec métastases viscérales (synchrones et métachrones)? *Gastroenterol Clin Biol* 1998; 22: S 168- S 176.
13. Nagorney DM. Opinion: Resection of hepatic metastasis for colorectal cancer. *J Surg Oncol* 1991 Suppl 2: 74.
14. Sheiner PA, Brower S T. Treatment of metastatic cancer to the liver. *Seminars in Liver Disease* 1994; 14: 169- 177.
15. Levi F, Zidani R, Misset JR. Randomised multicentre trial of chronotherapy with oxaliplatin, fluorouracil and folinic acid in metastatic colorectal cancer. *Lancet* 1997; 350: 681-686.
16. De Gramont A, Vignoud J, Tournigand et al. Oxaliplatin with high-dose leucovorin and 5-fluorouracil 48 hours continuous infusion in pretreated colorectal cancer. *Eur J Cancer* 1997; 33: 214-219.

17. Rougier P, Van Cutsem E, Bajetta E et al. Randomised trila of irinotecan versus fluorouracil by continuous infusion after fluorouracil failure in patients with metastatic colorectal cancer. *Lancet* 1998; 352: 1407-1412.
18. Geoghegan J G, Scheele J. Treatment of colorectal liver metastases. *Br J Surg* 1999; 86: 158-169.
19. Wallace J R, Christians K K, Pitt H A et al. Cryotherapy extends the indications for treatment of colorectal liver metastases. *Surgery* 1999; 126: 766-774.
20. Elias D, Goharin A, Taieb J et al. La radiofréquence peropératoire permet d'augmenter le nombre des hépatectomies pour métastases hépatiques. *Gastroentérol Clin Biol* 2000; 24: A21.
21. Nordlinger B, Guiguet M, Vaillant J C et al. Surgical resection of colorectal carcinoma metastasesto the liver. A prognostic scoring system to improve case selection, based on 1568 patients. *Cancer* 1996; 77: 1254-1262.
22. Doci R, Gennari L, Bignami P et al. One hundred patients with hepatic metastases from colorectal cancer treated by resection: analysis of prognostic determinants. *Br J Surg* 1991; 78: 797.
23. Rosen C B, Nagorney D M, Taswell H F et al. Perioperative blood transfusion and determinants of survival after liver resection for metastatic colorectal carcinoma. *Ann Surg* 1992; 216: 493-305.
24. Stephenson K R, Steinberg S M, Hughes K S et al. Perioperative blood transfusions are associated with decreased time to recurrence and decreased survival after resection of colorectal liver metastases. *Ann Surg* 1988; 208: 679-687.
25. Gayowski T J, Iwatzuki S, Madariaga J R et al. Experience in hepatic resection for metastatic colorectal cancer: Analysis of clinical and pathologic risk factors. *Surgery* 1994; 116: 703-711.
26. Younes R N, Rogatko A, Brennan M F. The influence of intraoperative hypotension and perioperative blood transfusion on disease-free survival in patients with complete resection of colorectal liver metastases. *Ann Surg* 1991; 214: 107-113.
27. Nuzzo G, Giuliante F, Giovannini I et al. Liver resections with or without pedicle clamping. *Am J Surg* 2001; 181: 238-246.
28. Barrat C. Traitement chirurgical des cancers coliques localement avancés et/ou métastatiques. Conférence de consensus: Prévention, dépistage et prise en charge des cancers du colon. *Gastroenterol Clin Biol* 1998; 22: S 265 - S 272.
29. Scheele J, Stangl R, Altendorf-Hofmann A et al. Indicators of prognosis after hepatic resection for colorectal secondaries. *Surgery* 1991; 110: 13.
30. Elias D, Rougier Ph, Mankarios H, et al. Metastasi epatiche e localizzazioni extra-epatiche sincrone e resecabili di origine colo-rettale. *La Presse Medicale* (it.ed.) 1993; 8: 239-244.
31. Elias D, Saric J, Jaeck D et al. Prospective study of microscopic lymph node involvement of hepatic pedicle during curative hepatectomy for colorectal metastses. *Br J Surg* 1996, 83: 942-945.
32. Rodgers M S, McCall J L. Surgery for colorectal liver metastases with hepatic lymph node involvement: a systematic review. *Br J Surg* 2000, 87: 1142-1155.
33. Nordlinger B, Jaeck D, Guiguet M et al. Résection chirurgicale des métastases hépatiques. Enquête de l'Association Française de Chirurgie. In: Nordlinger B, Jaeck D: Traitement des Métastases Hépatiques des Cancers Colorectaux. Rapport du 94e Congrès de l' Association Francaise de Chirurgie. Paris, Springer-Verlag 1992; p 141-159.
34. Kokudo N, Seki M, Ohta H et al. Effects of systemic and regional chemotherapy after hepatic resection for colorectal metastases. *Ann Surg Oncol* 1998; 5: 706-712.
35. Bismuth H, Adam R, Lèvi F et al. Resection of non resectable liver metastases from colorectal cancer after neoadjuvant chemotherapy. *Ann Surg* 1996; 224: 509-522.
36. Adam R, Laurent A, Azoulay D et al. Two-stage hepatectomy: a planned strategy to treat irresectable liver tumors. *Ann Surg* 2000; 6 : 777-785.

CHAPTER 8

HEPATIC METASTASES FROM NON COLORECTAL CANCER: WHICH ONES SHOULD BE RESECTED?

Angelo Benevento, Luigi Boni, Gianlorenzo Dionigi, Renzo Dionigi
Department of Surgery, University of Insubria, Varese, Italy

Keywords:
Liver resection, non colorectal metastases, survival.

Abstract

Background and objectives While liver resection for metastatic disease from colorectal cancer is likely to extend survival in selected patients, the efficacy of hepatic resection as treatment for metastases from other malignancies has not yet been defined.

Methods Between 1988 and 2000, 26 hepatic resections were performed on 24 patients (two patients underwent a double resection due to recurrence), as treatment of non-colorectal metastases. One, two, five years' overall and disease-related actuarial survival (sec. Kaplan-Meier) have been calculated.

Results No intraoperative or early post-operative deaths were reported. Seven minor (30%) and one major (5%) post operative complications occurred; the mean blood loss was 401 +/- 324 ml; in 75% of patients, no intra/post operative blood transfusion was needed. The mean post-operative hospital stay was 13.2 days (9-23).

The overall actuarial survival rate was 54% at one year, 42% at two years and 21% at five years (mean 38 ± 11 months). Survival is related to the primary tumor nature and stage.

Conclusions Hepatic resection for metastases from non-colorectal carcinoma is safe and feasible, with relatively low incidence of intra/post-operative complications, and short hospital stay. Although it achieves good results in terms of survival only in patients suffering from neuroendocrine metastases, it could also have a cytoreductive effect for other tumors.

A.M. Farinon (ed.), *Advances in Abdominal Surgery 2002*, 115-126.

INTRODUCTION

The efficacy of hepatic resection as treatment for metastases from malignancies other than colorectal cancer, has not yet been defined. [1-3]

Non-colorectal cancer liver metastases (NCLM) originate mainly from other abdominal primary tumors (50-75%), due to portal system drainage. However, results of post-mortem studies demonstrated hepatic involvement in 40% of patients dying of lymphatic, breast, kidney, endometrial, sarcomatosus and bone tumours [1-2].

The development of new techniques and technologies [3] to reduce bleeding (such as total and selective liver ischemia, the use of argon beam coagulator and harmonic scalpel), a decrease in intraoperative mortality to acceptable rates (2-3% in referring centre) [4], and improvement in anaesthetic management, have led to a more aggressive attitude towards surgical resection as a potential cure of liver metastatic disease.

We present the outcome of patients treated by liver resection for non colorectal metastases.

MATERIALS AND METHODS

Between 1988 and 2000, three hundred and ninety patients suffering from primary or metastatic hepatic tumors were observed at the Department of Surgery of the University of Insubria (Tab. 1). Eighty surgical resections for liver metastases were performed .

Table 1. Hepatic tumours observed and resected between 1988 and 2000

HEPATIC TUMOURS	OBSERVED	RESECTED
Hepatocarcinoma	115	71 (61%)
Biliary tract tumors	20	5 (25%)
Colo-rectal metastases	162	54 (33.3%)
Non Colo-rectal metastases	93	26 (27.9%)
TOTAL	**390**	**156 (40%)**

Metastases originated from colorectal cancers in 54 cases (67.5%), while 26 (32.5%) hepatic resections were performed on 24 patients (two patients underwent a double resection due to recurrence), as treatment of NCLM (Tab. 2).

This last group consisted of 12 males and 12 females, with a mean age at the time of first operation of 54.3 ± 11.8 years. Records of the liver resection registry were analysed retrospectively.

Table 2. Origin of liver metastases

PRIMARY TUMOUR	N. OF CASES
Breast carcinoma	4
Breast Lyposarcoma	1
Neuroendocrine Tumour	10
Gastric Cancer	5
Squamous Cells Lung Cancer	1
Kidney Tumour	1
Pancreatic Cancer	1
Endometrial Carcinoma	1
TOTAL	**24 Pts**

Operative techniques (Tab. 3) and amount of liver parenchyma to be resected, were selected considering patients' ages, general health conditions and hepatic reserve, evaluated by using the Child-Pugh score, and the indocianine green retention test.

Table 3. Surgical tecnique for treatment of noncolorectal cancer metastases

TECHNIQUE	N. OF CASES
Metastasectomy	7
Segmentectomy	7
Bisegmentectomy	8
Left hepatectomy + segmentectomy	1
Left hepatectomy	1
Extended right hepatectomy	1
Wedge resection	1

Intraoperative ultrasound scanning has also been used in order to locate deep lesions. Follow up evaluation consists of serial hepatic panels, tumor markers (alpha-fetoprotein, human gonadotropin and Ca 19.9), liver CT and ultrasounds.

One, two, five years' overall and disease-related actuarial survival (sec. Kaplan-Meier) have been calculated. Survivals were analysed with the log rank test and statistical significance was accepted at $p \leq 0.05$.

RESULTS

No intraoperative or early post-operative deaths were reported. Seven minor (30%) and one major (5%) post-operative complications occurred (Tab. 4).

Table 4. Major and Minor postoperative complications

MINOR COMPLICATION	NUMBER OF PATIENTS
Atrial Fibrillation	1
Wound infection	2
Disventilation	2
Bladder infection	2
MAJOR COMPLICATION	
Biliary fistula (drainage)	1
TOTAL	8

The mean operation time was 274.4 minutes, when hepatectomy was performed during resection of the primary tumor, and 168.5 minutes when resection of metastases was the only procedure performed.

Pringle's manoeuvre was used in 20 out of 26 cases, in order to reduce blood losses during the operation. Mean ischemia time was 25 minutes; mean blood loss was 401 ± 324 ml, and intra/post operative blood transfusion was needed in 25% of patients. The mean post-operative hospital stay was 13.2 days (9-23).

The overall actuarial survival (sec. Kaplan-Meier) rate is 54% at one year, 42% at two years and 21% at five years (mean 38 ± 11 months) (chart 1).

The disease-related actuarial survival, and differences among different tumours (log rank test) are described in chart 2 and Table 5.

Gastric Cancer Liver Metastases

Nine synchronous liver metastases were resected, during gastrectomy procedure in five patients (4 males and 1 female, mean age 57.8 ± 10.5 years) suffering from gastric cancer.

In 3 cases a single lesion coming from direct infiltration was found, and liver resection had to be performed in order to complete gastrectomy.

Six true liver metastases were surgically removed in the remaining two cases. In all cases, the pathologist's report revealed a 1-cm free margin of the liver specimens.

One year actuarial survival is 20 % (mean 12 ± 8 months) (Tab. 5), and only one patient survived more than one year.

Table 5. Primary tumours, number of lesions, diameter and survival

GASTRIC CANCER	NUMBER OF LESIONS	MAX. DIAMETER (mm)	ACTUARIAL SURVIVAL	
Adenocarcinoma	1*	21	1 YEAR	20%
Adenocarcinoma	2	20		
Adenocarcinoma	4	80	2 YEARS	-
Adenocarcinoma	1*	17		
Adenocarcinoma	1*	15	5 YEARS	-
	TOTAL	MEAN		
	9	30.6	MEAN (months)	12 ± 8
NEUROENDOCRINE TUMOUR				
Ileal carcinoid	1	25	1 YEAR	75%
Ileal carcinoid	1	15		
Gastrinoma	2	22	2 YEARS	50%
Broncogenic carcinoid	1	19		
Broncogenic carcinoid	1	22	5 YEARS	50%
Broncogenic carcinoid	8	40		
Ileal carcinoid	1	7	MEAN (months)	89 ± 26
Rectal carcinoid	2	25		
	TOTAL	MEAN		
	17	21.3		
BREAST TUMOUR				
Adenocarcinoma	3	20	1 YEAR	60%
Adenocarcinoma	1	27		
Adenocarcinoma	8	50	2 YEARS	40%
Adenocarcinoma	1	30		
Lyposarcoma	2	180	5 YEARS	-
	TOTAL	MEAN		
	15	73.4	MEAN (months)	23 ± 7
MISCELLANEA TUMOUR				
Pancreas Adenocarcinoma	1	12	1 YEAR	25%
Endometrial Carcinoma	1	50	2 YEARS	-
Squamous Cell Lung cancer	2	100	5 YEARS	-
Kidney Tumour	1	85	MEAN (months)	10 ± 3
	TOTAL	MEAN		
	5	61.7		

* Direct infiltration

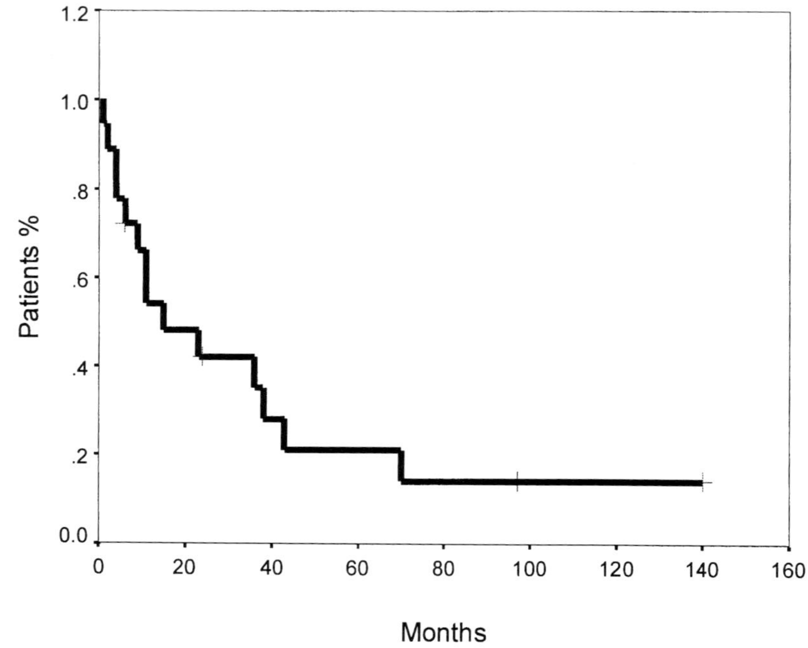

Chart 1. Actuarial Survival (sec Kaplan - Meier) for liver resection for non-colorectal metastases

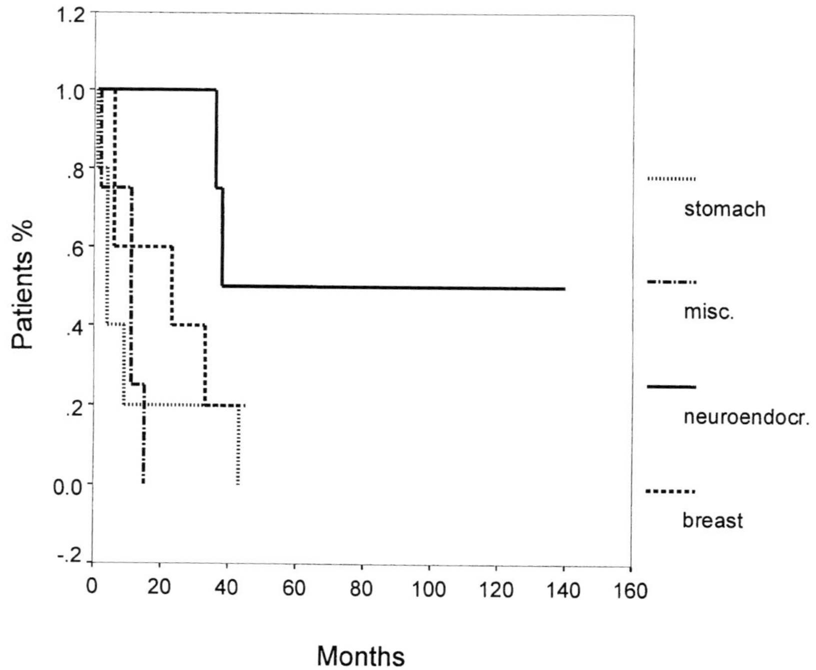

Chart 2. Lon rank test for liver resection for non colorectal metastases

Neuroendocrine Tumor Liver Metastases

Eight patients (4 males and 4 females) underwent ten hepatic resections, as treatment of neuroendocrine tumor liver metastases. One patient suffering from ileal neuroendocrine tumor, and one from atypical bronchogenic carcinoid, had to undergo a second liver resection forty and twelve months after the first operation respectively. The first patient is still alive after 140 months, the other died one year after the second operation.

In the remaining cases, two patients (broncogenic carcinoid) died 38 months after liver resection, while the others (3 ileal carcinoids and 1 gastrinoma) are still alive after 97 - 160 months.

The actuarial survival rate is 75% at one year, and 50% at two years and five years (mean 89 ± 26 months) (Tab. 5).

Survival for neuroendocrine tumour is significantly longer ($p \leq 0.05$) than for gastric and miscellanea tumors. Compared with breast tumor, although survival seems better, the survival rate doesn't reach a statistically significant difference ($p=0.1$) (Chart 2).

Breast Tumor Liver Metastases

Five patients (mean age 46 ± 9 years) suffering from breast tumor liver metastases were treated by liver resection. In 1 out of 5 patients the primary tumor was a breast lyposarcoma, while breast adenocarcinomas were reported in the remaining cases. Characteristics of the metastatic lesions and survivals are described in Table 5.

The actuarial survival rates at 1 and 2 years are 60% and 40% respectively (mean 45 ± 16 months).

In two cases intra-arterial catheter for post-operative local chemotherapy was positioned. One of these patients died 33 months after surgery, while the remaining is still alive 45 months after liver resection.

Difference between local chemotherapy group and surgery alone is significant ($p=0.05$).

Miscellanea Tumor Liver Metastases

In the remaining four patients (3 males and 1 female, mean age 63 ± 3 years) primary tumors were of different origin .

One unsuspected twelve mm liver metastases was revealed by intraoperative ultrasound scan in a 62 years old male patient, during distal pancreasectomy procedure for carcinoma of the tail of the pancreas.

Sub-segmentectomy of the IV was performed, without any post-operative complication. The patient died eleven months later due to neoplastic cachetia.

A 62 years old patient underwent hystero-annessectomy procedure for Muller's tumor. Although systemic chemotherapy regimes were undertaken, sixteen months later one fifty mm hepatic lesion was revealed by ultrasound scan across the II and the III segment.

US-guided bi-segmentectomy was performed without any post-operative complication, but the patient died of cardio-respiratory failure two months later.

Eighteen months after the nefrectomy procedure for white cell renal tumor, one 85 mm hepatic lesion was revealed at CT scan in a 67 years old patient. Resection of the VIII liver segment was performed after a single chemoembolization course, but the patient died eight months later.

Two liver metastases with a maximum diameter of 100 mm were reported in a 66 years old patient, previously operated for squamous cell lung cancer (upper lobectomy). After one chemoembolization course, resection of the II, III and IV segments was performed. Wound infection was the only post-operative complication reported; the patient died eleven months later.

The actuarial survival rate for this group is 25% at one year (mean 10 ± 3 months) .

DISCUSSION

Although the liver is the most common site for distant metastases, surgical resection is considered as gold standard only for colorectal cancer, with a reported five year survival in the range of 20 to 35% [3-4].

The effectiveness of surgical resection as treatment of liver metastases from other tumours is still to be debated.

Our experience demonstrates a one, two and five years overall actuarial survival of 54%, 42% and 21% respectively, and a median of 38 ± 11 months (Chart 1).

These results are not significantly different from those obtained in patients undergoing liver resection for metastases from colorectal cancer: in this group we reported 1, 2 and 5 years survival rates of 90%, 71% and 18% respectively (Chart 3). In the non-colorectal metastases group, survival seems to be strictly related to primary origin (Chart 2).

Good results (75% live at one year and 50% at two years and five years; mean 89 ± 26 months) were obtained when liver resection was performed as treatment for metastases from neuroendocrine tumours. In these patients survival is significantly longer ($p \leq 0.05$) than survival obtained for the gastric and miscellanea group .

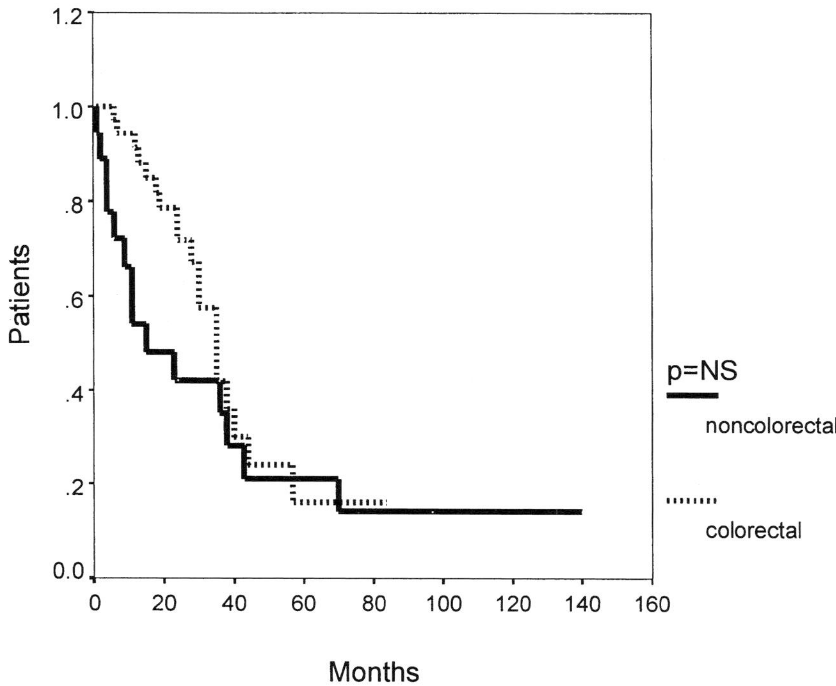

Chart 3. Comparison of actuarial survivals (sec Kaplan - Meier) for liver resection for colorectal versus non-colorectal metastases

In a retrospective study on 10 patients resected for non-colorectal metastases Wolf et al. [5] reported a mean overall survival time of 16 months, but, on considering the neuroendocrine liver metastases group, survival increased up to 20 months.

Describing their results on liver resection as treatment of NCLM, Mariette et al. [6] reported 50% of five years' survival in the neuroendocrine and Wilm's, versus 16% in the remaining patients.

In a recent study, Chen et al. [7] reported a significantly longer survival (p=0.003) in resected versus non-resected patients, suffering from neuroendocrine metastases.

Although surgical resection seems to be very effective, a variety of alternatives have been proposed for these patients: cryosurgery, liver transplantation, laparoscopic/percutaneous thermal ablation by radiofrequency, systemic and local chemotherapy, chemoembolization.

Cryotherapy has shown its efficacy in reducing hormone-related symptoms [8], but no evidences of prolonging survival has been demonstrated.

Two recent studies [9-10] reported a median survival rate of 30 and 55 months, but a high post-operative morbidity rate (19% - 25%).

Laparoscopic/percutaneous thermal ablation by radiofrequency [11] has also been used with preliminary but interesting results. On the contrary, systemic and local chemotherapy or chemoembolization have proved disappointing for this group of patients [12-14].

In a multicentre study, on the use of liver transplantation as treatment of neuroendocrine liver metastases, Le Treut and al. [13] reported a short five years survival rate (36%).

In the gastric cancer liver metastases group, we report a short actuarial survival (20 % at one year, mean 12 ± 8 months) . However 3 out of 5 metastases occurred from direct hepatic infiltration, and hepatic resection was performed only to complete the gastrectomy.

Ochiai et al. [15] suggest that hepatic resection should be attempted if no serosal invasion of the stomach is present, or if the primary tumour has neither venous nor lymphatic infiltration.

Although most reports have demonstrated that the type of liver resection does not affect postoperative prognosis and survival in patients suffering from colorectal liver metastases [3, 16-18], in a retrospective study Miyazaki et al. [19] reported longer survival in patients with a narrow-free margin (>10mm), when liver resection is performed as treatment for metastases from gastric cancer.

This different behaviour could be explained by the high incidence (67%) of micro-metastases around the macroscopic lesions in this group of patients, in comparison with a relatively low (25%) incidence of micro-metastases when they originate from gastric cancer [12].

In the breast cancer liver metastases group, we reported an actuarial survival rate at 1 and 2 years of 60% and 40% respectively (mean 23 ± 7 months) . These results are not significantly worse than those obtained for the neuroendocrine tumors group; the relatively small number of patients in both groups could explain this. Furthermore, liver resection for breast cancer metastases could play an important role if post-operative local chemotherapy regimes are undertaken. In fact, actuarial survival for this specific group of patients is significatively longer ($p=0.05$) than survival of patients where resection was the only therapy adopted. In other words, hepatic resection for breast metastases seems to be mainly a cytoreductive procedure capable of increasing the efficacy of chemotherapy.

Similar results have been achieved by Elias et al. [20], who reported a median survival of 38.2 months, and 2 and 5 years' survival rates of 78% and 24% respectively, when liver resection was combined with pre- and post-operative chemotherapy. Furthermore, better prognosis was reported for those patients with negative lymphnodes, where the median survival was at least three-times that of patients treated with standard non-surgical procedure [21].

Schneebaum et al. [22] compared three different treatments for patients suffering from breast cancer liver metastases. They reported a median survival of 5, 25 and 42 months in the systemic, local chemotherapy and surgery groups respectively.

In the miscellaneous group we reported an actuarial survival rate of 25% at one year (mean 10 ± 3 months) .

Liver metastases from Wilm's tumor and renal cell carcinoma have been resected with relative frequency. In a review Schwartz [23] collected 20 cases of liver resection for Wilm's tumour; of the 16 patients in whom survival could be assessed, seven (43%) were still alive 5 years after hepatic resection, without any evidence of recurrence.

In one review [5], only one out of eleven patients resected for liver metastases from cutaneous melanoma survived 5 years, although he subsequently died of recurrence. Schwartz [26] reported 8 cases described in the literature, but only one with long term survival.

CONCLUSIONS

Although this study examined a relatively small number of patients, it demonstrates that hepatic resection for metastases from non-colorectal carcinoma is safe and feasible, with relatively low incidence of intra/post-operative complications, and short hospital stay.

Although it achieves good results in terms of survival only in patients suffering from neuroendocrine metastases, it could also have a cytoreductive effect for tumors such as breast and gastric cancer, where also with the most recent chemotherapy regimes, median survival times of 7-14 and 3-9 months can respectively be achieved [24-26].

REFERENCES

1. Dionigi R, Benevento A. Il fegato. In Dionigi R. (eds):" Chirurgia" Milano: Masson, 1998:1261-1270.
2. Foster JH, Lundy J. Liver metastases. *Curr Probl Surg* 1981; 18: 161-201.
3. Dionigi R, Madiaraga J (eds.). "New technologies for liver resection". New York: Landes, 1998.
4. Hughes K, Simon R et al. Registry of hepatic metastases. Resection of the liver for colorectal carcinoma metastases: a multi-istitutional study for indication of resection. *Surgery* 1988; 103: 278-287.

5. Wolf RF, Goodnight JE, Krag DE et al. Results of resection and proposed guidelines for patient selection in instanced of noncolorectal hepatic metastases. *Gynec Obstet* 1991; 173: 454-460.
6. Mariette D, Fagniez PL. Hepatic metastasis of non-colorectal cancers. Result of surgical treatment. *Rev Prat* 1992; 42: 1271-1275.
7. Chen H, Hardacre JM, Uzar A et al. Isolated liver metastases from neuroendocrine tumors: Does resection prolong survival? *J Am Coll Surg* 1998; 187: 88-93.
8. Cozzi PJ, Englund R, Morris D. Cryotherapy treatment of patients with hepatic metastases from neuroendocrine tumors. *Cancer* 1995; 73: 501-519.
9. Lang H, Oldhafer KJ, Weimann A et al. Liver transplantation for metastatic neuroendocrine tumors. *Ann Surg* 1997; 225: 347-354.
10. LeTreut YP, Delpero JR, Dousset B et al. Result of liver transplantation for metastatic neuroendocrine tumors: a 31-case French multicentric report. *Ann Surg* 1997; 225: 355-364.
11. Siperstein AE, Rogers SJ, Hansen PD et al. Laparoscopic thermal ablation of hepatic neuroendocrine tumor metastases. *Surgery* 1997; 12: 1147-1155.
12. Frame J, Kelson D, Kemeny N et al. A phase II trial of streptocin and adriamycin in advanced APUD tumor. *Am J Clin Oncol* 1988; 11:490-495.
13. Moertal CG, Kvols D, O'Connell MJ et al. Treatment of neuroendocrine carcinomas with combined etoposide and cisplatin: evidence of major therapeutic activity in the anaplastic variants of this neoplasm. *Cancer* 1991; 68: 227-232.
14. Perry LJ, Stuart K, Stokes KR et al. Hepatic arterial chemoembolization for metastatic neuroendocrine tumors. *Surgery* 1994; 166: 1111-1117.
15. Ochiai T, Sasako M, Mizuno S et al. Hepatic resection for metastatic tumors from gastric cancer: analysis of prognostic factors. *Br J Surg* 1991; 78: 797-801.
16. Holm A, Bradley E, Aldrete JS. Hepatic resection of metastases from colorectal carcinoma: morbidity, mortality and pattern of recurrence. *Ann Surg* 1989; 209: 428-434.
17. Ekberg H, Tranberg KG, Andersson T et al. Determinants of survival in liver resection for colorectal secondaries. *Br J Surg* 1986; 73: 727-731.
18. Isono T, Miyazaki M, Udagawa I et al. The clinicopathological study of intrahepatic micro-metastases of gastric cancer and colorectal cancer. *J JPN Soc Cancer Therapy* 1992; 27: 893-898.
19. Miyazaki M, Itoh H, Nakagawa K et al. Hepatic resection of liver metastases from gastric carcinoma. *Am J Gastroenterol* 1997; 97: 490-493.
20. Elias D, Lasser PH, Montruccoli D, et al. Hepatectomy for liver metastases from breast cancer. *Eur J Surg Oncol* 1995; 21(5): 510-513.
21. Elias D, Lasser P, Spielmann M et al. Surgical and chemotherapeutic treatment of hepatic metastases from carcinoma of the breast. *Surg Gyncol Obstet* 1991; 172: 461-464.
22. Schneebaum S, Walker M, Young D et al. The regional treatment of liver metastases from breast cancer. J Surg Oncol 1994; 55: 26-32.
23. Shwartz SI. Hepatic resection for non colorectal non neuroendocrine metastases. *World J Surg* 1995; 19: 72-75.
24. Harris J, Morrow M, Norton L. Malignant tumors of the breast. In: DeVita VT Jr, Hellman S, Rosemberg SA, (eds) "Cancer: Principles and Practice of Oncology". Philadelphia: Lippiconcott-Raven, 1997: 1557-1616.
25. Fumoleau P. Treatment of patients with liver metastases. *Anticancer Drugs* 1996; 7: 21-23.
26. Alexander HR, Kelsen DG, Tepper JC. Cancer of the stomach. In: DeVita VT Jr, Hellman S, Rosemberg SA, (eds.) "Cancer: Principles and Practice of Oncology". Philadelphia: Lippiconcott-Raven, 1997; 1054-87.

CHAPTER 9

RADIOCHEMOTHERAPY OF LIVER METASTASES FROM BREAST CANCER: REVIEW OF LITERATURE AND PERSONAL EXPERIENCE

Ausili Cefaro G, Nardone L, Marmiroli G, Manfrida S, Salvi G
Institute of Radiology, Catholic University of the Sacred Heart, Rome, Italy

INTRODUCTION

Breast cancer, like several other solid tumors, has the capacity to metastasize to the liver, with a dismal prognosis.

A number of studies carried out on the natural history and therapy of liver metastases have contributed to an in-depth knowledge of this evolution ability, and to the development of new therapeutic approaches, to improve the patient's life both in terms of duration and quality of life.

Autopsy studies evidenced that liver metastatic involvement is present in a high number of cases, even if not detected clinically by instrumental examinations. This high incidence is to be correlated with the peculiarity of portal venous drainage, and the marked tropism of malignant cells towards the liver parenchyma, associated to the presence at this site of glycogen deposits. No specific relationships were instead evidenced between histological type and symptoms, since the series of clinical signs is associated above all to liver failure, caused by the progressive replacement of healthy parenchyma by metastases.

From a therapeutic viewpoint, the clinical distinction between solitary lesions and multiple lesions is of particular importance. Solitary lesions, present in approximately 5% of cases, are usually resectable to be cured. Multiple lesions are far more frequent, present in approximately 45% of cases, and accompanied by a series of different symptoms; they do not profit from surgery and require multidisciplinary therapies or symptom palliation alone.

The resection of solitary metastases has gained ground, since liver surgery widened its indications thanks to improved surgical procedures, anesthetic and

A.M. *Farinon (ed.), Advances in Abdominal Surgery 2002*, 127-139.

postoperative support. However, in liver metastases, due to their site and extent, the primary indication is rarely for operability.

The possible use of chemotherapy, alone or in sequential or concomitant combination with radiotherapy, opened up new therapeutic approaches, in terms of exclusive palliation as well as for cure.

Radiation therapy of liver parenchyma presents the problem of the hepatic tissue's limited tolerance to irradiation, associated with the possible risk of radiation-induced hepatitis. This is the reason why, in order to enhance the response to treatment, studies on the combination of radiotherapy with chemotherapy have been carried out, based on the synergism between the drugs and radiations and the principle of spatial cooperation.

However, experiences with locoregional intra-arterial and systemic chemotherapy, combined or not with radiotherapy, did not show definitively which was the most effective therapeutic modality.

Most reports where successes of different therapeuitc strategies are indicated are limited by the lack of phase III studies, that is, of patients included in control groups without treatment.

EPIDEMIOLOGY AND THERAPEUTIC OPTIONS

Liver metastases from breast cancer are frequent: they represent a very unfavorable event in the disease evolution. In fact, mean survival in untreated patients is approximately 6 months and survival at one-year follow-up is a mere 7% [1].

The appearance of liver metastases is above all correlated with the global disease aggressiveness, evidenced by some risk factors associated to its features and bio-pathology, such as cell ploidy, mitotic index, receptor expression and other parameters of cell proliferation.

Liver metastases from breast cancer rarely manifest as a solitary metastasis, multiple locations are more frequent, even if they are not always evidenced with the common diagnostic tools. This is evident when the difference between the number of metastases seen on diagnostic examinations is compared to that of those found at autopsy. This data should be kept in mind when treatment and outcome is considered. Mean survival of patients with small liver metastases is definitely better than that of patients with diffuse metastases (16.7 months vs. 3.1 months) [2].

For a long time, the inadequate performance of diagnostic imaging has limited the diagnosis and comparison of results. At present, the combination of the three main methods, US, CT and MRI allows a good assessment of the lesions, as well as of the achieved therapeutic result. The sensitivity and specificity of the various diagnostic procedures are reported in Table 1. PET should be added to these; it seems much more promising especially in minute lesions.

Table 1. Sensitivity and specificity of CT, MRI, US and their combinations in the diagnosis of liver metastases

Imaging	sensitivity	specificity
CT	72	95
US	50	100
MRI	55	98
US + CT	78	95
US + MRI	64	98
TC + MRI	74	93
US + CT + MRI	81	93

Surgical resection, where feasible, can be considered as the therapy of first choice, but it should be associated to systemic treatments.

Experiences with surgical resection of metastases from breast cancer, though limited in number, report 22-38% actuarial survival at 5 years [3-5]. Median survival is between 24 and 44 months.

In presence of a diffuse hepatic neoplasm, as well as in presence of metastases to other organs or apparatus, the commonly used therapeutic strategy is based on systemic intravenous chemotherapy. An alternative to the intravenous route, especially in the eighties, was the selective intra-arterial route, with bolus or continuous infusion administration by mechanical or electronic infusion pumps.

The most commonly used drugs are the antineoplastic antibiotics, antracyclines in particular, that were shown to be more effective in the control of breast cancer than other cytostatic agents, in terms of objective responses to treatment .

Vinorelbine, a mitotic spindle inhibitor, has also shown moderate efficacy against liver metastases, when used in monochemotherapy or in combination with anthracyclines [6-8].

More recently, taxans seemed to be able to control liver metastases from breast cancer better than other drugs [9-10]. Per cent responses and drugs used are reported in Table 2.

To-date, studies of the effectiveness of the different chemotherapy schedules did not show a significant improvement in overall survival, while evidencing a different percentage of objective responses and local control. However, a true comparison of reported results is very complex, because a uniform assessment of objective responses to treatment has not been used by the various authors.

Hormonotherapy is rarely used as a single therapy, also in cases where receptors are well represented [11].

The use of radiotherapy in the treatment of liver metastases is conditioned by the liver's limited tolerance of irradiation, apart from its combination with other therapies. Irradiation can be used for prophylaxis after surgery, or after a complete response to chemotherapy; as a cure in case of incomplete response to systemic therapy, or as a palliation for pain relief.

Table 2 Drugs active against metastatic breast cancer: objective response

Drug	**Mean dosage mg/sqm**	**% objective response**
Methotrexate	40	26
Fluorouracil	600-1000	28
Cyclophosphamide	600	36
Mitomicyn C	10	32
Doxorubicin	60-75	43-54
Vinorelbine	25-30	30-41
Cisplatin	60-100	9-50
Paclitaxel	175-250	29-63
Docetaxel	75-100	48-68

RADIOTHERAPY

The studies carried out in the fifties and sixties showed that hepatic tissue tolerance of irradiation was dose-dependent, that is, in relation to the dose for a single fraction, and to the total dose. With 3Gy daily fractions, the total dose that can be delivered to the liver is 18-24 Gy; with 2.5 Gy per fraction the total dose is approximately 25 Gy, while with 1.5-1,8 Gy daily fractions, the total dose can be higher, up to 30-35 Gy. If these doses are surpassed, but sometimes even at lower doses after resection, within a short time signs of toxicity appear: these are characterized by centrilobular liver necrosis, with portal hypertension and ascitis typical of radiation hepatitis, irreversible signs leading to death [12-13]. The incidence of radiation hepatitis, as a function of the dose administered, is reported in Table 3.

Table 3. Incidence of radiation hepatitis as a function of the dose

Dose : Gy	**N° pts (12)**	**N° pts (13)**	**Lethal damage**	**Persistent damage**
30	1/9	0/9	0	0
35	2/9	1/11	1	0
35-40	7/18	0/6	1	2
>40	3/4		2	2

The various symptoms of acute radiation hepatitis can vary from a transient increase in transaminase and alkaline phosphatase to hepatic coma from ingravescent liver failure.

Usually, symptoms and abnormal laboratory findings revert to normal within a few weeks or months, but sometimes they can last for years. There is no specific therapy for acute radiation hepatitis; usually patients are treated on an individual support therapy according to presenting symptoms. Where metastases are not predomiant in the patient's clinical evolution, symptoms of the late phase of radiation hepatitis are characterized by edema, ascitis, pleural soffusion with congestive heart failure, associated or not with low platelet levels and deficit of coagulation factors, at times with esophageal varices.

In the early eighties, the non-randomized RTOG -76-05 trial assessed liver tolerance to radiation in the palliation of liver metastases. The study doses were: 21 Gy in two fractions, 20 Gy in 10 fractions, 25.6 Gy in 16 fractions, 30 Gy in 15 fractions, 30.4 Gy in 19 fractions. A selected group of patients with a solitary metastasis received a 20 Gy buster dose in 10 fractions, provided that the total volume was not over 1/3 of liver parenchyma. There was good tolerance of radiation in the various groups with no cases of hepatitis. The study conclusions indicated that the total dose had to be decreased, with an increase in the dose for a single fraction [14].

The doses reported in the RTOG study are poorly able to control clinically evident liver metastases, that normally do not respond to doses lower than 30 Gy, a dose that is, however, adequate for symptom control. Palliative pain relief is obtained in approximately 90% of patients, and improved liver function indices in 40% of cases. Survival in good responders can be interesting [15-16].

Certainly, patient selection in relation to some prognostic variables acquires a peculiar significance in this setting, as far as the response to radiotherapy is concerned. The performace status, the presence of extrahepatic metastases and liver function expressed as bilirubin level only, have definitely a marked impact on prognosis.

An additional effort at improving the response to therapy and patient compliance, was made with accelerated hyperfractionation. With this modality the dose administration is accelerated with a shorter total time, and a reduced level among single fractions, of a single dose lower than the standard, so aiming to limit the repopulation of rapidly proliferating tumors. Hyperfractionation can increase the redistribution of proliferating cells, in parts of the cell cycle more sensitive to radiation, allowing a more efficient cellular death of the single fraction resulting from the sum, or more daily fractions. The dose reduction of single fractions, and thus of potential late toxicity, allows the hyperfractionated treatment to reach a higher total dose with a corresponding, if not lower, late side-effect on healthy tissues. [17-18]

From these assumptions, the RTOG 84-05 study carried out with graded doses, in an effort to increase the total dose delivered to the liver with hyperfractionation, leads us to conclude that the 33 Gy dose, even if delivered with hyperfractionation and 1.5 Gy single dose, does not involve any advantage in terms of survival, being on the contrary associated with high toxicity. Therefore the previous recommendation not to exceed the 30 Gy dose to the entire liver, is to be stressed again [19].

CHEMOTHERAPY

There are a number of experiences with the treatment of liver metastases from breast cancer, with chemotherapy and various protocols and modalities.

Numerous drugs have shown substantial activity (Tab. 1). Anthracyclines, mitomycin, cyclophosphamide, 5-fluoriuracil, vinblastine and vinorelbine, taxans and their combinations, are the most commonly used drug in clinical practice. Objective responses vary widely, with a range between 7% and 60% (taxans) with approximately 10-12 months median survival [6, 9-10]. The drugs can be administered by intravenous or intra-arterial route, as bolus or continuous infusion. In the latter case, external or implantable infusion pumps should be used [7]: The intra-arterial route of infusion, with miniaturized implantable infusion pumps, has been gradually abandoned in favor of intravenous infusion, because of the risks and problems related to the surgical implant of the pumps, and because the pharmacokinetics of intra-arterial infusion was not so advantageous as initially hypothesized. In fact, the rationale was based on the hypothesis that intra-arterial chemotherapy could be more selective of metastases, so preventing toxicity to healthy tissues. The observation of the physiopathology of liver metastases documented that they receive the infusion predominantly from the hepatic artery, differently from the healthy parenchyma that receives 80% of it from the vena porta [8].

Some drugs administered by hepatic arterial infusion have a high degree of extraction on the first liver passage, determining their high local concentration that was thought to correspond to an increased neoplastic destruction, with negligible systemic toxicity.

Actually, studies of comparison between intravenous systemic administration and arterial administration to metastases from breast cancer, contrary to what was observed for metastases from colorectal cancer, did not show a significant advantage of the latter administration modality, with respect to the side-effects related to the method's complexity.

Polychemotherapy schedules, with the combination of two or more drugs, have definitely shown higher efficacy than monochemotherapy ones, with

35%-75% response rates in terms of local disease control, and 13-24 months percentages of median survival.

However, after several decades of experience with the use of chemotherapy in liver metastases from breast cancer, it is still difficult to define its exact role and real outcomes, because of the limited goals the therapy should set. In fact, while it is true that chemotherapy plays an effective role in the palliation of liver metastases, its advantages, as far as survival is concerned, are of more difficult assessment, since survival may not be significantly improved.

Evaluation of the objective response to chemotherapy may be the cause of uncertainties, rather than clarity, in relation to the different evaluation indexes. Some authors use the regression of hepatomegaly as an index of response to palliation; other authors define as responsive patients who show improved subjective symptoms, and still others use diagnostico-morphologic or laboratory criteria.

With a lack of unambiguous evaluations, comparison of the different experiences is jeopardized. Chemotherapy is often associated with hormonotherapy in the treatment of liver metastases, based on the endocrine correlation of breast cancer, in case of positive receptor expression. Studies directed towards the assessment of the efficacy of this combination, with respect to chemotherapy alone, while evidencing a higher percentage of response did not show a significant improvement in survival [11].

CONCOMITANT RADIOCHEMOTHERAPY

The use of concomitant radiochemotherapy in liver metastases is based on the synergism between the antineoplastic drug and radiotherapy to enhance radiation efficacy on secondary lesions, while toxicity to healthy cells is not increased.

When radiation to the liver is combined with antineoplastic drugs there is usually lower parenchymal tolerance of higher radiation damage; therefore, total doses should be lower. However, this observation was shown to be untrue in the combination with fluoropyrimidines (5-Fu and FUDR), hydroxyurea, cyclophosphamide, procarbazine and mitomycin C. In particular, the concomitant combination of 5-Fu as intravenous or intra-arterial infusion, with radiotherapy to the entire liver volume with 24-30 Gy, has shown good tolerance and higher therapeutic efficacy than single therapies [20-22]. Most likely, the latter is to be attributed to spatial co-operation, cell recruitment and synergism with radiations [23-25], as well as to an amplification of the direct cytocidal effect of radiotherapy.

The first observations of enhanced therapeutic efficacy, from the combination of radiotherapy with 5-Fu and mitomycin, date back to the early seventies

[26]. Subsequently, a number of in vitro and in vivo experimentations confirmed that both drugs enhance the cytotoxic effect of radiotherapy, through an additivity and superadditivity mechanism, in relation to a cytostatic and cytotoxic action against the different cell lines and, at times, according to the higher or lower number of hypoxic cells [27-29].

In particular, since 5-Fu is a phase-specific antineoplastic, its administration before radiotherapy tends to reduce DNA synthesis, synchronizing the cells in a condition of higher radiosensitivity. Its administration after radiotherapy inhibits the repair of sublethal damage, already caused by ionizing radiations.These observations led to the use of 5-Fu continuous infusion, and to the subsequent demonstration of the reduced bone marrow toxicity of continuous infusion, as compared to the same dose of the drug as bolus injection [30].

In the subsequent two decades, considerable interest was directed towards the combination of concomitant radiation and chemotherapy, based on encouraging results. Initially, in the treatment of liver metastases from colorectal cancer, bolus or continuous infusion was used; subsequently, the combination was applied also in other solid tumors like breast cancer [22, 31-34].

Personal experience

In the "Department of Radiotherapy" of the "Policlinico A. Gemelli" of the "Università Cattolica del S.Cuore" of Rome, already from the early eighties a protocol of radiotherapy, including liver irradiation for palliation in presence of liver metastases, was applied.

The results of the study showed a certain ability of the treatment to relieve pain, but not to slow down its evolution. Radiation to the liver was well-tolerated, even if the dose delivered to the liver parenchyma was near to that considered toxic (30 Gy) [35].

Based on these results and those reported in literature, from January 1992 a protocol of radiochemotherapy in liver metastases from breast cancer, was applied.

The study rationale was to verify whether, by lowering the total dose of radiotherapy, enhanced by chemotherapy, better symptom improvement, interruption of evolution and prolonged survival could be achieved.

In the first year, only patients with secondary liver involvement at onset were included in the protocol; subsequently, the study was extended to patients with metastases to other organs and apparatus [36].

In this retrospective analysis, we report the results of treatment of 45 patients, with evaluation of feasibility, toxicity and survival.

Before radiotherapy, in all patients CT liver US and MRI were performed; the latter was started when it was available in our Institute. All patients were also examined with bone scintigraphy and various parameters were applied for the evaluation of liver function at the start of treatment. All examinations were repeated 45-60 days after the end of radiochemotherapy and during follow-up.

In 18 of 45 patients, two cycles of chemotherapy were administered before liver irradiation; in 22 patients, chemotherapy was performed after concomitant radiochemotherapy; in 6 patients chemotherapy was administered before and after radiochemotherapy.

The therapy protocol was as follows: radiotherapy to the liver with high energy beams, Co 60 or 10 MeV linac, by two opposed AP-PA beams, 160 cGy daily dose, to a total dose of 2400 cGy in 15 fractions.

During the first and third week of treatment, chemotherapy was administered as follows: mitomycin C, 10 mg/sqm, bolus, day one followed by 5-Fu, 1000 mg/sqm daily in 24 h continuous infusion on days 1-4 and 11-14.

Survival was calculated starting from the date of diagnosis of liver metastases.

RESULTS

The patients' mean age was 52 years (range: 32-70 years). The interval from breast cancer diagnosis to the appearance of solitary or multiple liver metastases was 35 months.

All 45 patients could be assessed for tolerance and survival.

Tolerance

Hepatic, gastrointestinal and hematologic toxicity was classified according to the WHO parameters. Treatment was well-tolerated and 41 of the 45 patients were able to complete the planned therapy. Four patients discontinued radiochemotherapy because of side-effects: they performed only radiation therapy with no drug addition on week 3. No patient showed symptoms of acute radiation hepatitis; no late damage to the liver was evidenced in long-survivors.

Altered liver function parameters (alkaline phosphatase, transaminase, gamma GT) were observed in all patients. These alterations were mild, and regressed after adequate support therapy. It should be stressed that in many patients, the altered liver function parameters were already present in association with the presence of metastases.

Grade 1 gastric pain and nausea appeared in 44 of the 45 patients, but regressed promptly after the administration of antiemetics and agents coated for stomach protection. One patient showed grade 3 stomatitis that required temporary therapy discontinuation.

Hematologic toxicity was more marked, also due to the fact that 28 patients had already received at least two cycles of chemotherapy before combined therapy.

Hematologic toxicity appeared in 11 of the 45 patients treated, of whom 9 with grade 2 leukopenia and 2 with grade 3 leukopenia. Low platelet levels were observed in 3 patients: 2 grade 2 and 1 grade 3. Two patients had grade 2 anemia, but therapy was completed with no need for blood transfusion.

Survival

Survival was calculated for the entire series starting from the diagnosis of liver metastases. The results of radiochemotherapy were also evaluated, as a function of whether liver metastasis was solitary or combined with other metastases, and of timing with systemic chemotherapy performed before and/or after radiochemotherapy.

Overall survival was 22.1 months (range: 5-98 months). Six patients were still alive when this report was prepared.

Survival in relation to the appearance of metastases was as follows: the 24 patients who showed the first liver metastasis had a mean survival of 27.5 months and a median survival of 24 months. The six survivors belong to this group. The survival of the 21 patients with multiple metastases besides the liver metastasis was 15.8 months with an 11-months median survival. The 6 patients who performed chemotherapy before and after concomitant radiocheotherapy had a 31-months survival and 20.5 –months median survival respectively.

Discussion and conclusion

The therapy of liver metastases is still controversial and not standardized. Surgery, contrary to what occurs in colorectal tumors, is poorly feasible in breast cancer. This is due to the fact that rarely are metastases solitary and when it is so, most probably the spread is more extended than what was evidenced on radiography. PET rather than CT or MRI will certainly contribute to the identification of still invisible locations.

Chemotherapy alone was shown to be unable to achieve high objectives, and long-lasting responses. Controlled studies concerning the treatment of liver metastases alone are lacking, and therefore results come from protocols of chemotherapy in disseminated forms.

Radiotherapy alone finds its major limitation in the total dose: if the total dose is not beyond 30 Gy, liver tolerance is good but disease control is poor. If the dose is beyond 30 Gy, control is better but tolerance is worse.

Radiochemotherapy had not been considered in breast cancer and therefore our results, even if derived from a retrospective analysis, do acquire some interest. The combined treatment we administered did not involve excessive toxicity. Hematological and liver toxicity was practically absent, and the patients who showed it had previously undergone chemotherapy.

As for radiotherapy, there were no particular technical difficulties, attention being paid only to previous irradiations, for example to the chest wall or vertebral bone metastases.

In terms of survival, the results appear interesting also because they are associated to a good quality of life as far as the liver is concerned.

The group with metastases as the first sign of disease had better survival, as compared to those present also at other sites (27.5 months versus 15.8 months). This result was expected, but it should be stressed that 15.8 –months survival in patients with multiple metastases was calculated from the time of the appearance of liver metastases.

The most diffult problem is that of the therapy that should be combined with liver radiotherapy, and its timing. Its being understood that radiochemotherapy should be combined with a systemic therapy, our results seem to indicate that therapy before and after radiotherapy represents a slightly better combination. However, there were only six patients in this group, and the difference in terms of survival was minimal as compared to the patients who received chemotherapy after radiotherapy (31 vs 29 months).

Considering the available data, we believe that the obtained results deserve confirmation based on a controlled study, with strict criteria of inclusion and standardization of chemotherapy to be combined with radiochemotherapy.

REFERENCES

1. Jaffe BM, Donegan WL. Factors influencing survival in patients with untreated hepatic metastasis. *Surg Gynecol Obstet* 1968; 127: 1-11.
2. Hoe AL, Royle GT, Taylor I. Breast liver metastases – incidence, diagnosis and outcome. J R Soc Med 1991; 84(12): 714-716.
3. Santoro E, Vitucci C, Carlini M, et al. Liver metastasis of breast carcinoma. *Chir Ital* 2000; 52 (2): 131-137.
4. Yoshimoto M, Tada T, Saito M, Takahashi K, Uchida Y, Kasumi F. Surgical treatment of hepatic metastases from breast cancer. *Breast Cancer Res Treat* 2000; 59(2): 177-1.
5. Selzner M, Morse MA, Vderenburgh JJ, Meyers WC, Clavien PA. Liver metastases from breast cancer: long-term survival after curative resection. *Surgery* 2000; 127(4): 383-389.
6. Joensuu H, Holli K, Heikkinen E et al. Combination chemotherapy versus single-agent therapy as first and second line treatment in metastatic breast cancer: a prospective randomized trial. *J Clin Oncol* 1998; 16(12): 3720-3730.
7. Barone RM, Bayfield JE, Goldfarb PB, Frankel S, Ginn C, Greer S. Inta-arterial chemotherapy using an implantable infusion pump and liver irradiation for the treatment of hepatic metastases. *Cancer* 1982; 50: 850-862.
8. Sullivan R. Systemic and arterial infusion chemotherapy for metastatic liver cancer. *Int J Radiat Oncol Biol Phys* 1976; 1: 973-976.

9. Trudeau ME. Phase I-II studies oh docetaxel as single agent in the treatment of metastatic breast cancer. *Semin Oncol* 1999; 28(Suppl8): 21-26.
10. Sparano J. Novel combination chemotherapy regimens for metastatic breast cancer. The 21st San Antonio Breast cancer Simposium. December 12-15, 1998.
11. Cocconi G, De Lisi V, Boni C, et al. Chemotherapy versus combination of chemotherapy and endocrine therapy in advanced breast cancer. *Cancer* 1983; 51: 581-588.
12. Ingold JA, Reed GB, Kaplan HS, Bagshaw MA. Radiation hepatitis. *Am J Roentgenol* 1965; 93: 200-208.
13. Phillips R. Roentgentherapy of hepatic metastases. *Am J Roentg Ther Nucl Med* 1954; 71: 826-834.
14. Borgelt BB, Gelber R, Brady LW, Griffin T, Hendricksson FR. The palliation of hepatic metastases: Results of the Radiation Therapy Oncology Group pilot Study. *Int J Radiat Oncol Biol Phys* 1981; 7: 587-591.
15. Heimdal K, Hannisdal E, Fossa SD. Survival after palliative radiotherapy of liver metastases. *Acta Oncol* 1988; 27: 63.
16. Kagan AR. Dose-time relationships in the palliation of metastases to liver, lung, brain and bone metastases. *Front Radiat Ther Oncol* 1988; 22: 165-
17. Thames HD, Peters LJ, Withers RH, Fletcher GH. Accelerated fractionation vs hyper fractionation. Rationale for several treatments per day. *Int J Radiat Oncol Biol Phys* 1983; 9: 127-138.
18. Thames HD, Withers RH, Peters LJ, Fletcher GH. Changes in early and late radiation response with alterated dose fractionation. Implication for dose-survival relationships. *Int J Radiat Oncol Biol Phys* 1982; 8: 219-226.
19. Russell AH, Clyde C, Wasserman TH, Turner SS, Rotman M. Accelerated hyperfractionated hepatic irradiation in the management of patients with liver metastases: results of the RTOG dose esclating protocol. *Int J Radiat Oncol Biol Phys* 1993; 27: 117-123.
20. Lokich J, Kinsella T, Perri J Malcom A, Clouse M. Concomitant hepatic radiation and intraarterial pyrimidine therapy: correlation of liver scan, liver function test and plasma CEA with tumor response. *Cancer* 1981; 48: 2569-2574.
21. Kinsella TJ. The role of radiation therapy alone and combined with infusion of chemotherapy for treating liver metastaes. *Sem Oncol* 1983; 10: 215-22.
22. Rotman M, Kuruvilla AM, Choi K, Bhutiani I, Aziz H, Rosentha J, Braverman A et al. Response of colo-rectal Hepatic metastases to concomitant radiotherapy and intravenous infusion 5-fluorouracil. *Int J Radiat Oncol Biol Phys* 1986; 12: 2179-2187.
23. Byfield JE, Calabro-Jones P, Klisak I, Kulhanian F. Pharmacological requirements for obtaining sensistization of human tumor cells in vitro to combined 5-fluorouracil or ftorafu and x-rays. *Int J Radiat Oncol Biol Phys* 1982; 8: 1923-1933.
24. Fu K, Rayner BS, Lam K. Modification of effects of continuous low dose irradiation by concurrent chemotherapy infusion. *Int J Radiat Oncol Biol Phys* 1984; 10: 1473- 1478.
25. Nakajima V, Miyamoto N, Tanabe M, Watanabe I, Terasima T. Enhancement of mammalian cell killing by 5-fluorouracil in combination with x-rays. *Cancer Res* 1979; 39: 3763-3767.
26. Nigro ND, Vaitkevicius VK, Considine B. Combined therapy for cancer of the anal canal: a preliminary report. *Dis Colon Rectum* 1974; 17: 354-357.
27. Dobrowsky W, Dobrowsky E, Strassl H, Braun O, Scheibers V. response to peoperative radio-chemotherapy with mitomycin C and 5-fluorouracil in advanced head and neck cancer. *Eur J Cancer Clin Oncol* 1989; 25:845-849.
28. Steel GG, Peckham MJ. Expoitable mechanism in combined radiotherapy-chemotherapy: the concept of additivity. *Int J Radiat Oncol Biol Phys* 1979; 5: 85-91.
29. Kennedy KA, Rockwell S, Sartorelli AC. Preferential activation of mitomycin C to cytotoxic metabolites by hypoxic tumor cells. *Cancer Res* 1980; 40: 2356-2360.

30. Seifert P, Baker LH, Reed ML, Vaitkevicius VK. Comparison of continuously infused 5-Fluorouracil with bolus injection in treatment of patients with colorectal cancer. *Cancer* 1975; 36: 123-128.
31. Peretz T, Freund HR, Isacson R et al. Treatment of primary and metastatic liver cancer using an implantable chemoinfusion pump. Isr J Med Sci 1988; 24: 562-567.
32. Mohiuddin M, Chen E, Ahmad N. combined liver radiation and chemotherapy for palliation of hepatic metastases from colorectal cancer. *J Clin Oncol* 1996; 14: 722-728.
33. Aray Y, Sone Y, Inaba Y, Ariyoshi Y, Kido C. Hepatic arterial infusion chemotherapy for liver metastases from breast cancer. *Cancer Chemother Pharmacol* 1994; 33S: 141-144.
34. Schneebaum S, Walker MJ, Young D, Farrar WB, Minton JP. The regional treatment of liver metastases from breast cancer. *J Surg Oncol* 1994; 55(1): 26-31.
35. Ausili Cefaro G, Smaniotto D, De Renzis C. Radiotherapy of hepatic metastases. *Acta Med Rom* 1986; 24: 143-148.
36. Nardone L, Salvi G, Brizi MG, Caspiani O, Abu Rumeileh I. Trattamento integrato radiochemioterapico concomitante per le metastasi epatiche da carcinoma mammario. In: Squillaci S: "Neoplasie epatiche e pancreatiche" – Monduzzi Editore, 1993, 253-257.

CHAPTER 10

CARCINOMA OF THE PAPILLA OF VATER: PROGNOSTIC AND THERAPEUTIC CONSIDERATIONS

Giovanni Serio, Calogero Iacono, Luca Bortolasi, Ettore Montresor
Department of Surgery, University of Verona, Verona, Italy

Abstract

Sixty-seven cases of pancreaticoduodenectomy for adenocarcinoma of the papilla were observed over the period from 1970 to 2000 for the purposes of assessing results, and identifying possible prognostic factors based on pathology and biomolecular criteria.
The surgical technique adopted was the Whipple operation. In the last decade the pylorus-preserving procedure was adopted. Eight patients operated on in the last decade were submitted to pancreaticoduodenectomy plus extended lymphoneurectomy.
The overall mortality was 5.9% (4 cases out of 67). The mortality rate decreased progressively from 16% in the first decade (1970-80) to 5% in the second (1981-90), and then to 0% in the third (1991-2000). The incidence of major morbidity was 38.5%.
The overall actuarial survival rate was 47% at 5 years and 34% at 10 years. In the group treated with pancreaticoduodenectomy plus extended lymphoneurectomy the 5-year actuarial survival rate was 80%.
At univariate analysis, tumour ulceration, T4 stage, lymph node metastases and combined scores of 5-7 (according to the system proposed by Talbot *et al.*) were negative prognostic factors. At multivariate analysis, however, only the T stage factor was found to be an independent prognostic factor.
In molecular study, 16% of cases presented microsatellite instability (RER-positive). These patients are all still alive, whereas in the RER-negative subjects the 5- and 10-year survival rates were 30% and 26%, respectively. Seventy-nine percent of the cases reviewed presented deletion of chromosome 17p. On combining the analysis of the status of this chromosome with tumour stage, it was found that in cases with undeleted chromosome 17p survival was 100% in stages 2 and 3 and 38% in stage 4, whereas in those in which deletion of chromosome 17p was present the survival rate dropped sharply to 18% in stages T II and T III and to 0% in stage T IV.
Pancreaticoduodenectomy remains the gold standard in the treatment of carcinoma of the papilla. Extended lymphoneurectomy confers a greater measure of radicality on the operation by curbing the lymphoneural spread of the tumour. The extent of local invasion and a number of molecular markers (microsatellite instability and deletion of chromosome 17p) offer more reliable prognostic evaluation criteria.

A.M. *Farinon (ed.), Advances in Abdominal Surgery 2002*, 141-158.

INTRODUCTION

Carcinoma of the papilla of Vater is a relatively uncommon tumour. Its incidence in non-selected autopsy series ranges from 0.028 to 0.04% [1-2] and it accounts for 1.5 to 2% of all gastrointestinal tumours [1, 3]. The term "carcinoma of the papilla of Vater" would appear to be more appropriate than the more frequently used "ampullary carcinoma", in that it embraces not only carcinomas originating in the common duct (and thus in the ampulla), but also those arising in the epithelium, covering the papillary prominence of the duodenum and the intramural portion of Wirsung duct, and of the terminal common bile duct [4]. A thorough pathological examination with macrosections may enable this tumour to be distinguished from carcinoma of the terminal common bile duct, the duodenum and the pancreas. The term 'periampullary carcinoma' should therefore be adopted only when it is impossible to assign the tumour to one of the histogenetically different, but topographically very close, epithelial lines (papilla, common bile duct, pancreas). In this context, carcinoma of the papilla is unquestionably less frequent than cancer of the head of the pancreas, but more frequent than cancer of the terminal common bile duct and periampullary duodenum.

There is now a general consensus of opinion regarding the greater resectability rate (ranging from 60 to 100%), and better prognosis (up to 60% 5-year actuarial survival), of carcinoma of the papilla compared to carcinoma of the pancreas.

The evaluation of factors predictive of prognosis is a matter of some controversy, in that, with the exception of the criterion of local tumour spread (T stage), there is substantial divergence of opinion, with regards to the identification of other independent prognostic factors.

Recently, molecular investigation has come up with new criteria based on findings of chromosome deletions [5], oncogenes [6-7] and suppressor gene [5, 8] abnormalities, and mutations of DNA repair genes (RER phenotype) [8-9].

The aims of the present study were to analyze the results of pancreaticoduodenectomy (PD) in the radical treatment of carcinoma of the papilla, and to identify factors predictive of prognosis, in the light of pathology criteria and genetic factors, offered by the most recent advances in molecular biology.

PATIENTS AND METHODS

A retrospective study was conducted of 96 patients with tumours of the papilla of Vater, who were observed over the period from June 1970 to December 2000. Of these, 81 were submitted to resection (71 pancreaticoduodenectomies and 10 local resections of the tumour), and 15 underwent palliative surgical treatment (Tab. 1).

Table 1 Tumors of the papilla of Vater. Pathology and surgical treatments in 96 cases observed from 1970 to 2000

Pathology		**Surgery**
Adenoma	9	8 ampullectomies, 1PD
Carcinoid	2	2 ampullectomies
Adenocarcinoma	82	67 PD, 15 pall. surg.
Small-cell ca.	3	3 PD

PD: pancreaticoduodenectomy

The specific study population consisted of 67 patients (45 males, 22 females; mean age: 63 years; range: 35-78 years), operated on for adenocarcinoma. These accounted for 16.7% of all 401 pancreaticoduodenectomies, performed over the same period for pancreatic and periampullary tumors (Tab. 2). Four pancreaticoduodenectomies performed for adenoma (1) and for small-cell neuroendocrine carcinomas of the papilla (3), and the 10 local resections of adenoma and carcinoid tumors, were omitted from the study.

Table 2. Pancreaticoduodenectomy for pancreatic and periampullary tumors (1970 - 2000): (401 cases)

• Ca. Head of the pancreas	195	• PA (unrecognized site)	12
• Ca. Papilla of Vater	70	• Other tumors	7
• Ca. Common bile duct	39	• Papillary-cystic tumor	5
• Cystic t. (Serous, mucinous)	19	• Ca. acinar	2
• IMPT	18	• Adenoma of papilla of Vater	2
• Endocrine tumor	16	• Dermoid cyst	1
• Ca. duodenum	15		

PA = periampullary cancer, IMPT: intraductal mucinous producing tumors

Jaundice and subjaundice along with abdominal pain were the most frequent symptoms, being present in 90% of the patients operated on.

The preoperative diagnostic investigation up to 1980 was based on contrast radiography of the upper digestive tract, gastroduodenoscopy, and percutaneous transhepatic cholangiography (PTC). After 1980 the diagnosis came to be based on endoscopic retrograde cholangiopancreatography (ERCP), ultrasonography (US) and computed tomography (CT). Since 1999 magnetic resonance cholangiography (MRC) has also been used.

The surgical technique most commonly adopted up to 1990 consisted of the standard Whipple resection, while in recent years the pylorus-preserving procedure has tended to be the operation of choice.

Eight patients were submitted to extended lymphadenectomy. This involved removal of retroperitoneal and perivascular neural, lymphatic and adipose tissue, with skeletonisation of the vena cava, the mesenteric-portal axis, and the superior mesenteric artery for about 10 cm, the left renal vein, the common hepatic artery, and the vascular elements of the hepatoduodenal ligament, the coeliac trunk and the aortic tract, including the coeliac trunk and lower mesenteric artery, and the intercavo-aortic space [10, 12].

All the pathological specimens were grossly and microscopically reviewed, to confirm diagnosis, macroscopic aspect (ulcerated or non-ulcerated tumour), and precisely establishing the local tumour spread (classified from T1 to T4), according to Yamaguchi and Enjoji [4] (T-Stage I: intraductal tumors restricted to muscle of Oddi; T-Stage II: infiltration of duodenal submucosa; T-Stage III: involvement of muscolaris propria and T-Stage IV: infiltration of the periduodenal fat and pancreas), lymph-node status, tumour grading (low, grade 1; moderate, grade 2; high, grade 3), persistence of adenomatous residues, perineural and perivascular infiltration, and infiltration of the retroperitoneal margins. On combining the T-Stage data and tumour grades, a score was obtained ranging from 1 to 7, according to the criteria proposed by Talbot *et al.* [13].

In 44 patients operated on, the morphological examination was supplemented with a molecular investigation (RER-phenotype, chromosome 17p and 18q status), aimed at identifying factors predictive of prognosis.

The operative mortality as relating to the 30-day period immediately following the operation, and the postoperative morbidity, were calculated in all 67 patients.

The pathology findings (size, macroscopic appearance, grading, T-stage, lymph-node status, combined scores, presence of adenomatous residues) and the molecular variables (RER phenotype, chromosomes 17p and 18q) were assessed statistically, using univariate and multivariate analysis.

Survival probability was estimated according to the Kaplan-Meier method, whereas the long rank test was used for comparison of survival in different subgroups. Multivariate analysis was performed by the Cox regression model. Comparison of proportions was performed, using the Chi-square test and Fisher exact test. Means were compared using the Student t-test.

RESULTS

Pathology

On pathological examination the diagnosis of adenocarcinoma of the papilla was confirmed in 67 cases. The various macro- and microscopic characteristics and the tumour staging results are presented in Table 3.

Table 3. Pathological and molecular factors in 67 patients who underwent pancreaticoduodenectomy for adenocarcinoma of the papilla of Vater

	No. of patients
Size	
≤ 2 cm	44
> 2 cm	23
Gross aspect	
ulcerated	34
non ulcerated	33
Grading	
well	7
moderate	32
poor	24
not assessed	4
T-Stage	
I	3
II	17
III	15
IV	32
Lymph node status	
negative	42
positive	25
Score system	
2-4	15
5-7	48
not available	4
Adenomatous residues	
yes	30
no	37
RER status (in 44 pts)	
positive	6
negative	38
18q allele (in 44 pts)	
loss	15
retention	29
17p allele (in 44 pts)	
loss	23
retention	21

Lymph-node station involvement rates, for the 8 patients that underwent extended pancreaticoduodenectomy, are reported in Table 4.

Table 4. Lymph-node stations involved in 8 extended pancreaticoduodenectomy, for adenocarcinoma of the papilla of Vater

Lymph node station	Positive/negative
Posterior pancreaticoduodenal	4/8
Anterior pancreaticoduodenal	2/8
Mesenteric	2/8
Choledochal	1/8

Mortality and morbidity

Follow-up studies were completed for all the patients, with a mean time of 128 months (range: 6-240). The overall operative mortality was 5.9% (4 out of 67 patients that underwent pancreaticoduodenectomy). On dividing the 30-year observation period into three subperiods (1970-80, 1981-90, 1991-2000), a substantial difference in mortality rate is observed between the first (16%), second (5%) and third most recent decade (0%) (Fig 1).

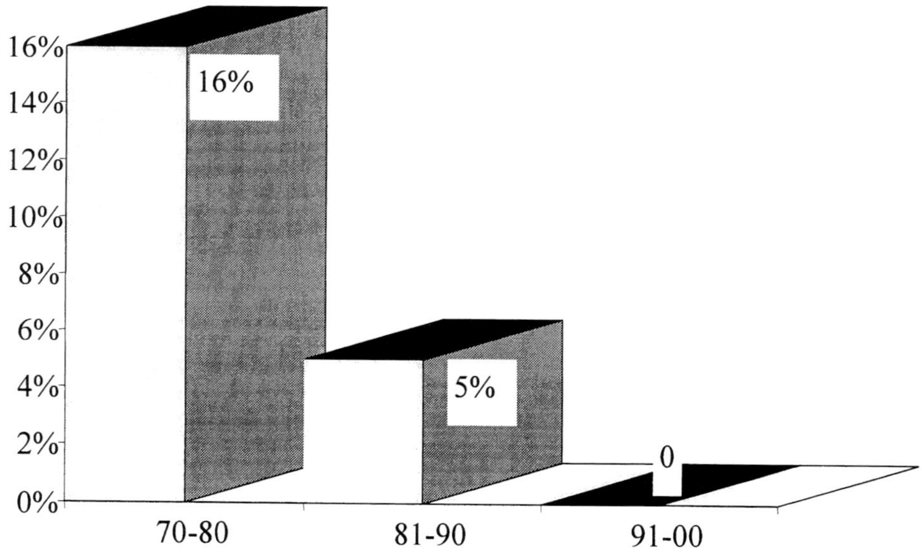

Figure 1. Operative mortality after PD for adenocarcinoma of the papilla of Vater, in three different decades of experience: 1970-80, 1981-90, 1991-2000

Major morbidity rate was 38.5%, and more frequent complications are listed in Table 5.

Table 5. Operative mortality and complications in 67 PD for adenocarcinoma of the papilla of Vater

• Operative mortality	4/67 cases	5.9%
• Global complication	35/67 cases	52%
• Medical complication	24/67 cases	36%
• Surgical complication	26/67 cases	39%
- *Pancreatic fistula*	*14.9%*	
- *Abdominal collection*	*10.4%*	
- *Hemorrhage* *	*7.4%*	
- *Biliary fistula*	*7.4%*	
- *Pancreatitis* *	*2.9%*	
- *Digestive fistula*	*2.9%*	
- *MOF* *	*1.4%*	

* Operative mortality (1/2 pancreatitis, 2/5 hemorrhage, 1/1 MOF)

Overall survival

The 5- and 10-year survival rates were 47% and 34%, respectively (Fig. 2).

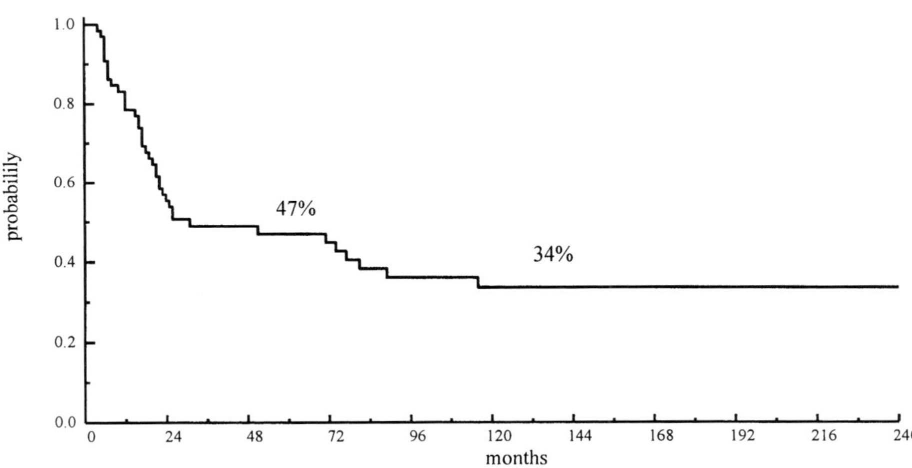

Figure 2. Survival curve (Kaplan-Meier method) after PD for adenocarcinoma of the ampulla of Vater

On comparing the patients treated before 1992 with standard pancreaticoduodenectomy (group A), with those treated after 1992 with extended lymphadenectomy (group B), 5-year survival was 42% in group A, versus 80% in group B (Fig. 3); even if there is a better trend in group B, the difference is not statistically significant for the small number of patients.

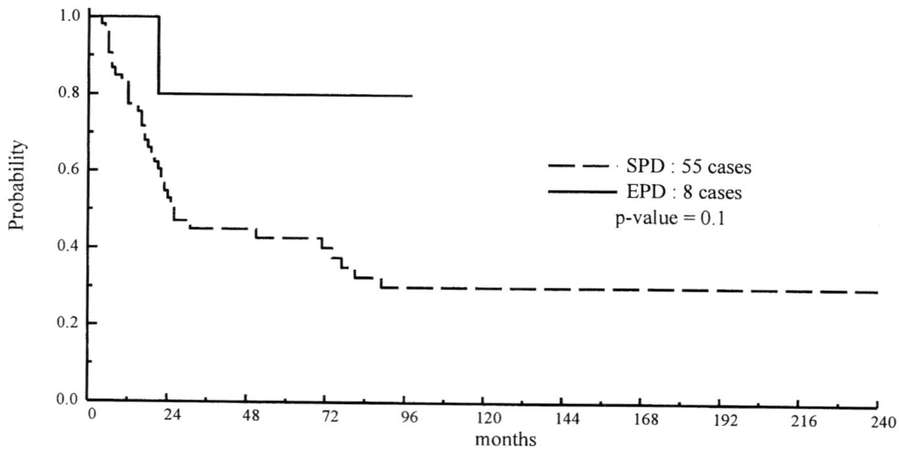

Figure 3. Survival curves (Kaplan-Meier method) after PD extended (EPD) or standard (SPD), for adenocarcinoma of the papilla of Vater.

PATHOLOGICAL AND MOLECULAR FACTORS

Analysis of survival revealed a better outcome in patients with non-ulcerated tumours than in those with ulcerated tumours, in patients with T-stages II and III, as compared to T-stage IV, in patients with low-moderate grade versus high grade of differentiation, in patients with no lymph-node metastases vs those with metastases, and in patients with combined scores of 2-4 vs those with scores of 5-7, whereas there were no differences related to tumour size, presence or absence of jaundice at the time of diagnosis, and presence or absence of adenomatous residues (Tab. 6).

Table 6. Adenocarcinoma of the papilla of Vater. Factors associated with poor prognosis: univariate analyses

Ulceration vs non ulceration	p<0.01
Poor differentiation vs well & mod	p<0.03
T-Stage IV vs T-Stage II & III	p<0.001
Lymph node positive vs negative	p<0.01
Score system 5 - 7 vs 2 - 4	p<0.01
Absence vs presence of RER phenotype	p<0.007
Chromosome 17p loss vs retention	p<0.001
Chromosome 18q loss vs retention	p<0.001

At multivariate analysis (Tab. 7), however, only the T-stage proved to be an independent prognostic factor. The 5 and 10-year survival was 61% and 42% for T-Stage I-II and 19% and 19% for T-Stage III-IV (p-value = 0.005), respectively. In the molecular study, 7 patients (16%) presented microsatellite instability (RER-positive). Survival analysis showed that all 7 were still alive (100% survival at 168 months) regardless of stage (these cases included 2 T-Stage III and 1 T-Stage IV cancers), while the RER-negative patients had 30 and 26% survival rates, at 5 and 10 years, respectively.

Table 7. Adenocarcinoma della papilla di Vater. Pathological and molecular factors in 44 patients: multivariate abalysis (Cox model)

Variable	RR	95% C.I.	p-value
T-Stage III vs II	1.79	0.46 - 7.00	< 0.001
T-Stage IV vs II	7.22	2.05 - 25.47	< 0.001
Loss vs retent. Chromosome 17p	5.77	2.18 - 15.29	< 0.001

Deletion of chromosome 17p was found in 23 cases (52%), deletion of 18q in 15 (34%) and deletion of both in 12 (27%). At multivariate analysis, however, only the 17p deletion proved to be an independent prognostic factor. Table 7 summarises the most significant indications furnished by multivariate analysis, with regards to the various pathological and molecular factors.

Seventy-nine percent (35 cases) of the patients examined presented deletion of chromosome 17p. On analyzing the survival of these cases in relation to T-Stage, we found that in the cases in which chromosome 17p was spared, survival was 100% in T-Stages II and III, and 38% in T-Stage IV, whereas in the cases in which it was deleted, survival drops to 18% in T-Stages II and III, and to zero in T-Stage IV.

DISCUSSION

Pancreaticoduodenectomy is the radical treatment of choice for carcinoma of the papilla of Vater. The 5-year actuarial survival rates with this procedure range from 24 to 60% [14-25], with mean values of around 35-46% [26-32].

Clinical (early onset of jaundice) and local factors (minor lymphatic diffusion, facility to achieve free margin of resection) allow a more radical resection to be obtained, determining a better prognosis than pancreatic cancer.

Operative mortality related to pancreaticoduodenectomy has shown a marked decrease in recent years, registering rates of less than 3-5% in referral Centres [14, 17, 19, 20-21, 24, 26-28, 30-34], as against the 11% to 25% mortality rates [15, 16, 35-38] registered up to about 15 years ago.

Our 30-years' experience shows an improvement regarding operative mortality, that has progressed from 16% in the seventies to 5% in the eighties, and in the nineties to 0%. This better result, which has also been confirmed for other pancreatic diseases, may be due to advances in operative and resuscitation techniques, and to the increased experience of the surgical team and high volume referral center [39-40].

Over the years, the undoubted drop in operative mortality following pancreaticoduodenectomy has not been accompanied by a proportional reduction in the incidence of complications, that remains still as high as 68% [20, 30, 41] , and shows the difficulties and risks of this procedure.

The reliability of the operative technique, and the oncological reliability of pancreaticoduodenectomy, have relegated to a subordinate rôle the local resection procedures (papillectomy, papilloduodenectomy), advocated in the past mainly by French surgeons [42-43]. The reasons for opting for limited resection, adduced by those authors, were based on the superior tolerance of local resection, as compared to the greater risks involved in pancreaticoduodenectomy, and on findings indicating satisfactory 5-year survival rates [15, 44-46]. Nevertheless, a critical review does not support this technique, due to the still high morbidity rate and frequent recurrence rate, when compared to pancreaticoduodenectomy [37, 47-48]. Up to now, there are very few indications for papilloduodenectomy: elderly and high-risk patients, patients with early-stage tumours (T-Stage I), as detected by accurate pre- and intraoperative staging [49].

Over the past two decades no substantial changes have been made in the standard pancreaticoduodenectomy procedure, for purposes of improving the quality of life and survival of patients with carcinoma of the papilla. Preservation of the pylorus was first accepted in the oncological setting, in periampullary carcinoma [50-52]. It was demonstrated that the technique does not have any adverse effect on long-term oncological results, also for carcinoma of the pancreas, and offers indubitable advantages in terms of patient postoperative nutritional recovery times [53].

Delayed gastric emptying, which is reported as being a frequent postoperative complication [54-55], was also confirmed in our experience, but with a less frequent incidence than in data reported in literature, and it is easily managed by maintaining a nasogastric tube in place.

Of considerable interest in the treatment of ductal adenocarcinoma of the pancreas, has been the introduction of lymphadenectomy extended to the 2nd level, with an intent to achieve a more radical procedure and to improve the poor outcome [12, 55-57]. Results in this regard have been discordant, and the procedure is still a matter of some controversy [58].

Over the past 10 years, we have analyzed the problem also in the case of periampullary carcinoma, with a view to establishing an optimal extent of lymphadenectomy for this type of tumour.

The most frequently involved lymph-node stations, after extended pancreaticoduodenectomy, were the posterior and anterior pancreaticoduodenal lymph nodes, the nodes of the inferior pancreaticoduodenal and mesenteric arteries, and less frequently the para-aortic lymph nodes, pericholedochal and retroportal lymph nodes, whereas pyloric, coeliac, medio-colic and hepatic artery lymph-node stations were never invaded. This type of distribution has been confirmed in similar studies conducted by other investigators [22, 59-61].

The Kaplan-Meier method revealed a significantly better survival, of the group treated with extended pancreaticoduodenectomy, than the group treated prior to 1992 with standard PD. Even within the limits of this study (not randomized, non-prospective, small series) some considerations may be deduced: in fact, considering 1st level lymphadenectomy as being an adequate treatment for the patients treated prior to 1992, how can we explain worse survival in this group of patients? In an effort to find clarification, some hypotheses can be advanced:

a) the non-availability of CT scans until 1980, and of spiral CT scans until 1990, might have limited the ability to establish a correct preoperative staging, with a poor selection of patients with extrapancreatic involvement;

b) the lymphadenectomy may not have been correctly performed. Pancreaticoduodenectomy, as performed up to 1980, probably left a number of gaps for carcinoma of the pancreas, as was accurately demonstrated by Fitzgerald and Cubilla. In their investigation, the weaknesses of the technique were failure to remove the superior and inferior lymph nodes of the body, the perimesenteric lymph nodes and, to a lesser extent, the peri-aortal lymph nodes.

In carcinoma of the papilla, the superior and inferior lymph nodes of the body and the peri-aortal lymph nodes are hardly ever invaded, but the perimesenteric lymph nodes are metastatic in 11-17% of the cases [21-22, 61] (25% of the cases in the present experience) and up to 58% [62].

There are some oncological reasons to believe that combined clearance of perimesenteric lymphadenectomy and of perimesenteric plexus, associated to pancreaticoduodenectomy, offer a better chance of radical resection, owing to the suppression of two major pathways for tumour spread, namely the lymphatic and the perineural pathways [10-11, 61, 63].

The longer natural history of carcinoma of the papilla compared to pancreatic ductal adenocarcinoma, has led to the assessment of a number of prognostic factors, some of which are suggested by ductal adenocarcinoma and others by morphological and time-course affinities with colorectal cancer. Figuring among the variables most commonly proposed are macroscopic appearance, pathological characteristics, tumour grading, local invasiveness (T factor) and lymph-node status.

A non-ulcerated appearance of tumours suggests a better prognosis than the ulcerated and scirrhous forms [4, 22, 48]. Also in our experience, the survival of patients with ulcerated forms was significantly worse than that of patients with protruding forms.

A number of authors [35, 64] claim that tumours with the characteristics of papillary tumors present a better prognosis. In the course of time this has become a grading criterion, and has led surgeons to distinguish between low-grade or grade-1 well-differentiated tumours, medium-grade or grade-2 moderately-differentiated tumours, and high-grade or grade-3 poorly-differentiated or clearly-undifferentiated tumours. According to various reports, a high-grade tumour carries a very poor prognosis incompatible with 5-year survival [13, 18, 47, 65], whereas satisfactory survival rates of the order of 48-62% are reported for resections of low-grade carcinomas [47, 64].

Local tumour-spread is a variable which many investigators regard as an independent prognostic factor [29, 41]. A number of them believe that infiltration of the pancreas is incompatible with 5-year survival even in the absence of other negative prognostic factors [36, 66], and place the natural history of these tumours on a par with that of ductal carcinoma of the pancreas [19, 21, 24, 67]. Yamaguchi and Enjoi [4] also agree as to the importance of local invasion: on the basis of a study of 109 surgical specimens, they conclude that a decisive factor for the prognosis is whether or not the tumour has spread beyond the sphincter of Oddi.

The criterion of local invasion, related to the infiltration capability of the tumour, has relegated to second place that of the size of the tumour, with a limit of 2 cm, above and below which a good or poor prognosis was to be expected, respectively [68-69]. The size criterion may have a purely indicative significance, given that larger size is correlated with a greater frequency of other negative prognostic factors such as pancreatic, vascular, perineural and lymph-node invasion [19, 33, 44, 47].

The persistence of adenomatous residues, as reported for colorectal carcinoma, may be related to tumour size, in the sense that it is more frequent in tumours measuring less than 3 cm [38]. It is difficult, however, to attribute any precise prognostic significance to the presence or otherwise of adenomatous residues, and in our patients this variable is not statistically significant as a prognostic factor.

One debated aspect has to do with lymph-node infiltration, which is a factor taken into consideration by all authors dealing with this type of malignancy. Most of them report a significant difference in 5-year survival and median survival of patients undergoing resection without metastases [18, 23-24, 28, 33-34, 44, 65, 67, 69, 70]. In some cases the distinction even goes so far as to indicate no survival at 5-years in patients with metastases [36, 66], with a median survival rate not dissimilar to that of patients undergoing palliative treatment. A smaller group of authors do not attribute any meaningful rôle to lymph-node metastases, in that they do not regard them as being decisive with regards to patient survival [15, 20, 26, 29, 47, 71-72].

Critical assessment of the numerous pathology prognostic factors proposed leads us to conclude that, with the exception of the T factor, none of the other variables can be regarded as reliable prognostic factors. These conclusions are also reached by Yamaguchi and Enjoji [59], in their meticulous study of 36 cases, in which they test as many as 18 prognostic factors.

The multifactorial analysis aimed at evaluating prognostic factors in colorectal cancer [73] suggested the use of the same methodology in carcinoma of the papilla. Talbot *et al.* [13] have proposed a prognostic score, based on the sum of the number denoting the tumour stage (defined as 1 to 4) and that denoting the grade (from 1 to 3). On this basis, one can distinguish between two groups, one with a combined score ranging from 2 to 4, and the other with a combined score ranging from 5 to 7. A highly significant difference in 5-year survival has been found between these two groups (84% in the 2-4 group vs 26% in the 5-7 group).

Substantial importance has recently been attributed to the extent of perioperative transfusions for malignancies, as a prognostic factor. Talamini et al. [30] have documented that the absence of intraoperative transfusions is predictive of better patient-survival in carcinoma of the papilla. On the basis of mutivariate analysis, the authors deduce that, in carcinoma of the papilla the prognostic rôle of transfusions is more important than the biology of the tumors, which is the opposite of findings observed in carcinoma of the pancreas [74].

In univariate analysis of various prognostic factors in our 54 cases, the following factors were found to have an adverse effect on survival: ulceration of the tumour, T4 stage, lymph-node infiltration, and combined score of 5-7 according to Talbot. In multivariate analysis, however, only T stage proved to be an independent prognostic factor.

The difficulty encountered by all investigators in establishing pathological factors as reliable criteria for predicting prognosis, has directed research towards factors more closely correlated with neoplastic cell DNA biology. There has been great interest in recent years in biomolecular research, with new predictive markers being proposed for survival. Familial colorectal cancer, polypoid and non-polypoid [75, 76], and also sporadic colorectal cancer have offered a whole range of gene mutations, relating to the inactivation of oncosuppressor genes (APC, DCC, p53), the activation of oncogenes (K-ras), and RER phenotype.

Reports of such mutations in carcinoma of the papilla are relatively recent [5, 9], but early results have seemed promising, with a view to providing more reliable indications as to prognosis. In our present study, we tested for deletion of chromosomes 17p and 18q, and for instability of the microsatellite sequence (RER phenotype positive).

In multivariate analysis, deletion of chromosome 17p proved to be an independent prognostic factor. The actuarial calculation revealed 5 and 10-year survival rates of 74% and 67%, respectively, in cases with preserved 17p, versus 9% and 9%, respectively, in cases with 17p deletion. Tumour stage being equal, the loss of chromosome 17p has a significant adverse effect on survival. In our sample, T-Stage II and III tumours with preserved chromosome 17p, had 5 and 10-year survival rates of 100 and 38%, respectively, whereas in those cases with deletion of the chromosome, survival dropped sharply to 18% and 0%, respectively.

Only 7 patients out of 44 (16%) were RER-positive, and these were all alive after 5 and 10 years, despite the presence of 3 cases of local invasion (duodenum and pancreas), unlike the RER-negative subjects, who presented 5 and 10-year survival rates of 30% and 26%, respectively.

Microsatellite instability has also been found in Lynch syndrome and, as in the case of this syndrome [76], carcinoma of the papilla may also be associated with other synchronous or metachronous tumors (in some cases also by familial transmission as in familial neoplastic syndrome) in the intestines, stomach, lung, breast, and female genitalia [47, 71, 77]. Of the 7 cases of RER-positive tumours in this review, 4 were found to have had the following antecedent or synchronous neoplasms: transverse colon carcinoma (2 cases), endometrial carcinoma, duodenal leiomyoma, gastric leiomyoma, and lung cancer.

In addition to being prognostic factors, the molecular markers may also serve as indicators of the therapeutic strategy, in the sense that in those cases where gene investigation reveals deletion of chromosome 17p, one may expect that surgical therapy alone will fail to prove curative, and so contemplate the need to supplement it with adjuvant measures.

At present, the latter are related essentially to the use of chemotherapy and radiotherapy, the results of which appear anything but encouraging [19, 30, 41].

We can conclude by saying that the mainstay in the management of carcinoma of the papilla of Vater firmly remains pancreaticoduodenectomy with extended lymphadenectomy, including the posterior and anterior pancreaticoduodenal, pericholedochal, and hepatic arterial nodes, and, above all, the perimesenteric and para-aortic nodes.

The degree of local invasion of the tumour, and a number of molecular markers (deletion of chromosome 17p, microsatellite instability or RER-phenotype), are factors for prognostic assessment and for planning multimodality treatment.

REFERENCES

1. Howard JM, Jordan GL. Surgical diseases of the pancreas. Philadelphia, J B Lippincott, 1960.
2. Edmonson HA. Tumors of the Gallbladder and extra-hepatic bile duvts. Atlas of tumors pathology, Section III, vol 26. Armed Dorces Institutes of pathology, 1967.
3. Jordan GL, Simons BE. Carcinoma of the ampulla of Vater. *Tex Med* 1970; 66: 70-3.
4. Yamaguchi K, Enjoji M. Carcinoma of the ampulla of Vater clinicopathologic study and phatologic staging of 109 cases of carcinoma and 5 cases of adenoma. *Cancer* 1987; 59: 506-15.
5. Scarpa A, Di Pace C, Talamini G, Falconi M, Lemoine NR, Iacono C, Achille A, Baron A, Zamboni G. Cancer of the ampulla of Vater: chromosome 17p allelic loss is associated with poor prognosis. *Gut* 2000; 46: 842-8.
6. Scarpa A, Capelli P, Zamboni G, Oda T, Mukai K, Bonetti F, Martignoni G, Iacono C, Serio G, Hirohashi S. Neoplasia of the ampulla of Vater. *Am J Path* 1993; 142: 1163-72.
7. Scarpa A, Zamboni G, Achille A, Capelli P, Bogina G, Iacono C, Serio G, Accolla RS. ras-family gene mutations in neoplasia of the ampulla of Vater. *Int J Cancer* 1994; 59: 39-42.
8. Imai Y, Tsurutani N, Oda H, Inoue T, Ishikawa T. Genetic instability and mutation of the TGF-ß-receptor-II gene in ampullary carcinomas. *Int J Cancer* 1998; 76: 407-11.
9. Achille A, Biasi MO, Zamboni G, Bogina G, Iacono C, Talamini G, Capella G, Scarpa A. Cancer of the papilla di Vater: mutator phenotype is associated with good prognosis. *Clin Cancer Res* 1997; 3: 1841-7.
10. Iacono C, Bortolasi L, Facci E, Falezza G, Prati G, Mangiante G, Serio G. Does extended pancreaticoduodenectomy increas operative morbidity and mortality vs. standard pancreaticoduodenectomy? *J Gastrointest Surg* 1997;1:446-453.
11. Iacono C, Facci E, Bortolasi L, Zamboni G, Scarpa A, Talamini G, Prati G, Nifosì F, Serio G. Intermediate results of extended pancreaticoduodenectomy. Verona experience. *J Hepatobiliary Pancreat Surg* 1999; 6:74-78.
12. Iacono C, Accordini S, Bortolasi L, Facci E, Zamboni G, Montresor E, Marinello P, Serio G: Results of pancreaticoduodenectomy for pancreatic cancer: extended versus standard procedure. *World J Surg* in press.
13. Talbot IC, Neoptolemos JP, Shaw DE, Carr-Locke D. The histopathology and staging of carcinoma of the ampulla of Vater. *Histopathology* 1988; 12: 155-65.

14. Jones BA, Langer B, Taylor BR, Girotti M. Periampullary tumors: which ones should be resected? *Am J Surg* 1985; 149: 46-52.
15. Tarazi RY, Hermann RE, Vogt DP, Hoerr SO, Esselstyn CB, Coopermann AM, Steiger E, Grundfest S. Results of surgical treatment of periampullary tumors. A thirty-five-year experience. *Surgery* 1986; 100: 16.
16. Michelassi F, Erroi F, Dawson PJ, Pietrabissa A, Noda S, Handcock M, Block GE. Experience with 647 consecutive tumors of the duodenum, ampulla, head of the pancreas and distal common bile duct. *Ann Surg* 1989; 210: 544-56.
17. Trede M, Schwall G, Saeger H. Survival after pancrreaticoduodenectomy: 118 consecutive resection without an operative mortality. *Ann Surg* 1990; 211: 447-58.
18. Monson JRT, Donhoue JH, Mc Entee JP, Mcilrath DC, Van Heerden JA, Shorter RG, Nagorney DM, Ilstrup DM. Radical resection for carcinoma of the ampulla of Vater. *Arch Surg* 1991; 126: 353-7.
19. Willett CG, Warshaw AL, Convery K, Compton CC. Patterns of failure after pancreaticoduodenectomy for ampullaary carcinoma. *Surg Gynecol Obst* 1993; 176: 33-8.
20. Allema JH, Reinders ME, Van Gulik TM, Van Leeuwen DJ, Verbeek PC, De Wit LT, Gouma DJ. Results of pancreaticoduodenectomy for ampullary carcinoma and analysis of prognostic factors for survival. *Surgery* 1995; 117: 247-53.
21. Shirai Y, Ohtani T, Tsukada K, Hatakeyma K. Patterns of lymphatic spread of carcinoma of the ampulla of Vater. *Br J Surg* 1997; 84: 1012-16.
22. Kayahara M, Nagakawa T, Ohta T, Kitagawa H, Miyazaki I. Surgical strategy for carcinoma of the papilla of Vater on the basis of lymphatic spread and mode of recurrence. *Surgery* 1997; 121: 611-7.
23. Su CH, Shyr YM, Lui WY, P'Eng FK. Factors affecting morbidity, mortality and survival after pancreaticoduodenectomy for carcinoma of the ampulla of Vater. *Hepatogastroenterology* 1999; 46: 1973-9.
24. Beger HG, Treitschke F, Gansauge F, Harada N, Hiki N, Mattfeldt T. Tumors of the ampulla of Vater: experience with local or radical resection in 171 consecutively treated patients. *Arch Surg* 1999; 134: 526-32.
25. Warren KW. Corrent concepts in management of periampullary carcinoma. *Ann Surg* 1982; 195: 152-61.
26. Matory JL, Gaynor J, Brennan M. Carcinoma of the ampulla of Vater. *Surg Gynecol Obstet* 1993; 177: 366-70.
27. Serio G, Iacono C, Zamboni G, Scarpa A, Talamini G, Facci E, Mangiante G. Carcinoma of the papilla of Vater. In: Hepato-Biliary and Pancreatic Tumours. Serio G, Huguet C, Williamson RCN eds. Graffam press Ltd Edinburg 1994: 139-45.
28. Roder JD, Schneider PM, Stein HJ, Siewert JR. Number of lymph node metastases is significantly associated with survival patients with radically resected carcinoma of the ampulla of Vater. *Br J Surg* 1995; 82: 1693-7.
29. Klempnauer J, Ridder GJ, Pichlmayr R. Prognostic factors after resection of ampullary carcinoma: multivariate survival analysis in comparison with ductal cancer of the pancreatic head. *Br J Surg* 1995; 82: 1686-91.
30. Talamini MA, Moesinger RC, Pitt HA, et al. Adenocarcinoma of the ampulla of Vater: a 28-year experience. *Ann Surg* 1997; 225: 590-600.
31. Howe JR, Klimstra DS, Moccia RD, Conlon KCC, Brennan MF. Factors predictive of survival in ampullary carcinoma. *Ann Surg* 1998; 228: 87-94.
32. Yeo CJ, Sohn TA, Cameron JL, Hruban RH, Lillemoe KD, Pitt HA. Periampullary adenocarcinoma: analysis of5-year survivors. *Ann Surg* 1998; 227: 821-31.
33. Delcore R Jr, Connor CS, Thomas JH, Friesen SR, Hermreck AS. Significance of tumor pread in adenocarcinoma of the ampulla of Vater. *Am J Surg* 1989; 158: 593-597.
34. Sperti C, Pasquali C, Piccoli A, Sernagiotto C, Pedrazzoli S. Radical resection for ampullary carcinoma: long-term results. *Br J Surg* 1994; 81: 668-71.

35. Cooperman AM. Cancer of the papilla of Vater, bile duct and duodenum. *Surg Clin North A* 1981; 61: 99.
36. Lerut JP, Gianello PR, Otte JB, Kestens PJ. Pancreaticoduodenal resection. Surgical experience of evaluation of risk factors in 103 patients. *Ann Surg* 1984; 199: 433-7.
37. Neoptolemos JP, Talbot IC, Carr-Locke DL, Shaw DE, Cockleburgh R, Hall AW, Fossard DP. Treatment and autcome in 52 consecitove cases of ampullary carcinoma. *Br J Surg* 1987; 74: 957-61.
38. Hayes DH, Bolton JS, Willis GW, Bowen JC. Carcinoma of the ampulla of Vater. *Ann Surg* 1987; 206: 572-27.
39. Gordon T, Burleyson GP, Tielsch JM, Cameron JL. The effects of regionalization on cost and autcome for one general high-risk surgical procedure. *Ann Surg* 1995; 221: 49-53.
40. Liberman MD, Kilburn H, Lindsey M, Brennan MF. Relation of perioperative deaths to hospital volume among patients undergoing pancreatic resection for malignancy. *Ann Surg* 1995; 222: 638-45.
41. Lee JH, Whittington R, Williams NN, Berry MF, VaughnDJ, Haller DG, Rosato EF. Outcome of pancreaticoduodenectomy and impact of adjuvant therapy for ampullary carcinomas. *Int J Radiation Oncology Biol Phys* 2000; 47: 945-53.
42. Vayre P, Hureau J. Les tumeurs vatériennes. *J Chir* 1997; 97: 447-78.
43. Chatelin CL. Techniques de l'ampullectomie. *J Chir* 1969; 97: 465-8.
44. Wise L, Pizzimbono C, Dehner LP. Periampullary cancer: a clinico-pathologic study of 62 patients. *Am J Surg* 1976; 131: 141-8.
45. Isaksson G, Ihse I, Andrén-Sandberg A, Evander A, Löfgren B, Millbourn E. Local excision for ampullary carcinoma: an alternative treatment for patients unfit for pancreatectomy: *Acta Chir Scand* 1982; 148: 163-5.
46. Knox RA, Kingston RD. Carcinoma of the campulla of Vater. *Br J Surg* 1986; 73: 72-3.
47. Robertson JFR, Imrie CW, Hole DJ, Carter DC, Blumgart LH. Management of periampullary carcinoma. *Br J Surg* 1987; 74: 816-9.
48. Futakawa N, Kimura W, Wada Y, Muto T. Clinicopathological characteristics and surgical procedures for carcinoma of the papilla of Vater. *Hepato-Gastroenterology* 1996; 43: 260-7.
49. Rattner DW, Fernandez-de Castillo C, Brugge WR, Warshaw AL. Defining the criteria for local resection of ampullary neoplasms.
50. Tsao JI, Rossi RL, Lowell JA. Pylorus-preserving pancreatoduodenectomy: Is it an adequate cancer operation? *Arch Surg* 1994; 129: 405-12.
51. Traverso LW. Preservation of the pylorus during pancreaticoduodenectomy-Evolution and current indications. *J Hep Bil Pacr Surg* 1994; 4: 329-34.
52. Shirai Y, Tsukada K, Ohtani T et al: Carcinoma of the ampulla of Vater: histopathologic analysis of tumor spread in Whipple pancreatoduodenectomy specimens. *World J Surg* 1995; 19: 102-7.
53. Hunt DR, McLean R. Pylorus-preserving pancreatectomy: functional results. *Br J Surg* 1989; 76: 173-6.
54. Warshaw AL, Torchiana DL. Delayed gastric emptying after pylorus-preserving pancreaticoduodenectomy. *Surg Gynecol Obstet* 1985; 160: 1-4.
55. Grace PA, Pitt A, Longmire WP. Pyrolus preserving pancreatoruodenectomy: an overview. *Br J Surg* 1990; 77: 968-74.
56. Ishikawa O, Oshigashi H, Sakai Y, Kabuto T, Fukuda I, Furukawa H, Imaoka S, Iwanaga T. Pratical usefulness of lymphatic and connective tissue clearance for the carcinoma of the pancreas head. *Ann Surg* 1998; 208: 215-20.
57. Imaizumi T, Hanyu F, Harada N, e at. Extended eadical Whipple resection for cancer of the pancreatic head: operative and results. *Dig Surg* 1998; 15: 299-307.
58. Pedrazzoli S, Di Carlo V, Dionigi R, Mosca F, Pederzoli P, Pasquali C, Kloppel G, Dhaene K, Michelassi F. Standard versus extended lymphadenectomy associated with pancreatoduode-

nectomy in the surgical treatment of adenocarcinoma of the head of the pancreas. A multicenter, prospective, randomized study. *Ann Surg* 1998; 228: 508-17.
59. Yamaguchi K, Nishihara K. Long and short-ter survivors after pancreaticoduodenctomy for ampullary carcinoma. *J Surg Oncol* 1992; 50: 195-200.
60. Nakao A, Harada A, Nonami T, et al. Prognosis of cancer of the duodenal papilla of Vater in relation to clinicopathological tumors extension. *Hepatogastroenterology* 1994; 41: 73-8.
61. Yoshida T, Matsumoto T, Shibata K, Yokoyama H, Morii Y, Sasaki A, Kitano A. Petterns of lymph node metastasis in carcinoma of the ampulla of Vater. *Hepatogastroenterology* 2000; 47: 880-3.
62. Fernàndez-Cruz L, Sabater L, Ardid J, Navarro S, Kuriansky J, Cardona V. Radical lymphadenectomy for patients with carcinoma of the ampulla of Vater: evaluation of the extent of lymph node metastasis. *HPB* 1999; 1: 79-83.
63. Shirai Y, Tsukada K, Ohtani T, Hatakeyama K. Carcinoma of the ampulla of Vater: is radical lymphadenectomy beneficial to patients with nodal disease? *Surg Oncol* 1996; 61: 190-4.
64. Makipour H, Cooperman A, Danzi J, Farmer R. Carcinoma of the ampulla of Vater: review of 38 cases with emphasis on treatment and prognostic factors. *Ann Surg* 1976; 183: 341-7.
65. Akwari O, Van Heerden J, Adson M. Radical pancreatoduodenectomy for cancer of the papilla of Vater. *Arch Surg* 1977; 112: 251-6.
66. Sato T, Saitho Y, Noto N, Matsuno S. Follow up of radical resection for pancreaticoduodenal cancer. *Ann Surg* 1977; 186: 581-6.
67. Mori K, Ikei S, Yamante T, Yamaguchi Y, Katsumori T, Shibata Y, Arai T. Pathological factors influencing ssurvival of carcinoma of the ampulla of Vater. *Eur J Surg Oncol* 1990; 16: 183-8.
68. Nix G, Wilsonj, Schmitz PI. Carcinoma of the ampulla and papilla of Vater. *Ftsch Roentg* 1983; 138: 531.
69. Buchler M, Rampf W, Backzaco K, Lobeck H, Merkle P, Bittner R, Karautzberger W, Beger HG. Klinik und feinstrukture des papillenkarzinoms. *DMW* 1984; 109: 43-50.
70. Bakkevold KE, Kambestad B. Staging of carcinoma of the pancreas and ampulla of Vater. Tumor (T) lymph node (N) and distant metastasis (M) as prognostic factors. *Pancreatol* 1995; 17: 249-59.
71. Schlippert W, Lucke D, Anuras S. Carcinoma of the papilla of the Vater. *Am J Surg* 1978; 135: 763-70.
72. Walsh DB, Eckhauser FE, Cronenwett JL, Leremiah G, Turcotte MD, Martin Lindenauer S. Adenocarcinoma of the ampulla of Vater. Diagnosis and treatment. *Ann Surg* 1982; 195: 152-7.
73. Jass SR, Morson BC. Reporting colorectal cancer. *Clin Pathol* 1987; 40: 1016-20.
74. Cameron JL, Crist DW, Sitzmann JV, et al. Factors influencing survival after pancreaticoduodenectomy for pancreatic cancer. *Am J Surg* 1991; 161: 120-5.
75. Vogelstein B, Fearon ER, Kern SE et al. Genetic alterations during colorectal tumors development. *N Engl J Med* 1988; 319: 525-32.
76. Lynch HT, Smyrk T, Watson P, Lanspa SJ, Lynch JF, Lynch PM, Cavalieri J, Boland RC. Genetics, natural history, tumor spectrum, and pathology of hereditary nonpolyposis colorectal cancer: an updated review. *Gastroenterology* 1993; 104: 1535-59.
77. Robertson JFR, Boyle P, Imrie CW. Patients with ampullary carcinoma are prone to other malignant tumours. *Br J Cancer* 1988; 58: 216-8.

CHAPTER 11

SPLENECTOMY IN HAEMATOLOGICAL PATIENTS

Roberto Vecchioni, Elda Baggio, Claudio Zardini
Department of Surgical and Gastroenterological Sciences, University of Verona, Verona, Italy

SUMMARY

In the period from January 1990 to July 1998 we performed splenectomy on 129 patients of whom 77 were males and 52 females. The average age of patients was 41.7 years, ranging from 7 to 76 years old. 38 of these (equal to 29.4%) underwent emergency operation owing to trauma (25 males and 13 females). In 3 patients (2.3%) splenectomy was necessary owing to the existence of localised enlargements (aneurysms) of the splenic artery. This particular motivation has gradually been reduced because of the growing possibility of embolizing a peripheral enlargement,or aneurysms in one of the branches of the subdivisions of the splenic artery.

In 88 patients (68.3%) splenectomy was necessary due to the manifestation of splenomegaly in the development of spherocytosis, idiopathic thrombocytopenic purpura, or Werlhof's disease, fibro-congestive splenomegaly or in the presence of haemolytic or auto-immune diseases, or other pathology.

Patients affected with lymphomata or chronic myeloproliferative disorders are a case apart. For these patients the advisability of performing splenectomy is relative, and strictly connected to their clinical histories, and to the accuracy of diagnoses. In our group 48 male patients and 40 females were involved.

Many laparosplenectomies performed in the past have been rendered useless, owing to the accuracy of clinico-pathology diagnostic systems such as TAC and RMN in confirming the presence or not of splenic infiltration and in diagnosing splenic lesions of uncertain nature. We chose to operate using median laparotomy, which allows good exposure of the whole abdominal cavity, even if technical difficulties can sometimes be met with at the level of the upper sector, in the case of a voluminous spleen attached to the diaphragm.

A.M. *Farinon (ed.), Advances in Abdominal Surgery 2002*, 159-172.

Complications which mainly occur are:

Haemorrhage, which may appear within the first 24-48 hours and be of such gravity as to necessitate re-operation.

High temperature, due to unknown causes, when not clearly correlated to the basic illness or connected with pleuro-pulmonary complications, which occur in a high percentage of cases. In particular outflow of pleural liquid is often present even in asymptomatic patients without high temperature.

Suppuration in the splenetic compartment, with formation of abscess,is a dangerous complication, particularly in a haematological patient whose basic conditions may be at risk; this never occurred in our case histories.

Over the years an increase has been observed in the choice of splenectomy as e therapeutic course of action in cases of haematological disorders, or at one point in the staging of lymphomata, forms of leukaemia and in Hodgkin's disease.

The history of splenectomy being used in therapeutic treatment of haematological disorders began by chance in 1887, when Sir Spencer Walls successfully removed the spleen of a 24-year-old girl who was being operated on for suspected fibroid of the womb. She was found, however, to be suffering from splenomegaly (Debove's disease, or enlargement of the spleen).

After removal of the spleen, the chronic jaundice she had suffered from for years, caused by hereditary spherocytosis, disappeared.

The spleen is a combined organ, consisting of red pulp which functions as a filter, and white pulp, responsible for immune reaction to various circulating antigens. It carries out numerous important physiological functions, in particular [2]:

- **Filtration**: in concentration of cellular elements, slowing down of bloodflow in cords, and in prolonged contact with macrophages.
- **Phagocitosis**: elimination of abnormal cells, capture of ageing cellular elements which are blocked in the meshes of the reticular macrophagical system.
- **Hemopoiesis**, only active in the foetus.
- **Antibody poiesis and production of immuno-competent lymphocytes**; complications of infection that may appear in patients undergoing splenectomy are due to the failure of this function, especially when operation occurs at a very early age.

However, under certain pathological conditions, the spleen performs excessive haemocatheretic functions and takes on a syndromc pattern known as Hypersplenism.

In agreement with Ellis [3], the criteria for defining hypersplenism are:

1. Splenomegaly - but it is to be remembered that not all instances of splenomegaly cause hypersplenism, which in itself, however, may be present even in cases of non-palpable spleens.

2. Anaemia, leukopenia, platelet deficiency (piastrinopenia), present singularly or in combination with each other.

3. Normal or increased medullary cellularity.

4. The improvement of the clinical picture after splenectomy.

The most important "haematological" situations for which splenectomy is recommended include:

- Haemolytic diseases
- Platelet alterations
- Myeloproliferative disorders
- Lymphoproliferative syndrome

Among haemolytic diseases, **hereditary spherocytosis**, known also as congenital haemolytic jaundice or icterus or Chauffard-Minkowski syndrome, of dominantly autosomal transmission, is the most common form of haemolytic anaemia. By general agreement, splenectomy is the accepted course of treatment to be taken for this disease. It is characterised by a defect in the membrane of red blood cells, which become less pliable and therefore more easily subject to being trapped in the spleen.

The main clinical symptoms include anaemia, reticolocytosis and varying degrees of splenomegaly, of 2 to 10 times the normal volume [2].

Splenectomy is the most frequently selected and practically imperative form of treatment for hereditary spherocytosis. After operation the survival of red blood cells is almost normal.

In **Thalassanaemia**, or **Mediterranean hereditary microcytic anaemia**, which is characterised by defects in haemoglobin synthesis, the red blood cells are microcytic and hypochromic. Since splenic sequestration tends to reduce survival of red blood cells, in some cases where serious splenomegaly, pain caused by splenic infarct, and increased transfusion requirements are all associated, splenectomy is necessary.

It is also indicated in all those cases of anaemia (such as "Sinckle cell disease") where splenic sequestration can be proved. In **autoimmune haemolitic anaemia**, the average life of erithrocytes is reduced. We can distinguish between more frequent chronic forms and rarer acute forms.

Steroid therapy is the first choice treatment, while splenectomy is to be taken into consideration for those patients with warm-reacting antibodies, for whom the therapy is hardly efficient, or who need such massive doses of cortisone as to cause serious side-effects. In these cases a positive outcome may be expected in 50-80% of cases [4].

- Among forms of platelet alteration, **Idiopathic Thrombocytopenic Purpura (I.T.P.)** or **Werlhof's disease** is the most common haematological motivation for performing splenectomy.

The average survival of platelets is about 10 days, and if this decreases we have a variable form of platelet insufficiency, in relation to the gravity of reduced survival and the capacity of medullary compensation. In most cases the aetiology is immunological (such as autoimmune disease, pharmacological reaction, or provocation by iso-antibodies) But in the case of I.T.P. we are dealing with an acquired syndrome of unknown cause and severe onset, where spontaneous recovery is more frequent; if it is subacute or chronic, recovery is less common [2].

Its pathogenesis is to be found in immunity, linked to circulating Immuno globelins (IgG), which act as anti-platelet auto-antibodies. W herlhof's disease is the most common form of thrombo cytophenic purpura, with a ratio between female and male patients of 3:1.

In infancy and adolescence a severe form of the disease is usually the case, which almost always heals and rarely needs splenectomy, while the chronic form is more frequent in adults.

The clinical picture is characterised by ecchymosis, purpura, gastrointestinal bleeding, bleeding from the gums, vagina and the urinal tract. These signs, however, appear in slow and insidious progression and often diagnosis is reached only after a clinical history which has lasted for years.

The patient is generally in good health and maybe shows only some petechial marks, some ecchimoses and brown pigmentation on the surface of the tibia (haemosiderin or haemozoin deposits) [2]. The platelet count is something less than 100-50,000. Coagulation tests are normal. There are also some immunological tests which in 80 % of cases show the auto-antibodies attached to the platelets.

First choice treatment consists of cortisone therapy which,even at a low dosage rate, reduces the destruction of platelets by decreasing the activity of macrophages. With stronger doses of cortisone an immunosuppressive activity is associated with reduction in the activity of macrophages, which causes a lower production of auto-antibodies.

Splenectomy must be taken into consideration as treatment for patients with complications arising from prolonged cortisone therapy, or suffering from serious piastrinopenia (platelet deficiency) - count inferior to 30,000 PTL/mm^3. Splenectomy is an efficient cure in 81-90% of cases [2-5], resulting in platelet counts which return to normal levels within 7 days after operation. In 10% of cases splenectomy is not followed by a permanent increase in the platelet count.

Over the last 10 years it must be noted that an increasing number of cases of I.T.P. in patients suffering from acquired immunodeficiency, show less response to cortisone therapy. Surgical treatment is necessary for cases of severe thrombocytopenia if response to cortisone therapy, and even more so to AZT, is lacking. Treatment with high dosage rates of immunoglobulin brings about a temporary increase in the platelet count; therefore, as in all cases of thrombocytopenic purpura, doses to be used in preparation for surgical operation are 1-2 gr/Kg, for 3-5 days [6].

In the case of **thrombotic thrombocytopenic purpura (TTP)**, the thrombocytopenia is the consequence of platelets being trapped in the arterioles, which appear to be full of hyaline material composed of platelets and fibrin. Immunoflorescence has clearly shown that immunoglobulins and addiment are present inside them.

Thrombocytopenia, haemolitic anaemia, high temperature, neurological symptoms, initially of mental confusion, delirium, altered state of consciousness, with various combinations of hemiparasi, aphasia and impaired vision are characteristic aspects of the clinical situation. Alterations in values such as proteinuria and increases in azotaemia and creatinin occur at the beginning, and may develop towards kidney failure.

Until a short time ago the disease evolved fatally towards death, in spite of cortisone therapy, anti-aggregates and splenectomy. Today, high volume plasmapherisis is a form of treatment which meets with 60-80% success, and splenectomy remains as a high-risk optional therapy, considering the general conditions of patients in cases of non-response to plasmapherisis. When **thrombocytopenia is associated with splenomegaly** in patients suffering from portal hypertension, splenectomy increases the platelet count on one hand, but worsens the situation of portal hypertension, so that portal decompression is necessary,with distal splenorenal shunt or with splenectomy and central shunt [4].

- In **myeloproliferative disorders** classifiable as acute, subacute or chronic, there is often a form of splenomegaly associated with thrombocytopenia,in 30% of cases, and with thrombocytosis in 25%. For some cases splenectomy may be advisable, especially for idiopathic myelofibrosis when there is evident splenomegaly associated with platelet deficiency (piastrinopenia). Splenectomy improves the life quality of patients, who need fewer transfusions, without however influencing prospects of survival.
- In lymphoproliferative diseases, which include neoplastic pathology of lymphocites, whether leukaemic or lymphomatoid (Hodgkin's disease and non Hodgkin lymphoma), splenectomy can be a therapeutic step in the protocol of treatment.

Table 1 is an outline of possible resort to splenectomy in various forms of diseases.

Table 1. Lymphoproliferative Syndromes

Pathology	Sigla	Splenectomy
LEUKAEMIC EXPRESSION		
Acute		
Acute lymphatic leukaemia	ALL	never
Chronic		
Chronic lymphatic leukaemia	CLL	sometimes
Chronic Polylymphocytic leukaemia	PLCL	often
Hairy cell leukaemia	HCL	sometimes
LYMPHOMATOID EXPRESSION		
Hodgkin's lymphoma	HL	sometimes
non-Hodgkin lymphoma	NHL	sometimes

Splenectomy is a palliative treatment for **chronic lymphatic leukaemia**, but it can however permit improvement of the citopenia and so allow for carrying out treatment with chemio-therapeutics.

In **chronic proliferative leukaemia** splenectomy achieves definite improvement of anaemia and piastrinopenia (platelet deficiency), providing satisfying results with time.

In the past splenectomy was the only therapy available for treatment of **Tricholeukocytes leukaemia (Hairy cell leukaemia)**; apart from some cases in which no treatment is required, it is now reserved for cases which do not respond to medical therapy.

The advisability of carrying out splenectomy as treatment for lymphomata is controversial; persistent cytopenia is frequently also a result of hypersplenism, which often responds well to splenectomy.

In the past,before the availability of diagnostic potentials provided today by TAC, surgical staging of Hodgkin's lymphoma (which is rare nowadays) was often carried out in order to define the actual stage of disease and program the therapy. Surgical staging consisted of biopsies of the liver, splenectomy, biopsies of intraperitonial lymphonodi, and bone biopsy. The spleen was involved in about 40% of cases.

Preparation of the patient undergoing splenectomy requires antipneumococcic vaccination, to be carried out at least 7-10 days before surgical operation, and in the case of children also anti-Hemophilus influenza vaccination [4]. Intravenous injection of massive doses of immunoglobulins is necessary for patients suffering from serious idiopathic thrombocytopenia (I.T.P.).

In our opinion a cycle of respiratory physiokinesitherapy is also useful in preparing the patient for surgery, by reducing to a minimum respiratory complications present in these patients.

Platelet transfusions are to be carried out at the moment of operation, and not before, since platelets are rapidly destroyed by the spleen, thus rendering the transfusion useless.

ANATOMY AND SURGICAL TECHNIQUES

Situated in the upper mesocolic region of the abdomen and occupying the left hypercondrium, the spleen is totally covered by the peritoneum which on a level with the hilus bends back over surrounding organs to form those folds or peritoneal ligaments which serve to hold the spleen fixed in position.

- The gastrolienal ligament, inside which the short gastric arteries (vasa brevia) and the left gastroepiploic arteries pass.
- The pancreaticosplenic ligament, inside which is the tail of the pancreas and the vascular pedicle of the spleen, which varies in length from 2-3 5-6 cm, or on the contrary is very short. In this case, the tail of the pancreas comes into contact with the splenic hilus. In carrying out splenectomy these differences are significant,in so much as they condition the use of different surgical tactics to control the splenic ducts.
- The phrenosplenic or supporter ligament of the spleen extends from the upper end of the organ to the diaphragm, and may contain a branch of the lower diaphragmatic artery, which in the case of its not being visualised could be a cause of haemorrhage.
- The phrenocolic ligament extends from the lower end of the organ to the splenic flexure (flexura coli sinistra) or to the left extremity of the transverse mesocolon.

The splenic artery (arteria lienalis) usually runs along the upper edge of the pancreatic body as far as the level of the tail, then passes onto the front side of the gland, and at the extremity of the organ divides into two branches, an upper one and a lower one; after a short passage in the pancreaticosplenic ligament, they subdivide and fan out into secondary and tertiary branches of the splenic artery.

The splenic artery may be rectilinear or accentuate its tortuosity; instead of running along the upper edge of the pancreas (in 90% of cases) it may be behind the pancreas (8% of cases), or in front of the pancreas (3% of cases), or occasionally within the pancreas. Furthermore, it may divide on contact with the spleen at an angle of 180° between the two limbs, and consequently the two branches of the bifurkation proceed attached to the hilar side of the organ. These different situations involve specific surgical implications, as for example the difficulty of isolating an artery if it passes behind the pancreas, or of fastening it to the hilus if it has a T subdivision.

Particular attention must be paid to checking the upper polar artery,which varies in its source position; it may initiate towards the periphery of one of the branches of the splenic artery, or in closer proximity, even springing directly from the celiac trunk (accessory splenic artery).

The short gastric arteries pass through the gastrolienal ligament and reach the large gastric tuberosity. The length of the pedicle is determined by the point at which the gastric collaterals detach from the splenic artery; if this occurs close to the hilus, the pedicle is short, if it is at some distance from the hilus the pedicle is long.

Although one way of surgical access described is by left subcostal laparotomy, and in some cases even left thoracophrenolaparotomy when the spleen is enormous, we used a median zipho-subumbilicol laparotomy.

Two classical techniques of laparotomy exist; one is frontal with anterior ligature of the pedicle, and the other is posterior or typical splenectomy. In anterior splenectomy, which we reserved for cases of medium-sized spleens with firm adhesions to surrounding organs, the first stage consists in cutting the gastrolienal (gastrosplenic) ligament, so opening up the retro-cavity. Successively, isolation of the vascular pedicle is commenced, beginning from the lower edge. Having identified the blood vessels, and carrying out ligation, first the artery and then the vein are cut. Procedure then continues by liberating the spleen from the ligaments connecting it with the paries (wall) and the diaphragm.

In posterior splenectomy with the retro-cavity open, and by opening the gastric ligament and the higher-up gastrolienal ligament, liberation of the spleen is begun from the lower pole by cutting the splenocholic ligament. At this point the surgeon's hand dislocates the spleen, gently drawing it out towards the midline. This manoeuvre allows the exposure of the splenorenal ligament which is then cut, so completing the extenorisation of the organ.

Procedure continues with the possible detachment of the tail of the pancreas and the vascular pedicle, followed by ligation and cutting of the splenic artery and vein.

The **laparoscopic technique** which we adopted in 9 cases,requires that after inducing general anaesthesia and placing endotracheal intubation, the patient must be placed in gynaecological position with the principal operator between the lower limbs of the patient, both the assistants on the right of the patient and the instrumentalist on the patient's left.

Exposure of the spleen is facilitated by rotation of the operating table about 35° towards the right, and the definite anti-Trendelemburg position of the patient. Closed method aeroperitoneum (pneumoperitoneum) is induced, using a Verres needle.

The number of trocars introduced through 4-5 openings of 5-12 mm diameter depends on the conformation of the patient and the presence or not of adhesions.

Procedure begins with exploration of the abdominal cavity to search for accessory spleens. It continues with the opening of the gastrosplenic ligament, and tying and sectioning the short arteries by means of clips, or endo-GIA. At this point there is access to the retro-cavity of the greater omentum (epiploa), and to exploration of the vascular pedicle and the pancreatic tail. The splenic vessels are tied and cut separately, to avoid formation of arteriovenous fistulas. Ligation is carried out with clips on divided branches, and with endo-GIA in the case of a single trunk.

Liberation of the lower end of the spleen is obtained by tying and cutting the vessels existing in this area. The upper pole of the spleen is the last point to be liberated, to avoid its overturning downwards towards the visual plane (opticals), so obstructing successive manoeuvres.

After having been placed in a nylon collecting bag,and possibly broken into several pieces, the spleen is then removed from the upper left quadrant of the abdomen,and the bag is guided towards the abdominal wall. There follows accurate control of the haemostosis of the splenic compartment and the abdominal cavity, and drainage is placed in position.

CLINICAL CASISTICS

Between January 1990 and July 1998 we performed surgical operations of splenectomy for haematological reasons, on 88 patients, 48 of whom were males and 40 females. The ages ranged from 19 to 67 years (an average of 49.3 years) for females, and from 7 to 72 years (an average of 46.6 years) for the males.

In almost all of the patients splenectomy was based on therapeutic motivations. Table 2 illustrates the incidence of haematological pathologies at the basis of surgical necessity for splenectomy; Werlhof's disease in 29.5% of cases, and non Hodgkin lymphomas in 27.27% are the most commonly represented pathologies, followed by idiopathic myelofibrosis which prevails in about 16% of cases. The other 27.5% of cases include haemolitic anaemia, Hodgkin's lymphoma, gastric lymphomas, hypersplenism, and spherocytosis.

Thalassanaemia (Mediterranean hereditary microcytic anaemia), Cooley's disease and some forms of leukaemia are only minimally represented.

Table 2. Splenectomy for haematological reasons

	Number of cases	Percentage
Werlhof's disease	26	29.54
non Hodgkin lymphoma	24	27.27
Idiopathic Myelofibrosis	14	15.9
Autoimmune haemolitic anaemia	6	6.8
Hodgkin's lymphoma	4	4.5
Gastric lymphoma	2	2.3
Hypersplenism	3	3.4
Idiopathic Thrombocytopenic purpura	2	2.3
Spherocytosis	2	2.3
Thalassanaemia	1	1.1
Coole 's disease	1	1.1
Chronic myeloid leukaemia	1	1.1
Hairy cell leukaemia	1	1.1
Chronic lymphoid leukaemia	1	1.1
TOTAL	**88**	**100**

Analysis of Table 3 reveals greater frequency of Werlhof s disease in women - in agreement with data from literature (4-8) - and major incidence of cases of non Hodgkin lymphoma and idiopathic myelofibrosis in male patients.

The weight of the spleen varied considerably in relation to the basic pathology, and in most cases also in relation to the sex of patients.

Splenomegaly was of modest dimensions in Werlhof s disease, weighing an average 261 males (ranging form 170 to 340 gr) and an average 199 females (ranging from 60 to 500 gr). In patients suffering from autoimmune haemolitic anaemia splenomegaly was equally limited.

In case of non Hodgkin lymphoma splenomegaly was of greater dimensions, with an average weight of 1,452 gr (ranging from 385 to 3,250 gr) in males, and 1,277 females (ranging from 270 to 2,500 gr). Splenomegaly of the largest proportions occurred in patients affected by idiopathic myelofibrosis, when the average weight of the spleen was 2,545 gr (ranging from 900 to 5,450 gr.) in males, and 1,350 gr (ranging from 800 to 2,500 gr.) in females.

As can be seen in the table all other cases of splenomegaly were of modest proportions, except in the patient suffering from thalassanaemia and the one affected by chronic myeloid leukaemia. In our casuistics (case histories) respiratory system complications are frequent, but their occurrence has increased since 1993, when we started carrying out routine chest X-rays 5 or 6 days after operation. So it is possible to demonstrate the presence of slight pleural discharge (outflow) in patients without painful symptoms or high temperature.

Table 3. Average weight of the spleen in relation to sex and pathology

	Males	**Average weight**	**Females**	**Average weight**
Werlhof's disease	7	261	19	199
Non Hodgkin lymphoma	16	1452	8	1277
Idiopathic myelofibrosis	10	2545	4	1350
Autoimmune haemolitic anaemia	2	725	4	343
Hodgkin's lymphoma	2	260	2	200
Hypersplenism	2	220	1	860
Gastric lymphoma	2	145		
Idiopathic thrombocytopenic purpura	1	110	1	170
Spherocytosis	1	850	1	1130
Thalassanaemia	1	1640	-	
Cooley's disease	1	900	-	
Chronic myeloid leukaemia	1	1750	-	
Chronic lymphoid leukaemia	1	250	-	
Hairy cell leukaemia	1	430	-	
TOTAL	**48**		**40**	

Total occurrences of pleuro-parenchymal complications are 43% (in 38 cases), but if the valuation is made by separating off patients with spleens weighing over 1,000 gr., the percentage varies conspicuously. Out of 22 patients with splenomegaly of over 1,000 gr., incidence of respiratory complications rises to 81%, while in patients with spleens weighing less than 1,000 gr. the percentage of incidence falls to 33% (Table 4).

In 3 cases (3.4%) re-operation was rendered indispensable because of bleeding from the splenic compartment.

Mortality occurred in 2.2% of cases, one concerning a patient with BPCO who died the day after operation from a crisis of respiratory insufficiency. In the second case death occurred on the 11th day due to cardiac circulatory arrest.

Table 4. Pleuro-parenchymal complications

	66 cases of splenomegaly less than 1,000 gr	**22 cases of splenomegaly more than 1,000 gr**
Moderate pleural outflow	14	7
Bilateral pleural outflow	2	3
Parenchymal thickening	1	1
Parenchymal thickening associated with monolateral pleural outflow	2	5
Parenchymal thickening associated with bilateral pleural outflow	1	3
TOTAL	**20**	**18**

We have also taken into consideration 13 cases of thrombocytosis with a platelet count of over 750,000, representing an incidence of about 15%.

In all these cases, treatment with Oncocarbide was applied together with antiaggregating therapy until the platelet count returned to normality. In 5 cases (equal to 5.7%) an accessory spleen was reported.

Prior to operation, for all patients broad spectrum antibiotic therapy was set up, and was always continued until the fifth day for those without signs of general or respiratory complications. In cases of serious platelet deficiency (less than 30,000) and non reaction to cortisone therapy, endovenous drip treatment with immunoglobulins was applied for at least 5 days.

Surgical operation of **splenomegaly** is common for haematological disorders whether malign or not.

Considering that the general condition of these patients is often at risk, it is also burdened with morbidity of 14-52% [9, 11] and mortality of 2-10% [8, 10].

In our experience the most important complications affected the respiratory apparatus,with a total incidence of 43%.

According to MacRae and colleagues the frequency of respiratory complications concerns 21% of patients. Particularly in very serious splenomegalies, and in cases of adhesions to the diaphragmatic dome, surgical manipulation of the splenic compartment favours the appearance of respiratory complications.

Unlike experiences reported in the literature [4, 6, 9-10], in our series of patients there was no suppuration in the splenic compartment, as is usually reported in 2-10% of cases.

We usually leave splenic drainage in position until the third or fourth day, and even longer if there is any secretion, although there is a general tendency to leave drainage in place for 24-48 hours,and in some cases not use it at all [8]. Patients affected by idiopathic myelofibrosis, also in association with platelet deficiency, are at greater risk of bleeding. In the 3 cases of re-operation (relaparotomy) for bleeding, one single source of bleeding was never confirmed, but rather an oozing from the surface of the diaphragm, the pancreas or the splenic floor. We emphasise the fundamental importance of meticulous surgical technique, with ligation of even the smaller vessels and minimum use of electro-surgical knives. The greater the dimensions of the spleen the more important all this is, especially in cases of associated coagulopathy.

Scrupulous surgical technique and extremely careful haemostasis, permitted us on one hand to by-pass the presence of serious platelet deficiency, and on the other to have an average intra-operative haematic defluvium of 250 cc.

It is not always possible to have patients undergo surgical operation in good general health conditions, but we believe that careful preparation with respiratory physiokinesitherapy together with correction of any disionia or metabolic changes, permit the patient to be brought to operation in the best possible conditions to reduce morbidity and mortality to a minimum.

REFERENCES

1. Wells TS. Remarks on splenectomy with a report of successful case. *Med Chir Trans* 1988; 71:255.
2. Tura S. Lezioni di ematologia. Ed. Esculapio 1997; 429.
3. Ellis LD, Dameshek HL. The dilemma of Hypersplenism. *Surg Clin North Am* 1975; 55:277-285.
4. Schwartz SI. Role of splenectomy in hematologic disorders. *World J Surg 1*996 Nov-Dec; Vol l, 20 (9): 1156-9.
5. Chirletti P, Cardi M, Barillari P, Vitale A, Sammartino P, Bolognese A, Caiazzo R, Ricci M, Muttillo I, Stipa V. Surgical treatment of immune thrombocytopenie purpura. *World J Surg* 1992; 16:1001-1005.
6. Alonso M, Grassot D, Bourstyn E, Galera MJ, Oksenhendler E, Celerier M, Clot P. Splenectomy in human immunodeficiency virus-related thrombocytopenia. *Br J Surg* 1993; 80 (3) : 330-3.
7. Schwartz SI, Cooper RA. Surgery in the diagnosis and treatment of Hodgkin disease advance in surgery. Year Book 1972; (vol.6) Chicago.
8. Musser G, Lazar G, Hocking W, Busuttil RW. Splenectomy for hematologic disease. *Ann Surg* 1984; 1 : 40.
9. Mac Rae HH, Yakimots WW, Reynolds T. Perioperative complication of splenectomy for hematologic disease.JCC 1992; 35 (4) : 432-436.
10. Wobbes T, van der Sluis RF, Lubbers EJ.Removal of the massive spleen: a surgical risk?. *Am J Surg* 1984; 174 : 800-802.
11. Amaral JF, Meltzer RC, Crowley JP. Laparoscopic accessory splenectomy for recurrent idiopathic thrombocytopenic purpura. *Surg Laparosc Endosc* 1997; 7 (4): 340-4.
12. Hofkes HG, Weber F, Uppenkamp M, Meusers P, Teschendorf C, Philipp T, Brittinger G. Recovery by splenectomy in patients with relapsed thrombotic thrombocytopenic purpura and treatment failure to plasma exchange. *Semin Thromb Hemost* 1995; 21 (2) : 161-5.
13. Humphrey JS, Conley CL. Durable complete remission of macroglobulinemia after splenectomy: a report of two cases and review of the literature. *Am J Hematol* 1995; 48 (4) : 262-6.
14. Naouri A, Feghail B, Chabal J, Boulez J, Dechavanne M, Viala JJ, Tissot E. Results of splenectomy for idiopathic thrombocytopenic purpura. Review of 72 cases. *Acta Haematol* 1993; 89 (4) : 200-3.
15. Rodeghiero F, Frezzato M, Schiavetto C, Castaman G, Dini E. Fulminant sepsis in adults splenectomized for idiopathic thrombocytopenic purpura. *Haematologica* 1992; 77 (3) : 253-6.
16. Tyler DS, Shaunak S, Bartlett JA, Iglehart JD. HIV-1-associated thrombocytopeina. The role of splenectomy. *Ann Surg* 1990; 211 (2) : 211-7.
17. Vevon PA, Eleison EC, Carey LC. Splenectomy for hematologic disease. *Adv Surg* 1989; 22 : 105-39.
17. Vevon PA, Eleison EC, Carey LC. Splenectomy for hematologic disease. *Adv Surg* 1989; 22 : 105-39.
18. McAneny D, LaMorte WW, Scott TE, Weintraub LR, Beazley RM. Is splenectomy more dengerous for massive spleens? *Am J Surg* 1998; 175 (2) : 102-7.
19. Stephens BJ, Justice JL, Sloan DA, Yoder JA. Elective laparoscopic splenectomy for hematologic disorders. *Am Surg* 1997; 63 (8) : 700-3.
20. Cusack JCJr, Seymour JF, Lerner S, Keating MJ, Pollock RE. Role of splenectomy in chronic lymphocytic leukemia. *J Am Coll Surg* 1997; 185 (3) : 237-43.
21. Lee WJ, Kim BR. Laparoscopic spenectomy for chronic idiopathic thrombocytopenic purpura. *Surg Laparosc Endosc* 1997; 7 (3) : 209-12.

22. Tsiotos G, Schlinkert RT. Laparoscopic splenectomy for immune thrombocytopenic purpura. *Arch Surg* 1997; 132 (6) : 642-6.
23. Fiedman RL, Hiatt JL, Facklis K, Cymerman J, Philllips EH. Laparoscopic or open splenectomy for hematologic disease: which approach is superior? *J Am Coll Surg* 1997; 185 (1): 49-54.
24. Bohner H, Tirier C, Rotzscher VM, Heit W. Indications for and results of splenectomy in different hematological disorders. Langenbecks Arch Chir 1997; 11 (2) : 79-82.
25. Delaitre B, Pitre J. Laparoscopic splenectomy versus open splenectomy: a comparative study. *Hepatogastroenterology* 1997; 44 (13) : 45-9.
26. Winde G, Schmid KW, Lugering N, Fischer R, Brandt B, Berns T, Bunte H. Results of prognostic factors of splenectomy in idiopathic thrombocytopenic purpura. *JAm Coll Surg* 1996; 183 (6) : 565-74.
27. Smith CD, Meyer TA, Goretsky MJ, Hyams D, Luchette FA, Fagelman EJ, Nussbaum MS. Laparoscopic splenectomy by the lateral approach: a safe and effective alternative to open splenectomy for hematologic diseases. *Surgery* 1996; 120(5) : 789-94.
28. Jameson JS, Thomas WM, Dawson S, Woodd JK, Johnstone JM. Splenectomy for haematological disease. *JR Coll Surg Edimb* 1996; 41 (5) : 307-11.
29. Schlinkert RT, Mann D. Laparoscopic splenectomy offers advantages in selected patients with immune thrombocytopenic purpura. *Am J Surg* 1995; 170 (6) : 624-6.

SECTION III

COLO-RECTAL SURGERY

CHAPTER 12

ISCHEMIC COLITIS: AN ATTEMPT TO DEFINE THE SPECTRUM OF DISEASE.

Attilio Maria Farinon, Michele Grande, Francesco Rulli, Italo Stroppa
Department of Surgery, University of Rome "Tor Vergata", Rome, Italy

Abstract

Ischemic colitis encompasses a wide spectrum of pathologic and clinical findings, ranging from a mild self-limiting form to bowel infarction and perforation.
Although in some patients, more often in younger ones, a precipitating factor or a presumed etiologic condition may be established, in others, mainly elderly patients, the ischemic injury may be considered "spontaneous"; it develops in absence of major vasculature occlusion, and in presence of viable intestine elsewhere.
Ischemic tissue damage (including necrosis, ulcerations, submucosal edema and hemorrhage, or transmural infarction as common manifestations) more frequently shows patchy or segmental distribution, but can affect the entire colon. The severity of the tissue damage appears strictly related not only to hypoxia during the ischemic period, but mainly to subsequent reperfusion injury when blood-flow returns.
Basically two forms of ischemic colitis are recognized: nongangrenous, comprising transient reversible and chronic types (chronic persistent segmental colitis, ischemic stricture), and gangrenous, as the result of transmural progression of the ischemic necrotizing damage, leading to perforation and peritonitis.
Diagnosis is generally confirmed by colonoscopy, but caution should be exercised in advancing the scope beyond areas of marked necrosis, for fear of iatrogenic perforation of the bowel.
Management and outcome are mainly dependent on the severity of ischemic damage: nongangrenous ischemic colitis usually requires only conservative treatment followed by complete recovery, whereas surgery may be occasionally required to correct the sequelae of persistent segmental colitis and ischemic stricture; gangrenous ischemic colitis requires urgent surgical treatment, that happens to be associated with high postoperative mortality (60% in personal experience).

A.M. *Farinon (ed.), Advances in Abdominal Surgery 2002*, 175-189.

INTRODUCTION

Colonic ischemia without demonstrable occlusion of the inferior mesenteric artery was first described as a rare self-limiting disease ("reversible vascular occlusion") in five patients, by Boley and associates in 1963 [1]. Three years later, Marston and associates reported a similar disease spectrum in 15 patients, and coined the term "ischemic colitis", classifying the disease by severity into three different forms: transient ischemic colitis, ischemic stricture, and gangrene of the colon [2]. In 1975, Williams and Wittenberg reviewed 55 patients with ischemic colitis, concluding that prompt identification of disease and definition of its severity represented the most important factors affecting prognosis [3]. In 1978, one of us (A.M.F.) first published the endoscopic pictures of transient ischemic lesions, documenting their evolution towards healing, and emphasizing the prominent rôle of colonoscopy in the diagnosis of disease [4].

Since these early reports, numerous attempts to define the spectrum of ischemic colitis have been made, with little or no improvement on the original clinical classification proposed by Marston and associates 2, based on reversibility or non-reversibility of the lesions and grading the clinical forms of the disease according to their evolution. This is more true if we consider that ischemic colitis encompasses a wide spectrum of pathologic and clinical findings, ranging from a mild self-limiting form to bowel infarction and perforation, even if the cause of colonic ischemia often remains obscure.

We can, then, define ischemic colitis as a clinical entity characterized by necrotic-inflammatory segmental lesions, due to circulatory insufficiency of the colon by non-occlusive or occasionally occlusive causes; these lesions cannot be classically identifed as infarctual or inflammatory and infective in nature, resulting in varying degrees of local tissue necrosis and systemic manifestations.

Ischemic colitis represents the most prevalent form of intestinal ischemia, and accounts for approximately 50 to 60 percent of all gastrointestinal ischemic episodes [5]. Although it is generally believed that ischemic colitis affects elderly patients, there are reports of this form in younger patients, who may be inappropriately treated for inflammatory bowel disease [6]. Clinical features of the disease range from a transient episode of abdominal pain accompanied by rectal bleeding, to a fatal picture of colonic perforation with diffuse peritonitis. Treatment is generally supportive, but surgery may be indicated in the acute phase for colonic necrosis or perforation, as well as in the chronic phase to treat ischemic stricture [7].

BLOOD SUPPLY OF THE COLON

The blood supply of the colon is derived from branches of the superior mesenteric artery (SMA), inferior mesenteric artery (IMA) and internal iliac (hypogastric) arteries. An abundant collateral blood supply is usually present between the three systems, although flow variations in any of the above-mentioned vascular districts can lead to ischemic colitis, moreso if the connecting collaterals are absent or poorly developed. However, vascular collaterals connecting the SMA, IMA, and hypogastric arteries are of important clinical relevance.

Communication between SMA and IMA systems occurs *via* the meandering mesenteric artery (arc of Riolan), or the marginal artery of Drummond. The latter is the artery closest to the large bowel wall, from which end-arteries (vasa recta) originate and provide blood supply to the colonic wall. The marginal artery perhaps represents the most important collateral to the left colon, connecting the left branch of the middle colic artery, and the ascending branch of the left colic artery. However, at the splenic flexure there be no primary or secondary anastomotic arcades linking the two branches, therefore configurating a watershed area, the so called *Griffiths' point* [8]. The latter may further be defined as continuity of the left colic artery, with the marginal artery at the splenic flexure; 5% of the population with a diminished or absent marginal artery of Drummond is at particular risk of ischemia [9].

The meandering mesenteric artery (arc of Riolan), anatomically distinct from the marginal artery of Drummond, does not represent a constant collateral vessel, even if, when present, it joins the proximal middle colic with the left colic artery [10]. When SMA or IMA is occluded gradually, the arc of Riolan constitutes a dilated central anastomotic artery, and its presence connotes a chronic process [11].

The vascular anastomoses among terminal branches of IMA, the rectal arteries, and branches of internal iliac artery supplying the pelvis seem less clinically important. A watershed area at the junction of the lowest sigmoid branch and superior hemorrhoidal artery (*Sudek's point*), below which the ligature can lead to necrosis of the rectosigmoid is speculated to be caused by an incomplete marginal artery in the region [9].

Finally, the marginal artery of Drummond is also poorly developed in the right colon in nearly 50% of the population, explaining the frequent occurrence of right sided ischemic colitis [9]. In this region, the marked length of vasa recta, originating farther away from the mesenteric border of the bowel, and poor communication between vasa recta and vasa brevia, giving rise to a less well-developed microvascular plexus in the muscularis and submucosal layers, may be considered factors predisposing the colon to ischemia. This blood supply may accentuate a local vasospastic response to systemic hypotension, moreover considering that the colon has less blood flow per 100 g of tissue than does the remainder gastrointestinal tract [12], and that decrease in blood flow accompanies functional motor activity of the colon [13].

ETIOLOGY AND PATHOPHYSIOLOGY

The etiology of the disease is undoubtedly multifactorial and most often appears not so easily definable. This is justified by the acquired concept that colonic blood flow regulation is based on local regulatory mechanisms, extrinsic influences (autonomic nervous system, cardiocirculatory and ematologic factors), intrinsic factors (bowel wall metabolites, mechanic factors, derivative vascular factors), and circulating vasoactive humoral agents (catecholamines, angiotensin II, istamin, serotonin, vasopressin, prostaglandin (E_1), cations, plypeptides). Although ischemic colitis was considered in the past as resulting from major vascular occlusion, it is now felt to be due to a transient reduction in perfusion pressure, responsible for numerous biochemical alterations impairing the colonic circulation [14].

Although it appears unusual that a direct cause-effect relationship may be detected between the numerous conditions predisposing to ischemic colitis and the ischemic episode, the fundamental factor is an insufficient blood supply for the requirements of the mucosa. This is influenced by alterations in the systemic circulation, by anatomic and functional changes in the local mesenteric vasculature, and by the resistance of tissue to hypoxic injury.

The conditions predisposing to ischemic colitis can be broadly divided into occlusive and non-occlusive (Fig.1).

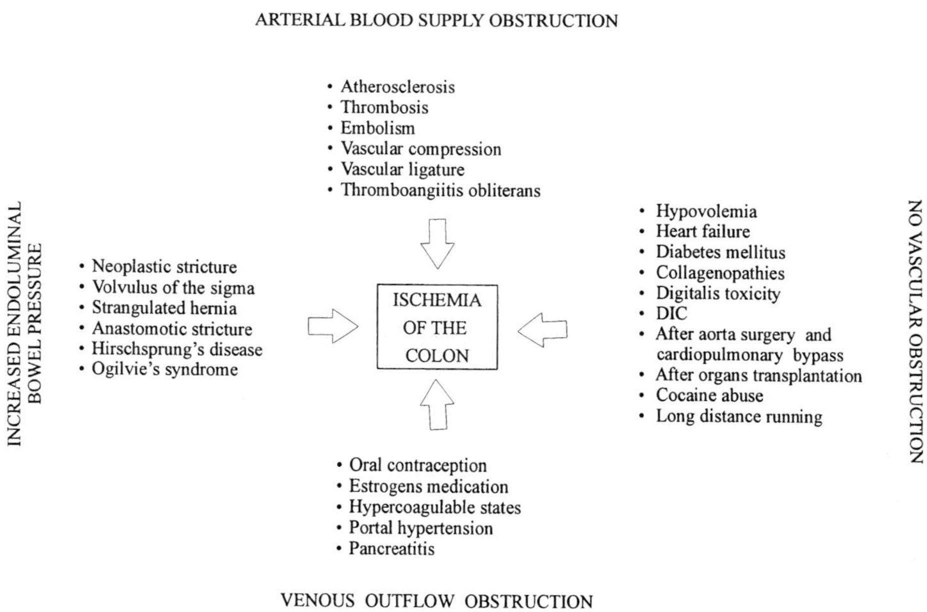

Figure 1. Ischemia of the colon: predisposing and precipitating etiologic factors

Occlusion can affect either arterial blood supply or venous outflow, involving large or small vessels. Large arterial vessels are mainly obstructed by atherosclerosis (atheromatous debris, atherosclerotic plaques dissection of the arterial wall), thrombosis, embolism, as well as by vascular compression or ligature (colectomy with inferior mesenteric artery ligation, postabdominal aortic reconstruction). Arterial blood flow can be also compromised by disorders of small arterioles, as occurs in diabetes, rheumatoid arthritis, or in systemic vasculitis disorders (autoimmune inflammatory arteritis, thromboangiitis obliterans), and radiation arteriopathy.

Venous outflow obstruction is commonly secondary to hypercoagulable states, oral contraception, estrogens medication, but also portal hypertension and pancreatitis [15]. Venous obstruction is, however, an extremely uncommon underlying pathologic condition.

Non-occlusive forms of ischemic colitis are due to low-flow states of any cause, responsible for intense mesenteric vasoconstriction especially in the right colon [16]. Severe vascular constriction is frequently related to hypovolemia, heart failure, diabetes mellitus, collagenopathies, and can also be secondary to certain medications (digitalis, diuretics, cathecholamines, non-steroidal antiinflammatory drugs, estrogens) or drugs, such as cocaine [17-19], and long-distance running in younger patients [20-21]. Colonic ischemia has been observed to occur in patients in the postoperative period following aortic surgery and cardiopulmonary bypass, and following abdominal organ transplantation [22]. Notwithstanding, a specific cause for the ischemic episode may be occasionally recognized, but, more typically, no clear cause for the ischemia is identified. Such "spontaneous" episodes are believed to be localized forms of non-occlusive ischemia, possibly in association with small vessel disease, as suggested by increased incidence of colonic ischemia in the elderly [11-12].

Increased endoluminal bowel pressure due to distal obstructing bowel lesion (carcinoma of the colon, volvulus of the sigma, diverticulitis, adhesions, fecal impaction) or secondary to massive distention of the colon in absence of any obstructing lesion, as in Ogilvie's syndrome and in Hirschsprung's disease, represents a possible cause of colonic ischemia, particularly of right-sided disease. This latter consideration, in contrast with earlier studies that demonstrated a preponderant left-sided colon involvement in ischemic colitis, is increasing, and probably reflects the prevalence of non-occlusive forms in current practice [11, 23].

Although the final pathway leading to colonic ischemia remains conjectural [23], ischemic tissue damage to the colon is mainly caused by two factors: hypoxia during the ischemic period and subsequent reperfusion injury when blood flow returns. Parks and Granger [24] have demonstrated that, paradoxically, reperfusion damage frequently exceeds the original ischemic insult.

When the ischemic period is brief, the injury caused by tissue hypoxia appears to be limited, but damage during the period of tissue reperfusion may be significant. With a lengthy period of ischemia, tissue hypoxia lead directly to cell death, and damage progresses transmurally from bowel lumen to serosal layer [25]. In addition to the local effects of ischemic injury on the colonic wall itself, ischemic colitis leads to systemic release of mediators of the inflammatory response, in large part due to endotoxemia and portal bacteremia resulting from the increase in mucosal permeability [26]; it may be particularly rapid owing to the large burden of intraluminal bacteria normally residing in the colon [15].

Reperfusion of ischemic intestine results in significant microvascular and parenchymal cell injury, and tissue injury appears to be mediated by both reactive oxygen metabolites and activated polymorphonuclear leukocytes. Xanthine oxidase, an enzyme present in the epithelial cells of the intestinal mucosal layer, is an important source of reactive oxygen metabolites in postischemic intestine; these may damage a number of molecules in tissue, such as nucleic acids, membrane lipids, enzymes, and receptors. Xanthine oxidase-derived oxidants initiate the production and release of proinflammatory agents, which lead to plymorphonuclear leukocyte adherence and emigration. Such adherent neutrophils, which in turn represent an additional source of oxygen free radicals, mediate microvascular injury either by release of proteases, physical disruption of the endothelial barrier, or both [25]. These considerations seem supported by data obtained in experimental models by using oxygen-free radical scavengers and xanthine oxidase inhibitors, to protect various organs against reperfusion injury [25], as well as by the observation that the severity of human intestinal reperfusion injury was attenuated by removal of activated neutrophils [27].

CLASSIFICATION AND CLINICAL PRESENTATION

Two main types of ischemic colitis are recognized: *nongangrenous* (Fig.2), including a reversible transient form and a nonreversible chronic form, and *gangrenous* [1-2]. The nongrangrenous form of ischemic colitis comprises 80-85 per cent of cases, whereas the gangrenous form encompasses the remaining 15-20 per cent [28].

Among nongangrenous ischemic colitis, the *transient reversible form* is characterized by the mildest pathologic changes in the colonic wall, which include edema, submucosal hemorrhage, with or without partial mucosal necrosis. The blood is gradually reabsorbed, or poured into the intestinal lumen through the overlying sloughed and then ulcerated mucosa, and complete recovery follows within two to three weeks.

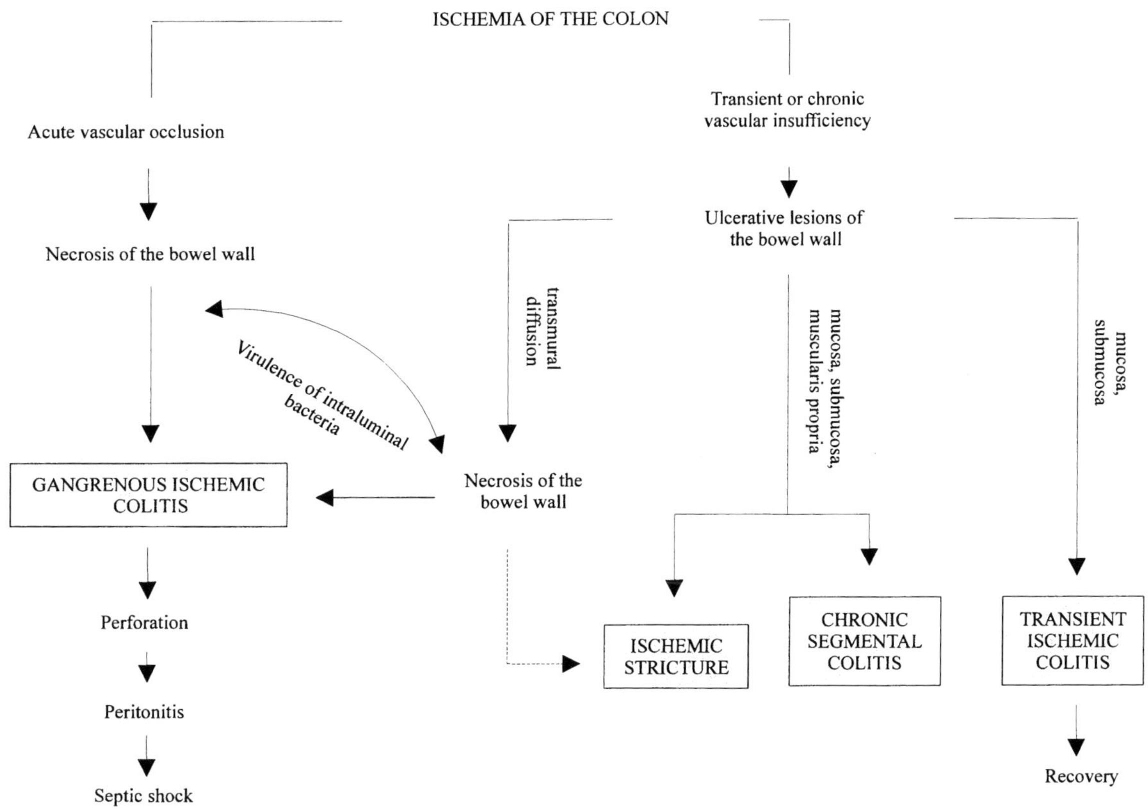

Figure 2. Schematic of involvement of the bowel wall by ischemic process and classification of various forms of ischemic colitis

When more severe injury occurs, the submucosa becomes difused and edematous, with abundant fibrous tissue and iron-laden macrophages. Often the damage penetrates the muscularis propria, which during a period of weeks to months may be replaced by fibrous tissue, and a *colonic ischemic stricture* may result [28]. In cases of moderately severe colonic ischemia, granulation tissue may replace the injured mucosa and submucosa, but, eventually, chronic ulcerations and persistent areas of *chronic segmental colitis* develop, due to mucosal regeneration over an edematous and extended submucosa [23]. The ulcerative areas appear interspersed among normal mucosa, mimicking Crohn's disease [11].

Gangrenous ischemic colitis results from the transmural progression of the ischemic necrotizing damage from the lumen outward, which promotes septic shock due to perforation and peritonitis.

Concerning clinical presentation, in the absence of specific pothognomonic signs and symptoms, ischemic colitis generally develops as an acute abdominal illness in patients over sixty years, without any history of previous colonic problems. Colonic ischemia affecting younger patients is being recognized more frequently, but is still rarely documented [17-21]. Most patients with colonic ischemia present with a sudden onset of mild, crampy, left-sided lower abdominal pain, followed by an urge to defecate. The passage of bright red or maroon blood mixed with stool commonly follows within twenty-four hours from th onset of symptoms; blood-loss in these patients is usually minimal, without any need for transfusion [29]. Physical examination generally shows only mild to moderate tenderness over the affected area of the colon; marked tenderness is unusual and suggests transmural necrosis necessitating surgical resection [11].

DIAGNOSIS AND MANAGEMENT

The diagnosis of ischemic colitis depends on early and repeated clinical evaluations of the patient, and serial roentgenographic or endoscopic studies of the colon [23]. If colonic ischemia is suspected, but signs of peritonitis are absent and abdominal plain films are normal or nonspecific, colonoscopy should be performed. Immediate surgical treatment is mandatory, when plain radiograms confirm the presence of worrisome signs of advanced ischemia or colonic infarction: free intra-abdominal air due to perforation, air within the bowel-wall or the portal venous system. [30] There are no sufficiently specific chemical or enzimatic markers of intestinal viability; serum acidosis, lactate dehydrogenase (LDH) levels, raised serum levels of phosphate, creatine phosphokinase (CPK), alkaline phosphatase, or diamine oxidase are nonspecific and relatively late findings [31-32]

Computed tomography (CT) scans, frequently employed in the evaluation of abdominal pain, may be fully normal in patients with early ischemic infarction, and may be abnormal in only one third of patients with established ischemic colitis [15, 33]. The conclusions of a study from Balthazar et al. [34] suggest that CT can be used to confirm the clinical suspicion of ischemic colitis, to suggest ischemia when it is unsuspected, and to diagnose complications. Thickened bowel wall represents the most common but nonspecific finding due to edema or hemorrhage [35], and color flow duplex imaging has been employed in the differential diagnosis between inflammatory and ischemic causes, even if absence of flow was found to be only 50% sensitive in diagnosing ischemia [36].

Magnetic resonance imaging (MRI) , not frequently used to diagnose ischemic colitis, has shown some promise in discriminating ischemic from nonischemic tissues [37]. Angiography, although frequently performed, is not indicated in the evaluation and management of patients with colonic ischemia, because it is rarely diagnostic; often major visceral vessels result patent, the vascular lesions responsible for ischemic colitis being extremely peripheral. Indium-111 white cell scans have been recently used in the early diagnosis of ischemic colitis, with encouraging results [38]. The definitive diagnosis of ischemic colitis is most frequently obtained by colonoscopy; only the endoscopic examination can permit evaluation of the severity of the disease, but not the depth of the involvement, in patients with suspected colonic ischemia who have no clinical and radiological signs of peritonitis. However, caution is requested in performing colonoscopy, moreover considering that distention of the bowel with room air to pressures greater than 30 mmHg decreases colonic blood flow [39], and may increase the severity of ischemic lesions. The insufflation of carbon dioxide, which in turn causes vasodilatation and increases blood flow, may minimize this hazard [39-40]. Several endoscopic examinations, in combination with serial observations of the patients' clinical course, are necessary to confirm the diagnosis of ischemic colitis, and to ascertain the outcome of the ischemic injury [23, 41]. The initial examination should be performed early in the course, because "thumbprints", visualized on barium enema, may disappear within days, as the submucosal hemorrhages are either reabsorbed or evacuated into the colonic lumen, when the overlying mucosa ulcerates and sloughs [4, 42]. In the acute setting, caution should be exercised in advancing the scope beyond areas of marked necrosis, for fear of iatrogenic perforation of the colon. However, the need to perform colonoscopy is related to the observation that failure to identify the patient with severe colonic ischemia continues to be a devasting problem: 62% mortality in patients requiring resection, as compared to 14% in patients not requiring resection [43].

In the differential diagnosis of ischemic colitis numerous clinical conditions should be considered, such as mesenteric arterial insufficiency, mesenteric venous thrombosis, inflammatory bowel disease, diverticulitis, and infectious colitis. Bowel obstruction, peptic ulcer disease, volvulus, and pancreatitis must also be excluded as causes of acute abdominal pain [5].

Once the diagnosis has been established, and clinical examination has excluded intestinal gangrene or perforation, the patients should be treated expectantly [23, 28, 41, 44- 45], and very mild cases can be managed as outpatients. In most cases optimization of cardiac function and oxygen delivery, as well as avoidance of medications that may contribute to ischemia, are appropriate, it being unknown whether pharmacologic improvement in local colonic blood flow can be attained. Signs and symptoms of the disease subside within 24 to 48 hours, and complete clinical resolution may follow within two weeks. More severe ischemic insults perpetuate necrosis and inflammation, with ulceration of the mucosa and development of chronic segmental colitis or strictures. Recurrent episodes of sepsis, in otherwise asymtomatic patients with unhealed areas of segmental colitis, and symptomatic strictures are indications for elective colon resection.

Clinical deterioration, despite conservative treatment, or endoscopic visualization of extensive gangrene, suggests colonic infarction and mandates urgent laparotomy. The extent of colon resection should be guided by the distribution of mucosal injury acquired on preoperative diagnostic studies, and by intraoperative assessment of colonic viability, that cannot be based on the appearance of serosal surface, in most cases appearing normal despite extensive mucosal damage. Several investigations have been proposed to solve this challenging problem for the surgeon, and among the most promising methods is tonometry, which is based on measurements of intraluminal pCO2, as an indirect assessment of intraluminal pH appears to be a reliable index of the metabolic status and cellular oxygenation of the colon, in relationship to its blood flow [46-47].

Outcome of spontaneous ischemic colitis is not so easily definable, because of marked variability in severity of the disorder and a limited number of clinical studies [41, 43, 48-49] comparing patients treated surgically with those managed by conservative measures (Tab.1). Recently, Longo and colleagues [49] reported the results of treatment of 43 consecutive patients with ischemic colitis, grouped into those with segmental ischemic colitis (n=31), and those with total colonic ischemia (n=12). In the patients with segmental colitis requiring surgery, the 30-day mortality rate was 22 percent, whereas it amounted to 75 percent among all 12 patients who underwent surgery for total colonic ischemia. These results confirm a worse prognosis related to total colonic ischemia, than to segmental colonic ischemia. The same group from St. Louis University [50], in a study concerning 47 patients with ischemic colitis, who were initially treated conservatively, demonstrated that duration of symptoms,

	Cases n.		Treatment			Mortality %
Reeders[41]	199	98	Conservative			57
		101	Surgical resection			
			66	elective		51
			35	urgent	(peritonitis)	100
Parish[43]	38	22	Conservative			14
		16	Surgical resection			62
Fitzgerald[48]	113	66	Conservative			
		47	Surgical resection			
			26	elective	(stricture)	
			21	urgent	(Gangrenous)	53
Longo[49]	43	31	Segmental colitis			
			11	conservative		
			20	surgical resection		22
		12	Total ischemic colitis			75

Table 1. Results of the management of ischemic colitis in the most consistent series available in literature: comparison of patients treated surgically with those who did not undergo surgery

coexisting medical disease, initial hemodynamic instability, and prolonged ileus were significant predictors of surgical management.

Personal experience, based on 42 cases of ischemic colitis (Tab. 2), confirms similar results. No mortality was registered in 12 patients with spontaneous ischemic colitis managed conservatively, and in 10 patients who underwent elective surgery for chronic segmental colitis (n=3) or ischemic stricture (n=7). Twenty patients underwent urgent surgery for gangrenous ischemic colitis (n=8), including two cases of total colonic ischemia, or occlusive ischemic colitis (n=12), the obstructing lesion being represented in one patient by a large biliary stone impacted in a diverticular sigmoid, and eleven died (60 percent).

CONCLUSIONS

Ischemic colitis is a heterogenous condition encompassing a wide spectrum of disease, in relation to numerous causative and precipitating factors. These latter are sometimes identifiable and then amendable, but more often they remain enigmatic. Despite the increased awareness of the disease, ischemic colitis still remains underdiagnosed.

	Cases n.	Treatment			Mortality %
Transient ischemic colitis	12	Conservative			–
Chronic persistent segmental colitis	3	Surgical resection (E)			–
Ischemic stricture	7	Surgical resection (E)			–
Gangrenous ischemic Colitis	8	Surgical (U)			
			Resection	6 [4]	
			Derivative + delayed resection	2 [1]	
Occlusive ischemic Colitis	12	Surgical (U)			60
			Resection	6 [2]	
			Exteriorization	6 [4]	

[ ] = patients died (E) = elective (U) = urgent

Table 2. Results of the management of ischemic colitis in personal experience

It is largely a disease of elderly people, although a minority may occur in relatively younger people; colonic ischemia affecting younger people is recognized more frequently, but still rarely documented. Transient forms of the disease commonly occur at an earlier age, are resolved more quickly and cause less of an acute phase response. In this patient population, identifiable causes include collagen-vascular diseases, hematologic disorders, long-distance running, and cocaine abuse.

The ischemic process may typically show a segmental involvement of the colon, even if all or most of the colorectal tract may be involved by a rare fulminating form of colonic ischemia. Right-sided ischemic colitis may prevalently affect a younger group of patients, and seems to have a relatively benign course, as compared to left-sided or total colonic involvement. Ischemic proctosigmoiditis, not accompanied by more proximal colonic involvement, is a rare condition because of excellent collateral supply in the region [51-52].

The most significant factors conditioning the improvement of outcome in the management of ischemic colitis are prompt recognition and aggressive treatment to avert disastrous sequelae. Early colonoscopic diagnosis and interval clinical and endoscopic evaluation, to ascertain progression or regression of ischemic process, should promote earlier diagnosis of full-thickness necrosis, warranting expeditious surgical intervention. Prompt recognition and resection can be lifesaving especially in patients with such a rare lethal condition as total colonic ischemia. Colon resection represents the elective operative treatment of chronic nongangrenous forms, including persistent segmental colitis and ischemic stricture, and the emergency management of gangrenous forms. In this latter instance, the most challanging problem for the surgeon is the amount of colon to be resected, and whether to perform immediate anastomosis.

REFERENCES

1. Boley SJ, Schwartz S, Lash J, Sternhill V. Reversible vascular occlusion of the colon. *Surg Gynecol Obstet* 1963; 116:53-60.
2. Marston A, Pheils MT, Lea Thomas M, Morson B. Ischaemic colitis. *Gut* 1966; 7:1-15.
3. Williams LF, Wittenberg J. Ischemic colitis: a useful clinical diagnosis, but is it ischemic? *Ann Surg* 1975; 182:439-48.
4. Farinon AM. Coloscopy: a necessary aid in the diagnosis of transient ischemic colitis. *Endoscopy* 1978; 10:112-4.
5. Stamos MJ. Colonic ischemia. In: Mazier WP, Luchtefeld MA, Levien DH, Senagore AJ, eds. Surgery of the colon, rectum, and anus. WB Saunders, 1995:705-13.
6. Arnott DR, Ghosh S, Ferguson A. The spectrum of ischemic colitis. *Eur J Gastroenterol Hepatol* 1999; 11:295-303.
7. Robert JH, Mentha G, Rohner A. Ischaemic colitis: two distinct patterns of severity. *Gut* 1993; 34:4-6.
8. Griffiths JD. Surgical anatomy of the blood suooly of the distal colon. *Ann R Coll Surg Engl* 1956; 19:241-56.
9. Harnsberger JR, Longo WE, Vernava AM. Vascular anatomy. *Semin Colon Rectal Surg* 1994; 108:641-50.
10. Kornblith PL, Boley SJ, Whitehouse BS. Anatomy of the splanchnic circulation. *Surg Clin North Am* 1992; 72:1-30.
11. Greenwald D A, Brandt L J. Colonic ischemia. *J Clin Gastroenterol* 1998; 27:122-128.
12. Kaminski DL, Hermann VM. Ischemic colitis. In: Cameron J, ed. Current surgical therapy. 2nd ed. Toronto: BC Decker 1986: 110-4.
13. Kvietys PR, Granger DN. Regulation of colonic blood flow. *Fed Proc* 1982; 41:2106-10.
14. Longo WE. The enigma of ischaemic colitis following cardiovascular surgery. *Ital J Gastroenterol Hepatol* 1997; 29:293-6.
15. Toursarkissian B, Thompson R W. Ischemic colitis. *Surg Clin N Amer* 1997; 77:461-470.
16. Landreneau R J, Fry W J. The right colon as a target organ of non-occlusive mesenteric ischemia. *Arch Surg* 1990; 125:591-594.
17. Niazi M, Kondru A, levy J, Bloom AA. Spectrum of ischemic colitis in cocaine users. *Dig Dis Sci* 1997; 42:1537-41.
18. Boutros HH, Paulter S, Chakrabarti S. Cocaine-induced ischemic colitis with small-vessel thrombosis of colon and gallbladder. *J Clin Gastroenterol* 1997; 24:49-53.
19. Papi C, Candia S, Masci P, Ciaco A, Montanti S, Capurso L. Acute ischemic colitis following intravenous cocaine use. *Ital J Gastroenterol Hepatol* 1999; 31:305-7.
20. Heer M, Respond F, Hany A, Sulser H, Kehl O, Jager K. Acute ischaemic colitis in female long distance runner. *Gut* 1987; 28:896-9.
21. Beaumont AC, Teare JP. Subtotal colectomy following marathon running in a female patient. *J R Soc Med* 1991; 84:439-40.

22. Groossmann EM, Longo WE, Solomon H, Presti ME, Dunphy FR. Ischemic colitis secondary to venous thrombosis following a previous orthotopic liver transplant. *Transplant Proc* 1999; 31:2135-7.
23. Gandhi S K, Hanson M M, Vernava A M, Kaminski D L, Longo W E. Ischemic colitis. *Dis Colon Rectum* 1996; 39:88-100.
24. Parks DA, Granger DN. Contributions of ischemia and reperfusion to mucosal lesion formation. *Am J Physiol* 1986; 250:G749.
25. Zimmerman BJ, Granger DN. Reperfusion injury. *Surg Clin North Am* 1992; 72:65-83.
26. Turnage RH, Guice KS, Oldham KT. Endotoxemia and remote organ injury following intestinal reperfusion. *J Surg Res* 1994; 56:571-8.
27. Sisley AC, Desai T, Harig JM, Gewertz BL. Neutrophil depletion attenuates human intestinal reperfusion injury.*J Surg Res* 1994; 57:192-6.
28. Brandt LJ, Boley SJ. Colonic ischemia. *Surg Clin North Am* 1992; 72:203-29.
29. ReinusJF, Brandt LJ, Boley SJ. Ischemic diseases of the bowel. *Gastroenterol Clin North Am* 1990; 19:319-43.
30. Scholtz FJ. Ischemic bowel disease. *Radiol Clin North Am* 1993; 31:1197-218.
31. Thompson JS, Bragg LE, West WW. Serum enzyme levels during intestinal ischemia. *Ann Surg* 1990; 211:369-73.
32. Jonas J, Bottger T. Diagnosis and prognosis of mesenterial infarct. *Med Klin* 1994; 89:68-72.
33. Smerud MJ, Johnson CD, Stephens DS. Diagnosis of bowel infarction: a comparison of plain films and CT scans in 23 cases. *Am J Radiol* 1990; 154:99-103.
34. Balthazar EJ, Yen BC, Gordon RB. Ischemic colitis: CT evaluation of 54 cases. *Radiology* 1999; 211: 381-8.
35. Philpotts LE, Heiken JP, Westcott MA, Gore RM. Colitis: use of CT findings in differential diagnosis. *Radiology* 1994; 190:445-9.
36. Teefey SA, Roarke MC, BrinK JA, et al. Bowel wall thickening: Differentiation of inflammation from ischemia with color Doppler and duplex US. *Radiology* 1996; 198:547-51.
37. Wilkerson DK, Mezrich R, Drake C, et al. MR imaging of acute occlusive intestinal ischemia. *J Vasc Surg* 1990; 11:567-71.
38. Moallem AG, Gerard PS, Japanwalla M. Positive In-111 WBC scan in a patient with ischemic ileocolitis and negative colonoscopies. *Clin Nucl Med* 1995; 20:483-5.
39. Brandt LJ, Boley SJ, Sammartano RJ. Carbon dioxide and room air insufflation of the colon: effects on colonic blood flow and intraluminal pressure in the dog. *Gastrointest Endosc* 1986; 32:324-9.
40. Wheeldon NM, Grundman MJ. Ischaemic colitis as a complication of colonoscopy. *BMJ* 1990; 301.1080-1.
41. Reeders JWAJ, Tytgat GNJ, Rosenbusch G, Gratama S. Ischaemic colitis. Boston: Martinus Nijhoff Publishers, 1984:113-6.
42. Farinon AM, Battistini C, Zanella E. Aspetti endoscopici delle coliti ischemiche. *G Clin Med* 1977; 58:339-58.
43. Parish KL, Chapman WC, Williams LF. Ischemic colitis. An ever-changing spectrum? *Am Surgeon* 1991; 57:118-20.
44. Zanella E, Farinon AM. Ischemic colirtis: a cause for vascular acute abdomen. *It J Surg Sci* 1981; 11:187-191.
45. Kaleya RN, Boley SJ. Colonic ischemia. *Perspect Colon Rectal Surg* 1990; 3: 62-81.
46. Fiddian-Green RG, Amelin PM, Herrmann JB, *et al.* Prediction of the development of sigmoid ischemia on the day of aortic ischemia. *Arch Surg* 1986; 121:654-60.
47. Poole JW, Sammartano RJ, Boley SJ. The use of tonometry in the early diagnosis of mesenteric ischemia. *Curr Surg* 1987; 44:469-72.
48. Fitzgerald SF, Kaminski DL. Ischemic colitis. *Semin Colon Rectal Surg* 1993; 4:222-8.

49. Longo WE, Ward D, Vernava III AM, Kaminski DL. Outcome of patients with total colonic ischemia. *Dis Colon Rectum* 1997; 40:1448-54.
50. Longo WE, Ballantyne GH, Gusberg RJ. Ischemic colitis: patterns and prognosis. *Dis Colon Rectum* 1992; 35:726-30.
51. Farinon AM, Sianesi M. Proctite ischemica. Presentazione di un caso clinico. *Chir Gastroent* 1978; 12:130-3.
52. Bharucha AE, Tremaine WJ, Johnson CD, Batts KP. Ischemic proctosigmoiditis. *Am J Gastroenterol* 1996; 91:2305-9.

CHAPTER 13

ADVANCES IN MOLECULAR GENETICS AND CLINICAL IMPLICATIONS OF SPORADIC COLORECTAL CANCER.

Giuseppe Midiri, Fabrizio Consorti, Enrico Giarnieri *, Alfredo Covotta, Lisa Luzzatto, Chiara Montana, Andrea Bertolotti, Aldo Vecchione *, Vanni Beltrami

*Department of Surgical Science, *Experimental Medicine and Pathology, University of Rome "La Sapienza ".*

Abstract

Genetic epidemiological studies have shown that the pathogensis of various neoplasias is due to defects in specific genes and the growth to multiple consequent genetic mutations.

In FAP (Famylial adenomatous polyposis) and HNPCC (Hereditary non polyposis colorectal cancer), compliant with Amsterdam and Bethesda criteria, the natural history procedes along with a set of rather well identified morfologic features to wich correspond genetic steps.

On the contrary very few is still known about the so called sporadic colorectal cancers, which account for the majority of instances.

Vogelstein reported a model of multistage carcinogenesis for sporadic colo- rectal cancer, in which an early mutation of genes of DNA repair system hMLH1 and h MSH2 could generate a mutational cascade.

The basic assumption as rationale of this research was that DNA repair genes (MMR system) are at beginning of the genetic mutational cascade causing the induction of oncogenesis of sporadic colorectal cancers as well as their multiclonal heterogeneity.

The AA randomly selected, from a serie of 256 patients, 29 patients up to the age of 60 years who underwent surgery for colorectal carcinoma with radical intent.

All the selected cases were considered as sporadic cancers from a clinical point of view, since none of them fulfilled the Amsterdam criteria for HNPCC and Familial adenomatous polyposis was escluded too.

Mismatch repair gene proteins expression and, in particular, gene hMSH2 protein, were investigated by immunohistchemistry analysis which allowed, in Authors' opinion, the direct linking of genetic aspects to morphologic features.

In 12 cases (41,4%) hMSH2 exhibited strong expression in the tumoral cells as well as in the surrounding mucosa and at distant mucosa.

In 14 cases (48,3%) loss of hMSH2 protein expression was observed in tumoral cells and low

A.*M. Farinon (ed.), Advances in Abdominal Surgery 2002*, 191-201.

immunoreactivity was detected in peritumoral mucosa while strong hMSH2 expression was observed in distant mucosa.

In a third small group of patients (10,3%) loss of hMSH2 protein expression was detected in tumoral, adjacent and at distance normal mucosa.
After a five years follow up, 100% of twelwe patients of first group are still alive vs 64,3% of fourteen patients of second group while in the third group only one patient survives .
These results support the hypotesis of an involvement of hMSH2 gene defect in development of a subset of sporadic colorectal cancers.
For the patients with strong expression of hMSH2 in the tumoral cells as well as in the surrounding mucosa and at distant mucosa, this parameter could represent an indipendent criterion for the prognostic value.
In conclusion the AA, revising the most recent literature about the topic, propose new criteria able to produce a dynamic multidimensional system by cross-matching the results of different kinds of bio – molecular and clinical evaluations.

Keywords
Sporadic colorectal cancer, mismatch DNA repair system, multidimensional staging and prognostic value

INTRODUCTION

In the last years genetic epidemiological studies have shown that the pathogensis of various neoplasias is due to defects in specific genes and the growth to multiple consequent genetic mutations.

As matter of fact about 5% of solid tumours can be to day considered hereditary.

BRCA 1 and 2 genes are identified as responsible for hereditary breast cancer.

p16 gene is involved in familial atypical multiple melanoma [32].

Medullary thyroid ancer can be developed at a very young age in children carrying a MEN 2 a syndrome with a RET gene mutation [13].

Hereditary in prostatic and ovaric tumours is under evaluation.

About colo - rectal cancer the correlation between genetic mutations, molecular carcinognesis and neoplastic growth has been extensively investigated.

Frequence of colorectal tumours in Italy is increasing at a 12% rate for females and 20% rate for males, with a prevalence of 200 new cases for 100.000 inhabitants and 60% rate patients aged between sixty and sixty-nine [5].

Moreover, the prevalence of this disease is expected to grow in the next five years.

So any effort in getting a deeper knowledge about molecular genetics and clinical features of this tumour is a worth.

The most updated hypotesis on the oncogenesis of colorectal cancer indicates a set of genetic and molecular events as responsible of neoplastic evolution of colonic mucosa [7].

As a matter of fact, in FAP (Famylial adenomatous polyposis) and HNPCC (Hereditary non polyposis colorectal cancer) cases, compliant with Amsterdam and Bethesda criteria, the natural history procedes along with a set of rather will identified morfologic features to wich correspond genetic steps [18].

In FAP the morpho – hystological sequence is represented by : - aberrant crypts (ACF) -, now existimated as the first morphologic step for oncogenesis, in which it is possible to evidence hyperplasia of the mucosa, frequent mitosis and alterations of cell lines, - adenomas -, at a various degree of dysplasia, - adenocarcinoma -, to which could be related aneuploid patterns and APC gene mutation by a stop-codon protein expression. [24, 26, 9].

Major advances in molecular genetics show that mismatch repair genes hMSH2 and hMLH1 are implicated in HNPCC's etiology [30].

Microsatellite instability that results from mutations in mismatch repair genes is referred to replication error repeat (RER) [14, 16].

On the contrary very few is still known about the so called sporadic colorectal cancers, which account for the majority of instance.

Oncogenesis, evolution from potential precursors, staging criteria and surgical planning are under deep re-consideration for these tumours.

In fact many dubts arise from the observation of differences in outcome of tumours which share the same staging and were treated in the same way [21].

The role of MMR system in sporadic colo - rectal cancer carcinogenesis is still an open question.

From a genetic point of view, Knudson's hypothesis seems to gain more and more consensus : beside hereditary forms with a dominant autosomic transmission pattern, the more frequent sporadic instances of colorectal cancer could be associated with a genetic polimorphism [22].

According to Vogelstein genetic model of colorectal oncogenesis, oncogenes and suppressors genes are mutated, leading to the synthesis of structurally and functionally altered proteins.

Vogelstein reported a model of multistage corcinogenesis for sporadic colo-rectal cancer, in which an early mutation of genes of DNA repair system hMLH1 and h MSH2 could generate a mutational cascade.

Subsequent mutations of oncogene K-Ras and four antioncogenes (APC, p53, DCC and NM23) could codify proteins with alterated structure and function.

From this point of view colorectal oncogenesis is considered a multisteep process in which multiple genetic alterations determine quantitative and qualitative abnormalities in cellular DNA content [33].

A sequence of chromosomal aberrations has been outlined in order to explain the mechanism of intratumoral DNA ploidy eterogeneity.

The result of genetc aberrations is a polyclonal pattern with different cell lines in different parts of the tumour.

The heterogeneity degree seems to depend on the balance between the genetic instability of proliferating cell lines and a continuing survival of the fittest cell lines [9, 20].

About sporadic colorectal cancer, as a supporting evidence to such criticism, recent findings, observed also with the contribution of our research group, showed that:

- clusters of aberrant crypts often are found in tracts of healty colonic mucosa far from sporadic cancer location [24];
- heterogeneous cellular clones are often detected with different cytometric patterns in the frame of the same tumour [9].
  This finding are confirmed by tumour multiple full thikness sampling and intranuclear DNA imaging analysis and it is likely to support an impredictable tumour spreading potentiality [23],
- alterations in DNA repair genes system (MMR system) are detected in over 60% of this tumour and it would be the starting point to sequential mutations leading to the expressions of structurally and functiunally altered proteins [14].
  These mutations could give to altered cells a selective advantage, thus leading to the expansion of new clones with different phenotypes inside the same tumour [9].

ALTERED EXPRESSION OF hMSH2 IN SPORADIC COLO-RECTAL CANCER

" Knowledge of the polyposis syndromes has spawned studies into the potentially heritable nature of sporadic adenomatous polyposis.

These findings will presumibly lead to the use of molecular diagnostics in the screening of familias susceptible to colon cancer, to strategies geared to the early detection of sporadic colon cancer and eventualy to the stratification of patients for adjuvant therapy".

This conclusion of a review of Rustgi on colon cancer was a rationale for our studies about sporadic colo - rectal cancer [27].

The basic assumption of the research is that DNA repair genes (MMR system) are at beginning of the genetic mutational cascade causing the induction of oncogenesis of sporadic colorectal cancers, as well as their multiclonal heterogeneity.

Considering also to the points highlighted in the introduction, we randomly selected, from a serie of 256 patients, 29 patients up to the age of 60 years (mean 52.7; 20 male and 9 female) who underwent surgery for colorectal carcinoma with radical intent.

All the selected cases were considered as sporadic cancers from a clinical point of view, since none or them fulfilled the Amsterdam criteria for HNPCC and Familial adenomatous polyposis was escluded too.

Mismatch repair gene proteins expression and, in particular, gene hMSH2 protein was investigated by immunohistchemistry analysis.

The expression of mismatch repair gene hMSH2 protein was evaluated in tumoral cells, in mucosa surrounding the tumour and in normal colonic mucosa far from the tumour.

Deparaffined an hydrated specimens were treated with hydrogen peroxidase.

A mouse monoclonal antibody against hMSH2 (clone FE11, Oncogene products, Cambrdge, Ma, USA) was used for the evaluation of hMSH2 protein expression.

Immunoperxidase test was performed using a streptavidin biotin universal detection system kit (Immunotech, France).

The hMSH2 protein expression was exclusively nuclear, both in the tumoral and in the normal tissue.

In normal epithelium nuclear positive staining was detected at the crypt base and in the germinal center of the lymphoid follicles.

On the basis of hMSH2 protein expression it was possible to subdivide all cases in three groups.

In 12 cases (41,4%) hMSH2 exhibited strong expression in the tumoral cells as well as in the surrounding mucosa and at distant mucosa.

In 14 cases (48,3%) loss of hMSH2 protein expression was observed in tumoral cells and low immunoreactivity was detected in peritumoral mucosa while strong hMSH2 expression was observed in distant mucosa.

In a third small group of patients (3 cases - 10,3%) loss of hMSH2 protein expression was detected in tumoral, adjacent and at distance normal mucosa (Fig 1).

There were no significant difference related to age, sex, location and staging between three groups.

Even if our clinical serie was limited, the results of this study confirm an involvment of hMSH2 gene defect in the pathogenesis of subset of sporadic colo-rectal tumours.

A possible explanation for the absent hMSH2 expression both in tumoral, peritumoral and distant normal mucosa in the patients of third group lead us to

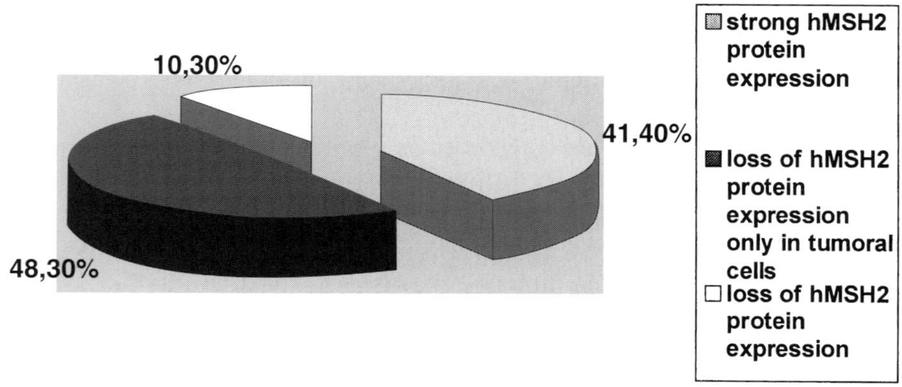

Figure 1. HMSH2 protein expression in sporadic colo-rectal cancer patients

consider them as HNPCC patients, even if their personal and family history was not compliant with the Amsterdam criteria [8].

PROGNOSTIC VALUE AND SURVIVAL

We already considered in our previous study the inadequacy of present colo-rectal cancer staging criteria that do not allow characterization of the effective biological activity of the disease which appears not to coincide with the neoplasm's natural history [6].

Unfortunately, up to day, in spite of recent findings about biology, citometric assay and genetics evaluations, only parameters concerning the neoplasia's anatomical extent are used for colon-cancer staging.

As a matter of fact over or understaging is still possible in colon cancer patients, so that treatment plannings, prognostic evaluation and follow up protocols are frequently inadequate.

We already reported a correlation between higly proliferative cell activity, aneuploid patterns and a severe prognosis, but it is very important to show the effective significance of these data [8-9, 21].

We must discover genetic alterations at the basis of the cell kinetic disorder.

Could hMSH2 protein espression be considered a parameter for prognostic value in resected colo-rectal cancer patients?

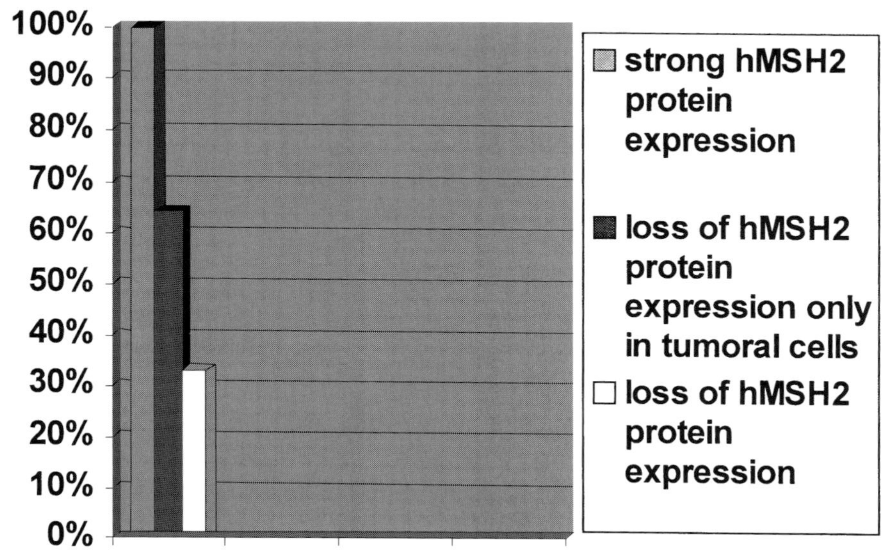

Figure 2. HMSH2 protein expression and survival in sporadic colo-rectal cancer patients

For 29 patients of this serie we performed a five years follow up by clinical examination and seric CEA evaluation every three months, hepatic ultrasonography every six months, endoscopy and TC yearly.

To day 100% of twelwe patients of first group are still alive vs 64,3% of fourteen patients of second group while in the third group only one patient survives [4] (Fig 2).

One of the patients of first group survived to a new surgical treatment for a methacronous neoplastic lesion, eight centimeters distant from previous lesion.

These data show, even if in a limited serie of patients, a possible correlation between hMSH2 espression and survival in sporadic colo-rectal cancer.

DISCUSSION

Recently two component of mismatch repair gene system were identified at chromosome 2p (hMSH2) and at chromosome 3p (hMLH1), both of which have been cloned [17].

Microsatellite instability that occurs from mutations in DNA repair gene system was evaluated in 500 sporadic tumours.

RER phenotype was revealed in 16,5% of 234 sporadic colorectal cancers, in 18% of 33 gastric cancers and in 22% of 18 endometrial carcinomas [12].

So MMR system alteration is not specific for colorectal cancer and there is no confirm that it is the only pathway for sporadic colorectal cancer oncogenesis.

Moreover mismatch system genes, as hMSH2 gene, have been described as responsible for the maintenence of genomic integrity and their inactivation results in an increased rate of mutation in genes that control cell proliferation and death [15].

Our results support the hypotesis of an involvement of hMSH2 gene defect in development of a subset of sporadic colorectal cancers ; but we can suppose other patways in sporadic colorectal cancers oncogenesis.

For the patients with strong expression of hMSH2 in the tumoral cells as well as in the surrounding mucosa and at distant mucosa, this parameter could represent an indipendent criterion for a good prognostic value.

Mismatch repair alterations, in turn, could be responsible for further inactivation of other oncosuppressor genes [8].

The role of immunohistochemistry requires consideration.

An himmunohistochemical approach to detect mismatch repair gene proteins has been used both in HNPCC and in sporadic tumours [14, 30].

Immunohistochemistry is an easy and unespansive approach.

Our findings too showed an added value for this technique because it allowed the direct linking of genetic aspects to morphologic features in sporadic colorectal cancer [8].

Recently many Authors explored new frontiers in molecular genetics about new pathways of colon cancer oncogenesis.

Bao noted that Hrad17, a human homologue of the Schizosaccharomyces pombe checkpoint gene rad17, is overexpressed in colon carcinoma [2].

Goss showed that, about APC and adenomatous polyposis, the role of APC seems to be related to its ability to regulate cytosolic levels of the signaling molecule beta-catenin and to affect the transcriptional profile in cell [10].

Takemasa evaluated a correlation between overexpression of CDC25B phosphatase, an oncogenic protein, and a poor prognosis of colo-rectal carcinoma [29].

Mariadason and Archer re-programmed genetic pathway of colonic cancer cell differentiation and highligthed the importance of short chain fatty acids as Sulindac and Butyrate to inhibit colon cancer cell growth [1, 19].

Watson showed a correlation between growth dysregulation and p53 accumulation in primary colorectal cancer [36].

Tominaga and Zirbes suppose a possible correlation between p21 expression and prognostic value through a pathway mediated by p53 alteration too [31, 38].

Yamamoto, Ciaparrone and Palmquist described the effects of p27 on growth and differentiation of colon carcinoma cells [3, 25, 37].

Handa and Watson investigated the role of cyclins in colon cancer tumorogenesis and proliferation and noted a possible correlation between cyclin expression and colon cancer stage and prognostic evaluation [11, 35].

Wang hiligthed autocrine TGFalpha and beta expression in the regulation of initiation of human colon cancer growth [34].

Sarela studied possible implications of ING1 gene in colorectal carcinoma [28].

In conclusion, up to day, anamnestic datas, clinical features, immunobiological parmeters and molecular genetics tests are not eunough to identify patients with sporadic colorectal cancer.

In order to highlight these very important questions we started a new protocol to evaluate the resected neoplastic lesions and their precursors (aberrant crypts, adenomas) both by cytometric DNA sequencing and by immunohistochemical genetic-molecular analysis starting to MMR systems and the subsequent cascade of genetic mutations.

Final objectives for this study are :

- to obtain new knowledge about the oncogenesis and " genetic epidemiology" of colorectal cancers;
- to better define groups of patients carrier of precancerous lesions and at different risk of development of subsequent colorectal cancer, in order to indications and limitations to endoscopic treatment of such lesions;
- to propose exact extension of resection in possibly different types of sporadic colorectal cancer for those patients which must undergone to surgical treatment;
- to evaluate a more precise prognostic value, closer to the natural history of sporadic colorectal cancers and their predictable biological evolution;
- to fit follow up plannings and adjuvant therapies protocols on possibly different patients' tumour features;
- finally to produce a dynamic multidimensional system by cross-matching the results of the different kinds of bio–molecular and clinical evaluations.

REFERENCES

1. Archer S, Meng S, Wu J, et al. Butytrate inhibits colon carcinoma cell growth through two distinct pathways. *Surgery* 1998; 124 : 248.

2. Bao S, Chang MS, Auclair D, et al. Hrad17, a human homologue of the Schizzosaccharomyces pombe checkpoint gene rad17, is overspressed in colon carcinoma. *Cancer Res* 1999; 59 : 2023.

3. Ciaparrone M,Yamamoto H,Yao Y, et al. Localization and expression of p27KIP1 in multistage colorectal carcinogenesis. *Cancer Res* 1998; 58: 114.

4. Consorti F, Midiri G, Giarnieri E, et al. Altered expression of hMSH2 in sporadic colorectal cancer, surrounding mucosa and at distance colonic mucosa. X Congr. ESSO in *Eur J Surg Onc* 2000; 26 : 296.
5. De Angelis R, Frova L, Capocaccia R, et al. Incidence and prevalence of digestive system tumors in Italy : estimates from mortality data. *Ann Ist Sup San* 1996; 32 : 537.
6. Di Paola M, Midiri G, Ramacciato G. Role of monoclonal antibodies in the management of colorectal carcinoma. In Current topics in surgical oncology ed. G.Fegiz Masson Milano 1991.
7. Fearon ER, Vogelstein B. A genetic model for colorectal tumorogenesis. *Cell* 1990; 61 : 759.
8. Giarnieri E, Consorti F, Midiri G, et al. Altered expression of hMSH2 in sporadic colorectal cancer, surrounding mucosa and at distant colonic mucosa. *Anticancer Res* 2000; 20 : 3829.
9. Giovagnoli MR, Giarnieri E, Midiri G, et al. Intratumoral heterogeneity in colorectal carcinoma : trucut sampling for DNA ploidy analysis. *Anticancer Res* 1999; 19 : 4577.
10. Goss KH, Groden J. Biology of the adenomatous polyposis coli tumor suppressor. *J Clin Oncol* 2000; 18 : 1967.
11. Handa K,Yamakawa M, Takeda H, et al. Expression of cell cycle markers in colorectla carcinoma : superiority of cyclin A as an indicator of poor prognosis. *Int J Cancer* 1999; 84 : 225.
12. Ionov YM, Perinado A, Malkhosyan S, et al. Ubiquitos somatic mutations in simple repeated sequences reveal a new mechanism for colonic carcinogenesis. *Nature* 1993; 363 : 558.
13. Kahraman T, Vermey A, Rouwe C, et al. Prophylactic total thyroidectomy in children with MEN-2a syndrome with a RET-gene mutation. X Congr. ESSO in *Eur J Surg Onc* 2000; 26 : 296.
14. Kim H, Piao Z, Kim JV, et al. Expression of hMSH2 and hMLH1 in colorectal carcinomas with microsatellite instability. *Pathos Res Pract* 1998; 194 : 3.
15. Kinzler WK, Vogelstein B. Landscaping the cancer terrain. *Science* 1998; 280 : 1036.
16. Leach FS, Polyak K, Burrell M, et al. Expression of the human mismatch repair gene hMSH2 in normal and neoplastic tissues. *Cancer Res* 1996; 56 : 235.
17. Lynch HT, Lynch JF. Clinical implications advances in the molecular genetics of colorectal cancer. *Tumori* 1995; 81 Suppl. : 19.
18. Lynch HT, Smyrk T. Hereditary nonpolyposis colorectal cancer. An update rewiev. *Cancer* 1996; 78 : 1149.
19. Mariadason JM, Corner GA, Augenlicht LH. Genetic reprogramming in pathways of colonic cell maturation induced by short chain fatty acid. *Cancer Res* 2000; 60 : 4561.
20. Midiri G, Giarnieri E, Tesoriere A, et al. It is possible to consider intranuclear DNA imaging as a new parameter for colorectal cancer prognostic evaluation ? 1th World Congr Surg Oncol March 1998 San Diego USA; 1 : 33.
21. Midiri G, Giovagnoli MR, Tesoriere G, et al. Immunobiological approach to colorectal cancer staging : biological markers, cellular " in situ " immunological response and intranuclear DNA imaging analysis. In Advances in abdominal surgery ed. E. Zanella Kluwer Ac. Publisher Dordrecht (NE) 1999.
22. Midiri G, Tesoriere A, Giarnieri E, et al. Fattori genetici e cancro del colon-retto: una nouva frontiera per la sperimentazione clinica. *Giorn Chir* 1999; 20 : 373.
23. Midiri G, Consorti F, Lorenzotti A, e Coll. D N A ploidy and prognosis in colorectal cancer patients : preliminary report. *It J Coloproct* 1999; 1 : 3.
24. Nucci MR, Robinson CR, Longo P, et al. Phenotypic and genotypic characteristics of aberrant crypt foci in human colorectal mucosa. *Hum Pathol* 1997; 28 : 1396.
25. Palmquist R, Stenling R, Oberg A, et al. Prognostic significance of p27 (kip1) expression in colorectal cancer: a clinico-pathological characterization. *J Pathol* 1999; 188 : 18.
26. Plyak K, Hamilton SR, Vogelstein B, et al. Early alteration of cell-cycle regulated gene expression in colorectal neoplasia. *Am J Pathol* 1996; 149 : 381. 27. Rustgi AK. Hereditary gastrointestinal polyposis and non-polyposis syndromes. *New Engl J Med* 1994; 331 : 1694.

28. Sarela AI, Farmery SM, Markham AF, et al. The candidate tumour suppressor gene, ING1, is retained in colorectal carcinoma. *Eur J Cancer* 1999; 35 : 1264.
29. Takemasa I, Yamamoto H, Sekimoto M, et al. Over expression of CDC25B phosphatase as a novel marker of poor prognosis of human colorectal carcinoma. *Cancer Res* 2000; 60 : 3043.
30. Thibodeau SN, French AG, Roche PC, et al. Altered expression of hMSH2 and hMLH1 in tumours with microsatellite instability and genetic alterations in mismatch repair genes. *Cancer Res* 1996; 56 : 4836.
31. Tominaga O, Nita ME, Nagawa H, et al. Expression of cell cycle regulators in human colorectal cancer cell lines. *Jpn J Cancer Res* 1997; 88 : 855.
32. Vasen HFA. Genetics and the role of the surgeon. X Congr. ESSO in *Eur J Surg Onc* 1999; 26 : 301 : 103.
33. Vogelstein B, Fearon ER, Hamilton SR. Genetic alterations during colorectal tumor development. *N Engl J Med* 1988; 319 : 525.
34. Yamamoto H, Soh JW, Shirin H, et al. Comparative effects of overexpression of p27Kipl and p21Cipl/Wafl on growth and differentiation in human colon carcinoma cells. *Oncogene* 1999; 18 : 103.
35. Watson DS, Brotherick I, Shenton BK, et al. Cyclin D3 expression, cell proliferation and pathological stage of human Primary colorectal cancer. *Oncology* 1999; 56 : 66.
36. Watson DS, Brotherick I, Shenton BK, et al. Growth dysregulation and p53 accumulation in human primary colorectal cancer. *Br J Cancer* 1999; 80 : 1062.
37. Wang D, Li W, Jiang W, et al. Autocrine TGFalpha expression in the regulation of initiation of human colon carcinoma growth. *J Cell Physiol* 1998; 177 : 387.
38. Zirbes TK, Baldus SE, Moenig SP, et al. Prognostic impact of p21/wafl/cipl in colorectal cancer. Int J Cancer 2000; 89 : 14.

CHAPTER 14

ANALYSES OF THE PROGNOSTIC FACTORS IN COLORECTAL CANCER. PRELIMINARY RESULTS OF A POSSIBLE NEW PROGNOSTIC FACTOR: MESENTERIC AND ANTIMESENTERIC TUMOR LOCATION.

Renzo Dionigi, Angelo Benevento, Gianlorenzo Dionigi, Luigi Boni, Luigi Albarello*, Carlo Capella*.
*Department of Surgery and *Pathology, University of Insubria, Varese, Italy*

Keywords
Prognostic factors, colorectal cancer.

Background

Colorectal cancer is the second cause of death from cancer in the world. In the USA 150.000 new cases per year have been reported, leading to 60.000 deaths per year [1].
It has already been demonstrated that clinical parameters (i.e. age, sex, symptoms, location of the tumors) are of very limited prognostic value [2] in colorectal cancer.
Other factors, mainly hysto-pathological, have been shown to be strongly correlated with the prognosis of patients suffering from colorectal cancer.
These factors can be stratified into 4 categories.

1. Category I prognostic factors

Factors that are definitively proven to be of prognostic value, on the evidence of well-designated robust multi-centric trial are routinely used in clinical practice.

A.M. Farinon (ed.), *Advances in Abdominal Surgery 2002*, 203-211.

1.1 Local extent of the tumor (T status)

The local extent of the tumor (T status) in colorectal cancer is one of the most important prognostic factors in pathological assessment [3]. T1 and T 2 tumors with no lymphnode or distant metastases have a 5 years' survival of 90%, while survival is significantly lower (up to 10%) for tumors with deeper infiltration of the bowel wall (T3/T4) [4].

Differences and variability in pathological examination and different sampling techniques can cause significant variations in evaluating the findings [5]. With a Consensus Statements (1999) the College of American Pathologists stated that standard techniques to define T status [6] proposed by the American Joint Committee on Cancer and the Union Internationale Contre le Cancer (AJCC/UICC) should be used [7].

1.2 Lymphnode metastases (N status)

The presence of lymphnode metastases (N status) is strongly related to the prognosis of patients resected for colorectal cancer [8].

Also for the N status, considerable inter-observers' variability has been demonstrated, and the College of American Pathologists has established the correct techniques that should be used, to analyse and stage, the presence of lymphnode involvement in colorectal cancer [6].

It is extremely important to examine all lymphnodes removed with the resected bowel: the presence of at least 12-15 negative lymphnodes defines the N0 status of the tumor [9].

The definitions and criteria decribed by the American Joint Committee on Cancer and the Union Internationale Contre le Cancer (AJCC/UICC) [7] should be followed.

While lymphnode metastases have been associated with poor prognosis, the value of identification of micrometastases in lymphnodes, by immunohistochemical or molecular techniques, is still controversial

1.3 Lymphatic and/or vascular invasion

It has already been demonstrated 3,5 that the degree of lymphatic and/or vascular invasion (both inside or outside the bowel wall), being associated with a higher level of lymphnodes or distant metastases, has to be considered as an independent prognostic factor.

Although its prognostic value has been widely studied, several techniques used to assess the vascular and/or lymphatic invasion of the tumor have been described, leading to a much higher variability in the results and findings reported in the literature .

The use of a standard hematoxylin/eosine staining on at least 3 (5 is better) sections of the resected bowel has been suggested by the College of American Pathologists 6, in order to standardize the hystopathological reports.

1.4 Presence of residual tumors (R status)

The presence of residual tumor, both microscopic (R1) or macroscopic (R2), has been shown to be of independent prognostic value 3,6. The classification of the R status of the removed specimens should follow the guidelines estabilished by the American Joint Committee on Cancer and the Union Internazionale Contre le Cancer (AJCC/UICC) 7, although misinterpretations might occur, when the R status is evaluated in patients who underwent neoadjuvant chemotherapic regimens.

1.5 Aster-Coller and the TNM classification

As described above, the prognostic value of the degree of infiltration of the bowel (T status) wall, and the local extension (N status), have already been demostrated. T and N status were used in 1935 by Duke and Kiklin to define a staging system for colorectal cancer. Dukes' staging system was later modified by Aster and Coller [10], and is still used during clinical practice.

This system is strictly related to post-operative survival: stage A tumor has a 5 year survival of 100%, which is reduced to 67% and 54% for B1 and B2 stages respectively. Stage C1 and C2 have an average survival of 43% and 23%, while less than 5% of patients at stage D survive more than 5 years.
The TNM classification of colorectal cancer is a more detailed version of the Aster-Coller classification, and its use should be preferred in clinical practice.

1.6 Preoperative CEA plasmatic level

Preoperative CEA plasmatic levels are the only "non hystopathological" prognostic factors that the College of American Pathologists 6 considered should be inserted in the category I group.
Several studies [11, 12] have already demonstred that a preoperative plasmatic level of CEA> of 5ng/ml, should be considered as a negative prognostic factor.

2. Category II prognostic factors

Category II are those factors that have been fully studied both clinically and biologically, demonstrating their prognostic value, but have not yet been confirmed by controlled clinical trial.

2.1 Hystological grading of the tumor (G status)

Hystological grading of colorectal tumor is related to the prognosis [13]: the higher the degree of differentiation the better the prognosis. Several grading systems have been proposed during the past decades, but none have been widely accepted. The College of American Pathologists 6 proposed a modification of the widely-used 4-grade system, grade 1 and 2 (well and moderately-differentiated), grade 3 and 4 (poorly or undifferentiated), with a 2 tiered grading system: Low Grade (G1/G2) and High Grade (G3/G4). This "higher" classification system could help to reduce inter-observer variability, and retain or improve the prognostic significance of the G status.

2.2 Host lymphoid response to tumor

2.3 Host lymphoid response to tumor

The presence of lymphoid infiltration close to the tumor has been associated with a better prognosis [14, 15]. Nevertherless, to date, no well-designated trial has been able to demonstrate its value as an independent factor, probably due to the high variability in the interpretation of hystological findings. The College of American Pathologists 6 stressed the importance of distinguishing a simple inflammatory reaction, often associated to colorectal cancer (e.i. medullary carcinomas), from a real host lymphoid response. Once guidelines are obtained for a standard interpretation of hystopathological findings, controlled clinical trials are needed to confirm its value as an independent prognostic factor.

2.4 Microsatellite instability (MSI)

Some colorectal cancers are distinguished by extensive nucleotide insertions, or deletions in numerous intrinsically unstable, repeated sequences in tumor DNA, termed microsatellite instability (MSI)6. MSI is defined as a change of any extent due to either insertion or deletion of repeating units in a microsatellite within a tumor, when compared with normal tissue. This instability could be of two kinds: low (MSI-L) or high (MSI-H).
MSI-H carcinomas are characteristic of the hereditary non-polyposis colorectal cancer syndrome (HNPCC), but sporadic forms of MSI-H colorectal cancer are also present (almost 15%),

and they are related to a better prognosis. Further studies and controlled trials have to be performed, to confirm the validity of MSI as a prognostic factor.

3. Category III prognostic factors

Category III includes factors not yet sufficiently studied to evaluate their prognostic value. Only preliminary studies have been performed, and their value has still to be confirmed.

3.1 Tumor cells DNA content [16, 17]

3.2 Oncogenes [18, 19]

- *Onco-suppressor genes (LOH 1p/p53; LOH 8p, LOH 1p, LOH 5q)*
- *Ongogenes (K-ras, c-myc)*
- *DNA synthesis genes*
- *Genes deputed to the production of transforming growth factors, epidermal growth factors, adhesion proteins, glycoproteins (CD44, Cadregin E), angiogenetic factors*
- *Allelic loss of chromosome 18q*

3.3 Perineural invasion [20]

3.4 Microvilli density [21]

3.5 Cellular proteins and carbohydrates

- *HLA I*
- *HLA II*
- *CA19.9*
- *Integrins*
- *C Phosfolipase C*
- *Cytokeratine 20*

3.6 Peritumoral Fibrosis (Desmoplasia) [22]

3.7 Purulent peritumoral inflammatory reaction [21]

3.8 Tumor proliferation indices [23]

4. Category IV prognostic factors

This category includes well-studied factors shown to have no prognostic significance:
Tumor size [5], gross tumor configuration [5], age [2], sex [2], symptoms [2, 5], bio-humoral parameters [2, 5], tumor location [2, 5].

INTRODUCTION

The most recent data from literature [24] on rectal cancer show that the incidence of local recurrence is lower when the mesorectum is completely excised. This is also true for colon cancer where the mesentery is always widely resected.

A multicentric clinical study has recently been proposed to evaluate whether colorectal tumors located on the anti-mesenteric (AM) site may have a better prognosis, if compared with tumors located on the mesenteric (M) site;

the hypothesis is that tumors on the M site, closer to blood and lymphatic vessels, could have easier and quicker diffusion.

Furthermore, the incidence of different locations of these tumors will be evaluated, since no data appear in the literature.

It will also be interesting to investigate whether location on the AM site of the colon and the high rectum could be responsible for coelomatic diffusion of the tumor, whereas location on the M site is responsible for haematogenous and lymphatic spread. This observation could not be valid for the medium and low rectum, where the type of diffusion is completely different. In this case, it will be interesting to see if the M implantation of tumor is related to a higher incidence of local recurrence, due to a diffusion to the mesorectum. Rectal tumors located on the AM site may have a better prognosis.

The first phase of the study will evaluate the incidence of lymphnodes' involvement, in relation to M or AM location. In the case of statistically significant differences, the study will continue for evaluation of recurrence and distant metastases.

PATIENTS AND METHODS

All patients operated for colorectal cancer are enrolled in the study. Clinical data are collected in a computerized designated form.

Once the tumor is resected, the specimen is opened on the anti-mesenteric site and sent for hysto-pathological evaluation.

The pathologist will perform at least 3 sections on different parts of the tumor, and the circumferential involvement of the bowel wall is reported in a specific diagram (Fig. 1), where mesenteric or antimesenteric location can be identified.

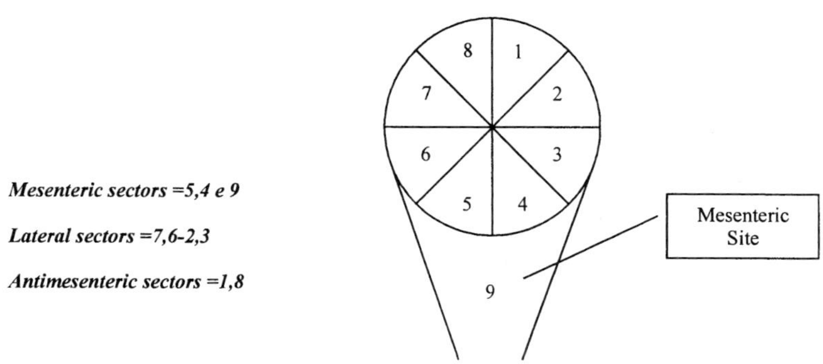

Figure 1. Identification of the involved sector at gross examination.

Hysto-pathological examination continues in the standard way, reporting the hystological type of the tumor, grading, T, N status as well as the presence of lymphatic, vascular or neural invasion, peritumoral lymphoid reaction, desmoplasia, MSI.

All the data are collected in a specifically designated computerized data base .

STATISTICAL ANALYSIS

It has been estimated that not less than 400 patients are needed to obtain uniform distribution for location and T status of M and AM tumors.

A chi-square Pearson's test was used to compare variables with "normal" distribution. A linear generalization test was used for variables with a Poisson's distribution. $P<0,05$ has been considered statistically significative.

PRELIMINARY RESULTS

From August 2000 to June 2001, 109 patients were enrolled in the study. Characteristics of patients and tumors are described in Table 1.

Table 1. Characteristic of patients and tumors

Sex	Mean Age	Location	
		Right colon	31
		Transverse Colon	2
M = 64	69 ± 13	Disc./Sigmoid colon	40
F = 45	(54 - 91)	High rectum	12
		Medium Rectum	13
		Low Rectum	11

There was no significant difference between the number of mesenteric and antimesenteric locations of resected colorectal cancer (Chart 1).

There was no statistically significant difference between the mesenteric and antimesenteric groups, regarding the degree of infiltration of the bowel wall by the tumor (T status) (Chart 2).

Comparing the mesenteric and the antimesenteric groups, for the degree of lymphnodes' involvement (N status), we found significantly ($p=0,03$) more lymphnode metastases for colorectal cancer located in the mesenteric side of the large bowel (Chart 3 and 4).

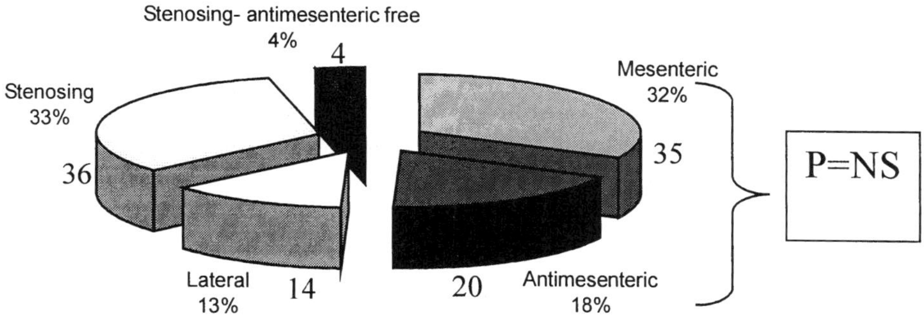

Chart. 1 Location and characteristics of the tumors

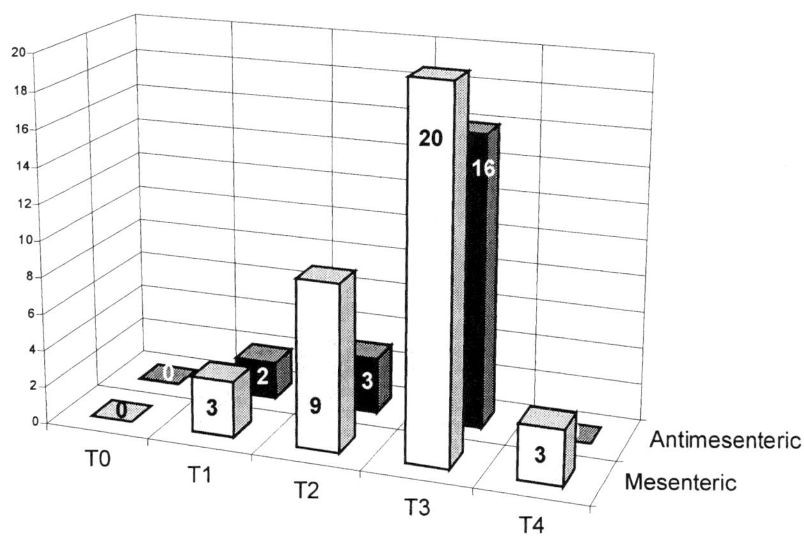

Chart 2. T distribution: mesenteric vs. antimesenteric

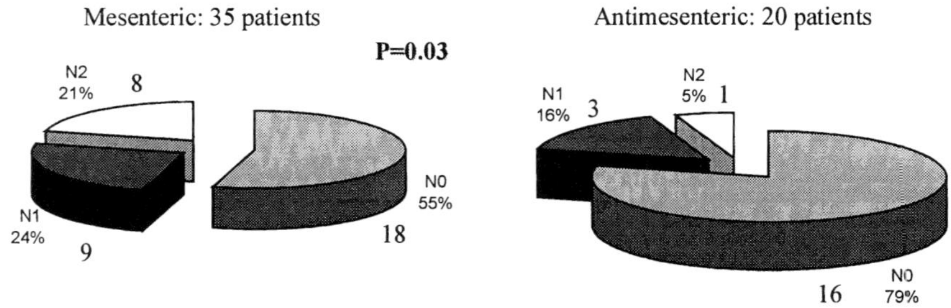

Chart 3 - 4. N status: Mesenteric vs Antimesenteric tumors

CONCLUSIONS

Although preliminary, our results show that almost 50% of the tumors are located on the mesenteric or antimesenteric site of the large bowel.

Tumors located on the mesenteric site of the large bowel, seem to have a more aggressive attitude in terms of lymphnode metastases, probably due to their closeness to blood and lymphatic vessels.

REFERENCES

1. Hannisdal E, Thorsen G. Regression analyses of prognostic factors in colo-rectal cancer. *J Surg Oncol* 1988; 37: 109-112.
2. Crucitti F, Sofo L, Foglietto GD et al. Prognostic factors in colorectal cancer: current status and new trends. *J Surg Oncol* 1991; 2: 76-82.
3. Hermanek P, Sobin LH. Colorectal carcinoma. In : Prognostic factors in cancer. New york, NY: Springer-Verlag NY inc; 1995.
4. Gordon DL. Malignant tumors of the colon. In Clinical practice of gastroenterology: Curchill Livingston Ph. 1999
5. Newland RC, Dent OF, Lyttle MN et al. Pathologic determinants of survival associated with colon or rectal cancer with lymph node metastases: a multivariate analysis of 579 patients. *Cancer* 1994; 73: 2076-2082.
6. Compton CC, Fielding LP, Burgart LJ et al. Prognostic factors in colorectal cancer. *Arch Pathol Lab Med* 2000; 124: 979-994.
7. Hermanek P, Henson DE, Hutter RVP et al. American Joint Committee on Cancer eds. Cancer Staging Manual. 5th ed. Philadelphia Pa. Lippincott Raven, 1997.

8. Jeffer MD, O'Dowd GM, Mulcahy H, Staff M et al. The prognostic significance of immunohistochemically detected lymph node micrometastases in colorectal carcinoma. *J Pathol* 1994; 172: 183-187.
9. Ratto C, Sofo L, Ippoliti M et al. Accurate lymph-node detection in colorectal specimens resected for cancer is a prognostic significance. *Dis Colon Rectum* 1999; 42 : 143-158.
10. Aster VB, Coller FA. The prognostic significance of direct extension of carcinoma of the colon and rectum. *Ann Surg* 1957;139:846.
11. Wolmark N, Fisher B, Wieand HS et al. The significance of preoperative carcinoembryogenic antigen levels in colorectal cancer. *Ann Surg* 1984; 199: 375-382.
12. Wanebo HJ, Rao B, Pinsky CM et al. Preoperative carcinoembryogenic antigen level as a prognostic indicator in colorectal cancer. *N Engl J Med* 1978; 299: 448-451.
13. Griffin MR, Bergstralh EJ, Coffey RJ, Beart RW et al. Predictors of survival after curative resection of carcinoma of the colon and rectum. *Cancer* 1987, 60: 2318-2324.
14. Jass JR. Lymphocytic infilatration and survival in rectal cancer. *J Clin Pathol* 1986; 39: 585-589.
15. Svennevig JL, Lunde OC, Holter J, Bjfrgsvik D. Lympgoid infiltration and prognosis in colorectal carcinoma. *Br J Cancer* 1984; 49: 375-377.
16. Nori D, Merimskky O, Saw D, Cortes E, Chen E et al. Tumor ploidy as a risk factor for disease recurrence and short survival in surgically treated Dukes B2 colon cancer patients. *Tumor Biol* 1996;17: 75-80.
17. Caruso ML, Pirrelli M, Armentano R. DNA content in colorectal carcinoma : application of image analysis to archival material. *Patologica* 1994;86:376-383.
18. Troungos C, Valvanis C, Kapranos N et al. K-ras mutation in Greek patients with poorly and moderately differentiated tumours of the lower intestinal tract. *Anticancer Res* 1997;17: 1399-1404.
19. Cerottini JP, Caplin S, Sarage E et al. The type of K-ras mutation determines prognosis in colorectal cancer. *Am J Surg* 1998; 175: 198-202.
20. Knudsen JB, Nilson T, Sprechler M, Johannsen A et al. Venous and nerve invasion as prognostic factors in post-operative survival of patients with resectable cancer of the rectum. *Dis Colon Rectum* 1983; 26 : 613-617.
21. Lindmark G, Gerdin B, Sundblerg C et al. Prognostic significance of microvascular count in colorectal cancer. *J Clin Oncol* 1996; 14: 461-466.
22. Halvorsen TB, Seim E. Association between invasiveness, inflammatory reaction, desmoplasia and survival in colorectal cancer. *J Clin Pathol* 1989; 42: 162-166.
23. Chi HJ, Jung IK, Kim SS, Hong SH. Proliferatine cell nuclear antigen expression and its relationship to malignancy potential in invasive colorectal carcinomas. *Dis Colon Rectum* 1997; 40 : 51-59.
24. Bolognese A, Cardi M, Irnerio AM et al. Total mesorectal excision for surgical treatment of rectal cancer. *J Surg Oncol* 2000; 1: 21-24.

CHAPTER 15

DIFFERENT ROLE OF THE COLONIC POUCH AFTER LOW ANTERIOR RESECTION OR COLOANAL ANASTOMOSIS.

Francesco Tonelli, Alessandro Garcea, Iacopo Monaci, Giacomo Batignani
Department of Clinical Physiopathology, Surgical Unit. University of Florence. Florence. Italy.

Abstract

Functional outcome after sphincter-saving operations can be improved by colonic pouch reconstruction, compared to the straight procedure. However, it is not clear whether the colonic pouch has a different behaviour in patients who underwent low anterior resection (LAR) or coloanal anastomosis (CAA).

Material and methods: 75 patients submitted to a sphincter-saving operation for rectal carcinoma or villous tumor of the middle or lower third of the rectum, were available for the study: 18 patients underwent coloanal anastomosis (CAA), 13 of whom had a colonic pouch construction (PCAA), 20 pts underwent low anterior resection (LAR), and 24 pouch low anterior resection (PLAR). The two groups of patients were similar in age and gender. Anorectal function was studied in 13 patients submitted PLAR, in 20 patients with straight LAR, in 7 with PCAA and in 18 with CAA. Patients were re-assessed 12 months after the initial operation, by an interview and anorectal manometry.

Results: The mean number of defecations/24h were significantly higher in LAR patients 4.1 ± 0.7 versus 2.0 ± 1.5 in CAA patients, 2.2 ± 1 in patients with PCAA and 2.3 ± 1.8 in PLAR patients ($p<0.05$ when LAR group is compared to the other groups). Fecal soiling was observed in all the groups except in the PLAR. Less degree of incontinence or urgency were present in PCAA than in CAA. There were no differences in anal resting pressure (ARP) and squeeze pressure among the various groups. A greater distensibility and compliance of the neo-rectum was observed in CAA, PCAA, and PLAR, compared to LAR, respectively 8.5 ± 7 mmHg/ml air for CAA, 8.7 ± 5 mmHg/ml air for PCAA; 6.3 ± 4 mmHg/ml air for PLAR versus 3.1 ± 2.7 mmHg/ml air for LAR. A significative inverse linear correlation was present between the mean number of defecations24/h and the compliance. No difference of sense of incomplete evacuation was observed among the group of patients.

Conclusion: Colonic J pouch provides an advantage over straight anastomosis in sphincter-saving operation, reducing the number of defecations, fecal soiling and urgency. The role of the pouch seems to be different in LAR compared to CAA. In fact in LAR the use of the pouch increases compliance and consequently decrease the number of defecations. In CAA the pouch does not improve the number of defecations and compliance, but reduces fecal soiling and urgency.

A.M. *Farinon (ed.), Advances in Abdominal Surgery 2002*, 213-223.

INTRODUCTION

Sphincter saving operations have recently increase and become the most common surgical procedures for the treatment of tumours of the middle and lower third of the rectum.

Total mesorectal excision provides local control of the disease, through resection of the primary tumor and of its regional spread. This is allows anal sphincter sparing if the section of the rectum is performed below the mesorectum just near the ano-rectal junction (low anterior resection; LAR). When the tumor is located in the lower third of the rectum, the excision of the last few centimeters of the rectal mucosa down to the dentate line could be performed and, according to the site and spread of the tumor, also the superior part of the internal sphincter may be excised. In this case, an endoanal anastomosis between colon and anal mucosa the dentate line level may be performed (coloanal anastomosis, CAA). Anatomical and surgical differences exist between LAR and CAA but functional outcome of these sphincter saving operations are considered together in several studies. We instead have evaluated differences in funtional results separately for each group of patients.

After both procedures, continence can be satisfactory but a variable percentage of patients may experience functional problems: high number of defecations, urgency and fecal soiling.

The use of the colonic "J" pouch has thought to be able in reducing the postoperative functional troubles, but controversies still remain about its role.

The aim of this study was to evaluate the clinical and manometric results of patients who underwent LAR and CAA with (PLAR and PCAA) or without (LAR and CAA) colonic pouch, trying to highlight the differences, if any among these surgical procedures.

MATERIAL AND METHODS

Between June 1989 and September 1998, 91 patients underwent a sphincter-saving operation for rectal carcinoma or villous tumor of the middle or lower third of the rectum. Sixteen of these patients were excluded because of anastomotic stricture [5], local tumor recurrence [2], pre or postoperative radiotherapy [2], presence of the stoma at the moment of the study [2], or because lost at follow-up [5]. Therefore 75 patients were available for the study: 18 patients underwent CAA, 13 underwent CAA with colonic pouch (PCAA), 20 underwent LAR and 24 LAR with colonic pouch (PLAR). The groups of patients were similar about age, and sex (Tab. 1).

The patients were studied by means of clinical and manometric assessment 12 months after surgery or after closure of the protective stoma.

Table 1. Clinical data of patients who underwent sphincter-saving procedures

	CAA (18)	PCAA (13)	LAR (20)	PLAR (24)
Mean age (years ±SD)	61 ± 9	61 ± 19	62 ± 10	61 ± 11
(range)	(47 - 75)	(47 - 87)	(41 - 78)	(40 - 84)
Sex ratio (M/F)	14/4	9/4	12/8	16/8
Temporary diversion	17/18	11/13	14/20	10/24
Anastomotic technique	Handsewn	Handsewn	Stapled	Stapled
Distance of the anastomosis from the anal verge (cm) (Means ± SD)	2.4 ± 0.8	2.5 ± 1.2	4.0 ± 1.5	4.5 ± 1.7
(range)	(2.2 - 2.7)	(2.1 - 2.8)	(3.2 - 4.3)	(3.5 - 5.3)

Operative technique

Total mesorectal excision and the nerve sparing technique were adopted during rectal dissection.

LAR: the rectum was transected just near the anorectal junction. A double stapling technique was performed using a linear stapler to close the rectal stump and a circular stapler, inserted transanally, to anastomose the rectum to the descending colon. The safety of the anastomosis was checked by the examination of the "doughnuts", and by air inflation with the pelvis filled with saline.

CAA: a short mucosectomy of the last 2 cm of rectal mucosa was usually performed. In two patients the upper part of the internal sphincter was excised. The descending colon was driven into the anal canal, and interrupted sutures (3/0 polyglycolic acid) were placed between the colon and the dentate line. Each suture incorporated the dentate line and a portion of the internal sphincter.

The colonic reservoir (7 cm in length) was constructed from two loops (J pouch) of the descending colon, using the GIA stapler device before placing the colon low in the pelvis.

The level of anastomosis was checked by means at endoscopy during follow-up.

A temporary loop ileostomy or transverse colostomy was performed if considered useful, and closed three months later.

Clinical assessment

The following parameters about anorectal function were evaluated: number of defecations/24 hours and those at night, presence of diurnal or nocturnal fecal soiling (defined as frequent if more than twice a week, and as occasional if less than twice a week), urgency (defined as an inability to defer defecation for at least 15 minutes) and incomplete evacuation (defined as an evacuation in many times or the need of going to the toilet again within 1 hour after the first defecation).

Continence was assessed according with Kirwan's classification [1].

Manometric assessment

Eighteen patients with CAA, 7 with PCAA, 20 with LAR and 13 with PLAR were evaluated by means of an anorectal manometry.

It was carried out by means of a polyethylene catheter (80 cm long and with external diameter of 2.7 mm) opened at the tip with four side holes of 0.7 mm diameter. This catheter was connected to a pressure transducer MK5-04 DTMVF (Sorenson Rescarch Co., Salt Lake City, UT) perfuse at a constant flow (3 ml/hour), with a saline solution using an "Intraflow" perfusion system (Abbott Labs, North Chicago, IL) that was connected to a polygraph recorder, "Honeywell RM 300" (Honeywell Medical Division, The Netherlands). The pressure rise-rate of the system was 50 mm Hg/second. The following parameters were evaluated: anal canal resting pressure (ARP), measured at 2 cm from anal verge, performing a station pull-through. Thus, withdrawing the catheter at 1 cm intervals (continuous pull-through) high pressure zone (HPZ) (cm) and the maximal resting pressure (MARP) (mmHg) were evaluated. With the catheter tip at 2 cm from anal verge, we measured the amplitude (mmHg) and duration (sec) of maximum voluntary contraction (MVC).

We then positioned a 5 x 6 cm latex balloon immediately above the anorectal ring, in order to verify the presence of rectoanal inhibitory reflex (AIR), and its volumetric threshold (ml of air). Then, by connecting this balloon to another pressure transducer, and inflating it with progressively increasing volumes (20 ml air every 30 seconds) we evaluated the volume (TV) and pressure (TP) at which the patient feels a transient sensation of rectal distension (threshold sensation) and the maximum tolerable volume (MTV) and pressure (MTP) (volume and pressure at which the patient feels the urge to defecate and is forced to do so). Neorectal compliance (NC) was expressed as the reciprocal of the slope of the straight-line, resulting from pressure/volume points thus obtained (ml air inflated/mm Hg measured, dV/dP).

STATISTICAL ANALYSIS

The results were expressed as a mean of the values + standard deviation (SD). The significance was calculated using Student's t-test for paired and unpaired samples. The correlation coefficient was determined using linear regression analysis (Pearson's test). Nominal variables were analysed, using chi-squared or Fischer's exact test when appropriate. We accepted $p<0.05$ as significant.

RESULTS

Clinical data are reported in Table 2. The mean number of defecations/24h after LAR resulted significantly higher compared to the other groups ($p<0.05$), whereas the number of nocturnal defecations did not varied significantly among the four groups. Frequent soiling (both diurnal or nocturnal) was never observed after PLAR, whereas similar incidence was found in the other groups.

Table 2. Functional outcome one year after sphincter-saving procedures

	CAA (18)		PCAA (13)		LAR (20)		PLAR (24)	
Number of defecations/24h (Means ± SD) (range)	2.0 ± 1.5 (1 - 5)		2.2 ± 1 (0.5 - 3)		4.1 ± 0.7* (3 - 7)		2.3 ± 1.8 (1 - 3)	
Number of nocturnal defecations (Means + SD) (range)	0.6 ± 1.5 (0 - 1)		0.1 ± 0.4 (0 - 1)		0.7 ± 0.4 (0 - 2)		0.5 ± 0.3 (0 - 1)	
	N	(%)	N	(%)	N	(%)	N	(%)
Urgency	4°	(22)	0°	(/)	8	(40)	2	(10)
Sense of incomplete evacuation	4	(22)	2	(29)	2	(10)	4	(20)

* $p<0.05$ with respect to the values of the other groups
° $p<0.05$

A significantly lower incidence of urgency was observed when the colonic pouch was employed; in particular it was never observed after PCAA ($p<0.05$).

There was no significant difference between the straight and pouch procedures about the sense of incomplete evacuation, although straight procedures were followed by a lower incidence (32% vs 49%). Suppositories, enemas or laxative drugs were never used from these patients.

Table 3 shows that the use of the pouch after sphincter saving operations may improve the degree of Kirwan's continence classification. In fact, 79% of patients with PLAR and 54% of the patients with PCAA had perfect continence with respect to 60% of the patients with LAR and 28% of those with CAA. Also the incidence of occasional soiling (degree III) seems to be improved by the use of a colonic pouch ($p<0.05$ CAA vs PCAA).

Table 3. Kirwan's classification after sphincter-saving procedures

		CAA (18)	PCAA (13)	LAR (20)	PLAR (24)
I	Perfect continence	5 (28%)	7 (54%)	12 (60%)	19 (79%)
II	Flatus incontinenece	0 (/)	0 (/)	0 (/)	0 (/)
III	Occasional soiling	9 (50%)*	3 (23%)*	6 (30%)	5 (21%)
IV	Frequent soiling	4 (22%)	3 (23%)	2 (10%)	0 (/)
V	Colostomy	0 (/)	0 (/)	0 (/)	0 (/)

* $p<0.05$

Manometric data are reported in Table 4. There were no statistical differences in the four groups, concerning the various parameters evaluated of internal (ARP, MARP, HPZ) (Fig. 1) and external (MVC) sphincter activity.

Table 4. Manometric data after sphincter-saving procedures

	CAA (18)	PCAA (7)	LAR (20)	PLAR (13)
ARP at 2cm (mmHg)	34 + 14	33 + 10	42 + 18	35 + 11
HPZ (cm)	2.2 + 1	2.8 + 0.6	3.1 +1.2	3.5 +0.4
MARP (mmHg)	56 + 23	55 + 12	58 + 21	56 + 18
MVC –amplitude (mmHg)	95 + 45	74 + 31	82 + 25	95 + 63
MVC- duration (sec)	59 + 42	32 + 21	49 + 19	68 + 35
MTV (ml air)	330 + 223	333 + 120	135 + 67*	313 + 226
NC (ml air/mmHg)	8.5 + 7	8.7 + 5	3.1 + 2.7*	6.3 + 4

*$p<0.05$

The study of neo-rectal capacity and compliance of the neorectum showed similar values of TS and TP after the four surgical procedures, and values of MTV, MTP and NC were significantly lower after LAR than after the other surgical procedures ($p<0.05$). A significant inverse correlation existed between the number of defecations/24h and values of MTV and NC in all the groups ($p<0.05$) (Fig. 2).

An absence of AIR was found in 8 patients with CAA (44%), 6 with PCAA (86%), 2 with LAR (10%) and 3 with PLAR (23%). No correlation was found between the absence of AIR and the presence of soiling.

The threshold of AIR was found lower after LAR procedures than after CAA procedures, this data did not reach statistical significance.

DISCUSSION

The functional outcome after sphincter saving operations is commonly reported related to the level of the anastomosis. Modifications of continence do

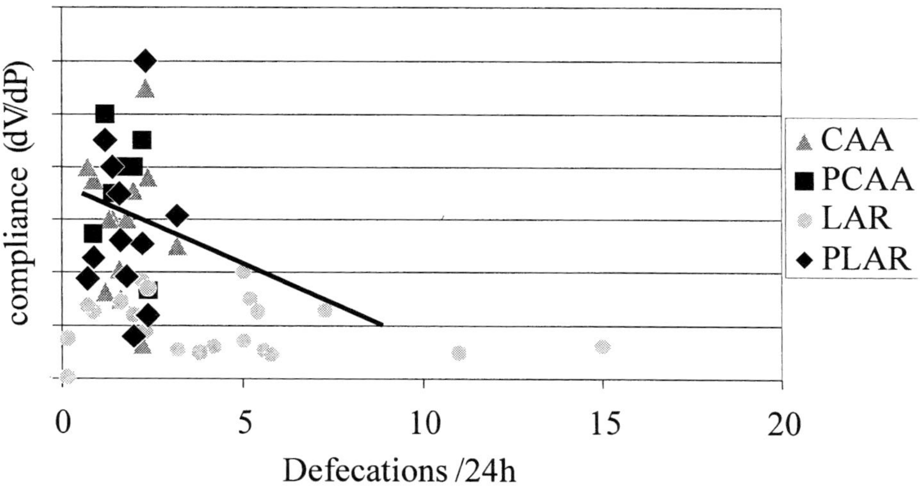

Figure 1. Inverse correlation between neorectal compliance and number of defecations/24h in sphincter-saving operations

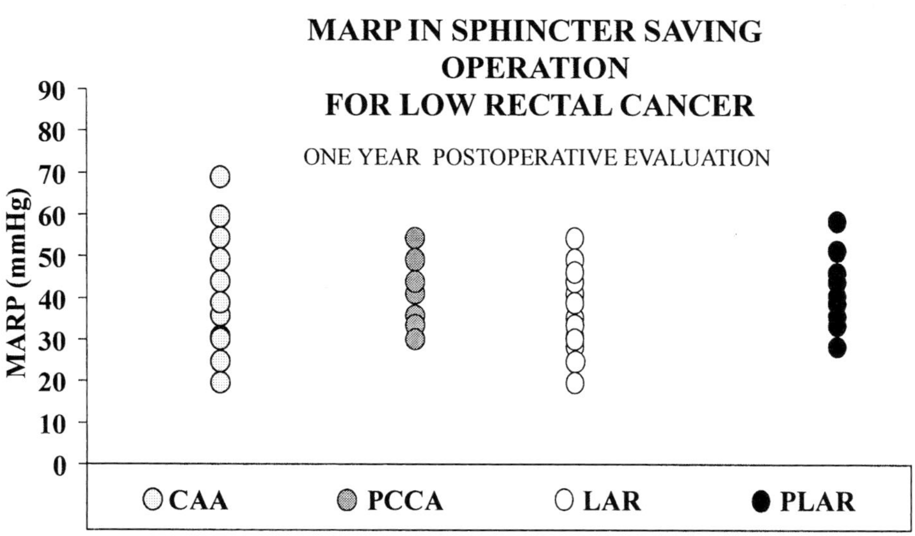

Figure 2. Distribution of the MARP in sphincter-saving operations

not usually occur when the residual rectum has a sufficient length of at least 6-8 cm. On the other hand, impairment of continence is frequent, if a total or near total rectal excision is performed [2-3].

The impairment of anorectal function after sphincter saving operations can be mainly due to two factors: the reduction of anal tone, and the loss of compliance and capacity of the neo-rectal ampulla.

When the length of the rectal stump is less than 6 cm the value of ARP is decreased in respect to preoperative evaluation [2]. This reduction is usually due to a reduced tone of the internal sphincter. It is controversial whether or not maintaining a few cm of the rectal stump or excising the whole rectum, might influence the anal resting tone. No differences in manometric values have been observed if the length of the residual rectum is less or more than 4 cm [2] or if the level of colorectal anastomosis is less or more than 6 cm above the anal verge [4]. Even when all the rectum is excised and a CAA is performed, some Authors [2] did not show any statistical difference in the values of ARP when compared to the LAR.

However, Deen et al [5], evaluating patients with stapled ileal pouch-anal anastomosis at different heights, showed that when the anastomosis is placed at the top of the anal columns (high anastomosis) the reduction in pressure is lower than when the anastomosis is placed at the level of dentate line (low anastomosis) [5]. This difference observed between the high and low anastomosis is explained by the excision of the proximal internal sphincter that occurs when a low anastomosis is performed. In the present study we did not observe any difference of anal tone in the four groups of patients (similar values of ARP and MARP). Only the length of HPZ was found higher, when the anastomosis was placed above the dentate line, but the difference between LAR and PLAR and with CAA and PCAA was not statistically significant.

It is also controversial if the decrease in anal tone might improves or not with time after surgery. Lane and Parks showed a reduction of ARP three months after LAR, with a progressive improvement within one year from surgery. [6] Hallbook et al, however, did not find any difference in ARP during the first postoperative year [7].

Even if it is clear that a sphincter saving operation is followed by a decrease of ARP, it is controversial if such decrease is related to a poor functional outcome. For example, patients with LAR complaining of fecal leakage have values of anal tone that are not different from those who do not complain of incontinence.

The other function which is impaired after sphincter saving operation is the capacity and compliance of the neo-rectal ampulla. In literature the values of MTV and NC after a straight reconstructive procedure (both LAR and CAA) are usually referred as significantly reduced in comparison to preoperative values and this reduction seem to be maintained at one year after surgery [7].

In some studies about manometric assessment and the functional outcome of sphincter saving operation, LAR and CAA surgical procedures are considered together while others LAR are named CAA. This makes results between the two procedures confusing and not comparable. In fact although the patients were similar about age, sex ratio and length of follow-up, many differences were noted among clinical and manometric data. Our study instead shows that LAR and CAA have many differences in manometric and clinical results.

The mean stool frequency was found significantly higher in LAR group when compared to CAA. It is also of interest that in our experience a straight CAA has a functional result similar to that of pouch procedures (either PCAA or PLAR). This is explained by the values of MTV and NC observed after CAA, which are significantly higher than after LAR and comparable with those observed when a pouch is performed.

A possible explanation of the higher capacity and compliance of CAA may lie in the absence of the residual rectal stump, having the colon directly sutured to the dentate line, and in the possibility of an optimal distensibility. In our opinion, the presence of a few cm of rectal stump above the dentate line and below the anastomosis may be the cause of the reduction in NC (and then of the high mean stool frequency), since fibrosis of the suture line may not allow a good distensibility. As in previous experience the values of MTV and NC were showed to be inversely related to the number of defecations 24/h [8]. High values of MTV and NC found after CAA do not match other studies in which lower values of these parameters are observed [2]. A possible explanation may be due to the different part of colon used for the reconstructive procedure. We used the proximal descending colon near the splenic flexure, a part of the colon with a larger diameter and probably higher distensibility than the sigmoid tract, whereas in most of the studies the sigmoid rather than the descending colon has employed to perform the anastomosis [6].

Therefore the use of a colonic pouch is able to increase the values of MTV and NC and thus to reduce significantly the mean number of defecations/24h after LAR, but does not change this parameters after CAA that is just characterised by high values of MTV and NC and thus by a low number of defecations/24h.

On the other hand CAA is followed by a higher incidence of soiling. We observed that the use of the pouch in sphincter saving operations may improve the functional outcome reducing the incidence of fecal soiling. In fact 54% of patients with PCAA e 79% with PLAR have perfect continence one year after the operation in compared to 28% of patients with CAA and 60% with LAR. The cause of the improvement in continence (that does not seem related to the values of ARP or MVC, being such values similar after the two procedures) is probably different in the two reconstructive procedures. In the present study

AIR has been found in almost all the patients operated by LAR. In LAR when the pressure in the residual rectum increases it could lead to a complete inhibition of the internal sphincter, causing fecal soiling. If this is the case, the construction of a pouch above the residual rectum increasing values in MTV and NC, may avoid that such total inhibition occur, since a critical endoluminal pressure is reached only in the presence of very great faecal volume. In CAA the MTV and NC are not further increased using a pouch. The improvement of continence can be probably due to the abolition or the reduction of the colonic peristaltic waves in the pouch. In patients without the pouch the pressure waves within the terminal colon could overcome anal sphincter pressure and consequently soiling may occur. When a pouch is performed the colonic muscular layers are sectioned, and as a consequence the colonic motility is altered if not reduced. The reduction in gradient pressure between the pouch and the anus may explain the lower incidence of soiling, when compared to straight procedures.

The size of the pouch is a key factor in avoiding defaecatory difficulties and faecal impaction. In a study by developing a mathematical model to quantify colonic reservoir capacity, a colonic pouch length of 8-10 cm was recommended [9]. The improved function of smaller volume colonic pouches may be similarly related to the interruption of propulsive movements in the J segment. In our study a 7 cm long pouch was used and there was no significant difference in sense of incomplete evacuation between straight and pouch groups.

In conclusion our study seems to stress that CAA and LAR are different procedures about the functional outcome and neorectal physiology. The association of a colonic J pouch may improve the functional outcome even if the pathophysiological mechanism seems partly different, in the two surgical procedures.

REFERENCES

1) Kirwan WO, O'Riordain MG, Waldron R: Declining indications for abdominoperineal resection. *Br. J. Surg.* 1989, 76: 1061-1063.

2) Lewis WG, Holdsword PJ, Stephenson BM, Finan PJ, Johnston D: Role of the rectum in the physiological and clinical results of coloanal and colorectal anastomosis after anterior resection for rectal carcinoma. *Br. J. Surg.* 1992, 79: 1082-1086.

3) Hida J, Yasutomi M, Maruyama T, Fujimoto K, Nakajima A, Uchida T, Wakano T, Tokoro T, Kubo R, Shindo K: Indications for colonic J-pouch reconstruction after anterior resection for rectal cancer. *Dis. Colon Rectum* 1998, 48: 558-563.

4) Jehle EC, Haehnel T, Starlinger MJ, Becker HD: Level of the anastomosis does not influence functional outcome after anterior rectal resection for rectal cancer. *Am. J. Surg.* 1995, 169: 147-152.

5) Deen KI; Williams JC, Grant EA, Billingham C, Keighley MR: Randomized trial to determine the optimum level of pouch-anal anastomosis in stapled restorative proctocolectomy. *Dis. Colon Rectum* 1995, 38: 133-138.

6) Lane RH, Parks AG: Function of the anal sphincters following colo-anal anastomosis. *Br. J. Surg.* 1977, 64: 596-599.
7) Hallbook O, Nystrom PO, Sjodahl R: Physiologic characteristics of straight and colonic J-pouch anastomoses after rectal excision for rectal cancer. *Dis. Colon Rectum* 1997, 40: 332-338.
8) Batignani G, Monaci J, Ficari F, Tonelli F: What affects continence after anterior resection of the rectum?. *Dis Colon Rectum* 1991, 34: 329-335.
9) Banerjee AK, Park K: Pediction of optimum dimensions of colonic pouch reservoir. *Dis. Colon Rectum* 1996, 39: 1293-1295.

CHAPTER 16

PRIMARY ANORECTAL RECONSTRUCTION AFTER ABDOMINOPERINEAL EXCISION BY COLOPERINEAL PULL-THROUGH AND ELECTRICALLY STIMULATED GRACILOPLASTY: EFFICIENCY AND LIMITATIONS OF A HARD-TO-CATCH-ON PROCEDURE.

Vincenzo Violi, Adamo S. Boselli, Renato Costi, Luigi Roncoroni
Department of Surgery of Parma Hospital, University of Parma, Parma, Italy

Abstract
After presentation of the historical background of graciloplasty for anorectal reconstruction, after abdominoperineal excision of the anorectum for cancer, and illustration of pathophysiological bases, techniques and results of "dynamic" graciloplasty, a 6-year experience is reported with twenty-one patients submitted to primary total anorectal reconstructions and temporary loop abdominal ileo- or colostomy.
Fourteen patients had activation of the neosphincter after abdominal stoma closure. Eleven of these patients had a pulse generator implanted, as delayed surgery in selected patients (5 cases) or during graciloplasty (6 cases). Early and 1-year clinical and manometric results were evaluated. Satisfactory results were recorded in eleven patients (78.5%) soon after stoma closure, and in 9 after 1 year (64.3%). Continuous electrostimulation proved effective on resting anal pressure, while voluntary contraction pressure seemed to be an independent variable.
Although primary total anorectal reconstruction involves a high complication level, and expenditure of economic and human resources, the good functional results which can be achieved in selected cases do not seem to justify the doubts and perplexities which still limit a wide acceptance of this procedure.

INTRODUCTION

In the last two decades, well-known oncological and technical reasons have promoted, sphincter-saving procedures in resective surgery for rectal cancer. Although surgeons have been prompted to perform intersphincteric

A.M. Farinon (ed.), *Advances in Abdominal Surgery 2002*, 225-246.

abdomino-transanal rectal excisions, with coloendoanal anastomosis [1-3], a limited number of patients must still undergo abdomino-perineal resection (APR), to fulfil correct oncological criteria.

A permanent colostomy involves serious physical disablement and psychological discomfort, as well as limitations in social life [4-6]. Several attempts at carrying out a continent perineal colostomy after APR have been performed in the past [7,8], but only in 1976 were anorectal neosphincters first constructed [9] by gracilis muscle transposition, adapting a technique originally described in 1952, for the treatment of faecal incontinence in childhood [10].

Nonstimulated graciloplasty

All myoplasty procedures obviously started out as static, that is, nonstimulated neosphincters. Various experiences in faecal incontinence in adults were reported as far back as the '80s [11-18]. Functional results were extremely conflicting, probably because of differences in indications, patients' preoperative conditions, surgical techniques, criteria and time of postoperative evaluation.

However, the principal issue of this procedure is that the muscle undertakes a different function, concerning anatomical site, cortical representation and physiology. The fast-twitch fatiguable fibres, which are predominant in the gracilis muscle, are incapable of prolonged contraction, and the natural evolution of a transposed, not adequately stimulated muscle is inevitably atrophy and fibrosis. Even if the muscle is constantly and correctly trained, it can contract only under voluntary control, while basal tone is determinant for continence.

These pathophysiological reasons fostered still greater doubts and perplexities about graciloplasty for total anorectal reconstruction (TAR) after anorectal excision, both in primary reconstruction, synchronous to excision of the anorectum, and in secondary, delayed reversal of abdominal into perineal colostomy, which involves loss of anorectal sensory function.

Thus, in spite of good results in 75% of 21 patients, the experience of Simonsen et al. [9], remained an isolated case, apart from one other report [19], until techniques of external-source, short-term intermittent electrical stimulation (IES) and biofeedback training (BFB) were adopted from 1985 on, by Cavina and co-workers [20-23]. These authors, who deserved the merit of reintroducing the use of this surgical procedure, reported a good degree of continence in 26 (65%) out of 47 patients, and at a later evaluation, in 71% of those still under study [24]. Other similar results, unfortunately not supported by longer-term evaluations, were reported by Italian surgeons in the following years [25-27]. However, according to an authoritative opinion [28] *"it is unlikely that the unstimulated graciloplasty functions in any way other than as a biological Thiersch wire"*. In effect, satisfactory results were also reported in most patients who underwent pseudo-continent perineal colostomy by Schmidt's [29] smooth muscle procedure [30-31], and static graciloplasty has not really stood the test of time, partly because the more recent possibility of using implantable pulse generators (IPGs) and performing a "dynamic" neosphincter, have led to higher probabilities of achieving satisfactory continence, thereby rendering obsolete the previous unstimulated reconstructions.

Dynamic graciloplasty and TAR

The physiological basis of the improved functional results obtained by means of dynamic graciloplasty lies in a demonstration in animals, dating back to the '60s [32], showing that, from a histological, histochemical and biochemical viewpoint, a continuous, long-term electrostimulation converts fast-twitch fatiguable (type II) into slow-twitch, fatigue-resistant (type I) muscular fibres [33-38]. This phenomenon has also been confirmed in the transposed electrically stimulated human gracilis muscle [39]. In practice, thanks to a chronic electrostimulation (CES) delivered by an implanted device, a dynamic neosphincter has a continuous basal tone, independent of voluntary actions, which would be a necessary, although not always sufficient, condition for continence. The patient may de-activate the stimulator by means of a magnet or, more recently, a hand radiotelemetry controller, thereby temporarily relaxing the neosphincter to evacuate the neorectum.

Apart from isolated cases operated on for restoration of intestinal continuity after excisional surgery of the anorectum [40-41], also dynamic graciloplasty was first investigated and developed in its application for faecal incontinence [24, 42-58]. A good degree of continence was achieved in 60-70% of the patients and it is now widely held that, in selected patients with severe faecal incontinence, dynamic graciloplasty may be effective.

Despite electrodynamic technologies doubts and perplexities still persisted concerning anorectal reconstruction after excisional surgery for cancer, and the first studies on a series of patients were not reported until some years later [24, 45, 53, 56-57, 59-65].

This application was considered a greater challenge, and, in effect, there would be reason to believe that functional results after TAR cannot be as satisfactory as after faecal incontinence in the presence of a native sphincter [28, 61, 66-67]: the surgical procedure is more complex and is prone to a higher early and late complication rate. Oncological evolution is a further unknown factor, and, above all, neorectal sensitivity and compliance, as well as defecatory sequence co-ordination, are lacking [68].

Techniques and procedure stages of primary TAR

After abdominoperineal excision, the colonic stump is brought down through the perineal wound. A straight coloperineal anastomosis is usually carried out. In a few cases a colonic pouch has been performed [26,49, 61, 64], but there is no evidence that this procedure improves the functional results.

The gracilis muscle is dissected and distally detached, preserving the proximal neurovascolar pedicle, and is then drawn through the inguinal groove into the perineum, to wrap the colon. Various surgical techniques and muscle arrangements have been described, although none of them have proved to be better than the others.

An initial distinction may be made between single (Williams' and Rosen's groups) and double graciloplasty (Cavina's and Baeten's groups). Each muscle may be wrapped according to alpha, gamma or epsilon configuration. In the technique described by Cavina and Seccia [21, 23], one gracilis is positioned behind the colonic stump so as to simulate a puborectalis sling, the other gracilis muscle surrounds the colonic stump more superficially, in "alpha" configuration.

In the techniques of Baeten and Geerdes [59-60] the two muscles surround the colon from behind and are anchored anteriorly, one to each other.

Rosen et al. [69] described a split-sling configuration, to prevent spiral working of the neoanus. The tendon of the gracilis may be fixed to the skin, to the ischiatic tuberosity or to the same or other muscle.

The procedure may be carried out in one or more stages: Mander and Williams [28, 61] complete it in three stages, the first consisting of APR, coloperineal pull-through and a "vascular delay procedure", which involves the division of the distal vascular pedicles to reduce the risk of muscle ischemia, the second one being inclusive of graciloplasty and pulse generator implantation, and the third stage involving the closure of the defunctioning stoma.

Geerdes and Baeten [59-60] also use a three-stage procedure, the first intended as APR+TAR+abdominal stoma, the second as pulse generator implantation, and the third as stoma closure.

Rosen and co-workers [57] report a single-stage procedure, which may, however, be considered as such, only if we do not take into account the closure of the diverting stoma, which they also performed in TAR.

Only Cavina and Seccia [62-63] gave up fashioning a diverting stoma, albeit after longstanding experience, and only their more recent procedure may therefore be properly considered as a single-stage one.

Finally, according to the modality of electrode implantation, the electrostimulation may be neural [61, 56], intramuscular [24, 57, 60] or both ("over the nerve plus intramuscular") [63]. Intramuscular electrostimulation would avoid the risk of intraoperative or chronic damage of the nerve trunk, and of lead displacement. Neural, as well as neural+intramuscular stimulation, would favour a complete recruitment of the muscle fibres, thereby increasing contraction efficacy, decreasing the contractility threshold and probably prolonging stimulator longevity, which is usually expected to be about five years but may be renewed by a very simple substitution technique.

Results and current opinions

Major reports showed: episodes of incontinence in all patients, controlled by constipating agents and neorectal irrigations [61]; a 57% rate of "reasonable continence" after primary and 42% after secondary TAR [60]; an 85% rate of continence for liquid and solid stool [63]; a 55% rate of continence for liquids and solids, solids alone, or occasional episodes for liquids [57], or for solids and liquids [64].

However, in many of these reports a specification is lacking as to whether continence was evaluated before or after the use of enemas, constipating or antimeteoric preparations, or proper diet. These measures might improve the "crude" functional results. It is also noteworthy that no patients of Mander's series wished to go back to abdominal stoma. Thus, it is likely that the functional evaluation of this condition has up to now been made with too restrictive criteria, or with unrealistic expectations of what a perineal colostomy can offer.

In previous reports [65, 70], we expressed the opinion that the two indications and postoperative conditions – graciloplasty supporting an incontinent native neosphincter and TAR – are not comparable, and that continence is the most important, but not the exclusive, issue in functional assessment after TAR, since other factors, some of them subjective, play an important role.

While coloperineal pull-through after a previous Miles resection is a risky procedure [71], which should be carried out only in very selected patients, by surgeons extremely skilled in primary graciloplasty, we wonder whether excessive criticism, in the evaluation of surgical and functional results after primary reconstruction, may account for the fact that, ten years after the first studies on dynamic neosphincters, this procedure does not seem to have caught on, although rectal cancer is very frequent and is usually treatable at any hospital.

This article was intended as a report on our experience in primary total anorectal reconstruction, as an attempt at evaluating its efficiency and limitations, and as a reading and interpretation of our results, according to criteria which we consider more relevant to the particular aspects of this condition.

PATIENTS AND METHODS

Management policy

When we started this type of surgery, in 1994, no substantial series of dynamic graciloplasty for TAR had been published. The use of stimulators still seemed to be at an experimental stage, while some reports on static graciloplasty were very attractive. In addition, in consideration of the high cost of the IPGs, we wondered whether their use would be unavoidable. For all these reasons, we decided that at least at an initial phase, until the verification of results, the IPG should be implanted only in selected cases; at a delayed stage, after preliminary IES plus BFB training of the neosphincter.

This phase, which lasted 3 years (1 April 1994 – 31 March 1997), enabled us to carry out a study which has been reported elsewhere [65]. In brief, with the only exclusion criteria being the palliative nature of the resection or gracilis muscle neuromuscular abnormalities, 13 patients underwent APR+TAR, defunctioning abdominal colo- or ileostomy, implantation of transitory cardiac electrodes, 4-6-month external-source intermittent electromyostimulation (IES), gracilis contraction exercises and biofeedback (BFB) training, with abdominal stoma closure (ASC) at least six months after initial surgery. Chronic, continuous electrostimulation (CES) via an implantable pulse generator (IPG) was used at a later time only in disease-free patients, when it was necessary from a functional viewpoint (1st protocol).

In the following period (1 April 1997 – 31 December 1999) a different policy was followed, which also included the T4 tumour category among the exclusion criteria. Eight patients underwent a one-stage procedure including APR, TAR, defunctioning abdominal stoma and IPG implantation. ASC was performed only after completion of the CES training protocol, which started a few days after surgery (2nd protocol).

Nineteen patients had rectal carcinoma, not eligible for a sphincter-saving procedure (lower margin of the tumor less than 5 cm from the anal verge) and 2 had recurrent, obstructing squamous cell carcinoma of the anal canal, previously treated by radiotherapy and local excision. We have never converted abdominal to perineal colostomy after previous APR.

General data, oncological features and outcome of all 21 patients are reported in Table 1. All patients with rectal cancer underwent preoperative colonoscopy+histological examination, CEA, chest x-rays, hepatic sonography and abdominopelvic CAT scan. From January 1995, the T3 or T4 rectal cancers, as judged by clinical examination and/or CAT scan, also underwent preoperative four-week 40 Gy radiotherapy. All procedures were carried out with the patient's informed consent, and in accordance with the standards of the Ethical Committee of our Institution.

Table 1. Twenty-one patients submitted to TAR. Cancer features and outcome (updated to January 31, 2000)

Patient	M/F	Age	pTNM	Grading	Outcome (months)
1. FF	M	70	T2N0M0	G2	alive, disease free (70)
2. GF	M	61	T2N1M0	G3	alive, disease free (70)
3. PI	F	75	T3N3M0	G3	local recurrence and inguinal metastases (9), dead (17)
4. AI	F	56	T3N2M0	G2	hepatic metastases (18), dead (36)
5. PL	M	68	T2N1M0	G3	hepatic metastases (6), dead (24)
6. ME	F	72	T3N1M0	G3	dead of myocardial infarction (2)
7. BI	F	73	T2N0M0	G2	alive, disease free (52)
8. FL	F	75	T3N2M0	G3	alive, disease free (50)
9 IN	F	54	T3N0M0	G2	alive, disease free (47)
10. SG	M	54	T2N0M0*	G1	alive, disease free (44)
11. BM	M	61	T3N0M0	G3	alive, disease free (41)
12. SG	M	46	T3N1M0	G3	resection of hepatic metastasis (19), alive, disease free (39)
13. SA	F	57	T4N0M0	G3	alive, disease free (34)
14. CS	F	67	T3N2M0	G3	alive, disease free (32)
15. BO	M	69	TXN0M0†	G2	alive, disease free (32)
16. FG	M	63	T2N0M0	G2	alive, disease free (30)
17. CL	M	64	T2N0M0	G2	alive, disease free (28)
18. BV	M	68	T2N0M0	G3	alive, disease free (20)
19. PA	F	73	T2N0M0	G2	alive, disease free (17)
20. BS	M	71	T2N0M0	G2	alive, disease free (12)
21. GP	F	66	T3N1M0*	G2	alive, disease free (2)

*: recurrent, obstructing anal carcinoma
†: totally downstaged after radiotherapy; pre-treatment endobioptic specimens: G2

Technical data

In all patients, surgery consisted of a procedure comprising:
1) APR;
2) coloperineal pull-through with "alpha-sling" double graciloplasty according to Cavina's technique [21, 23];
3) defunctioning abdominal colo- or ileostomy.

IES training, used only in patients of the 1st protocol, consisted of EMS, from the 4th or 5th day on, via two temporary electrodes (EP Temporary Pacing Wires, Ethicon), implanted into the gracilis muscle during TAR at the level of the branches of the nerve, and drawn up through the subcutaneous tissue and the skin of the left iliac area. The EMS was generated by an external stimulator (Urogyn™, In-Care Medical Products, Pabish, Milan, Italy). The time of training was increased from 5-10 minutes per day, up to 3-4 hours daily over 2 or 3 sessions, within about a four-week period. IES continued after the discharge of the patient, by means of a domiciliary device (Microgyn™, Pabish). In the absence of precise schedules, the parameters, conditioned by the characteristics of the devices, were chosen empirically, in order to evoke forceful but not painful contractions. They were usually as follows: frequency of 20 Hz, pulse width of 1 msecond, amplitude of 3-5 v, time «on» to time «off» ratio 1:2 seconds. Thus, the patient gradually learnt to identify and contract the muscles. This activity was reinforced by physical exercises and optimised by BFB training (Uromyogyn™, Pabish).

CES training was performed on all the patients who had the stimulator implanted, of both the 1st protocol, at a delayed phase (spinal anaesthesia), and the 2nd protocol. Two permanent intramuscular electrodes (model SP5548, Medtronic, Kerkrade, The Netherlands) were implanted, one in each muscle, crosswise to the branches of the nerve, connected to a quadripolar IPG (Itrel® II, model 7424, Medtronic), allocated to an abdominal subcutaneous pocket. The IPG was programmed under telemetry control (Itrel® Programmer Console model 7432, Medtronic) during surgery, and was activated 3-5 days after implantation.

The CES training schedule was the same as that used by other authors [24], who had previously given us personal information about the electrophysiological parameters. The amplitude was set individually, so as to evoke a forceful contraction at the start of training (usually 1 to 2 v are necessary) and to achieve at the end a valid neosphincter tone. This was considered acceptable when a difference of at least 25 cm H_2O between stimulated and unstimulated RAPs was recorded. Amplitude increments were later set only on clinical grounds, or at one-year manometry, to maintain the above pressure difference between IPG "on" and "off". The switch consisted of a magnet (Medtronic, model 7452) until July 1997; subsequently, a more recent IPG model was used (Interstim™, Medtronic), equipped with a hand controller.

Oncological and functional follow-up

Digital examination, CEA, chest x-rays and sonography (liver and pelvis) were scheduled every 6 months for 5 years. CAT scan (liver and pelvis) was scheduled at six months after surgery, and every 12 months.

A functional evaluation was performed only in patients who had, or were candidates for, ASC. It consisted of:

1. Clinical assessment on the basis of data obtained from a monthly diary, which were first expressed by a modified Jorge and Wexner [72] system, and were then recently re-assessed retrospectively by a personal scoring and grading scale (Table 2).

The clinical assessment was carried out in the patients of the 1st series 1-2 months after ASC, and in those who had stimulator implantation, also after CES training. In the patients of the 2nd protocol, clinical results were checked 1-2 months after ASC. Later on, all patients underwent yearly clinical assessments.

Table 2. Personal scoring and grading scale for functional result after TAR

	Never	Seldom	Often	Always
Incontinence for solid stool	0	1	2	3
Incontinence for liquid stool	0	1	2	3
Incontinence for flatus	0	1	2	3
Wears diaper	0	1	2	3
Needs for enema	0	0	1	2
Enema volume necessary >500 ml	0	0	1	2
Colonic voiding duration >30 min	0	0	1	2
Incomplete voiding / repeated enema	0	0	1	2

The continence score is determined by adding points from the above items.
Never: 0 (never); seldom: <1/week; often: <1/day, ^{3}1/week; always: ^{3}1/day.
Final grading into five categories:
Very good: 1-4; Good: 5-8; Fair: 9-12; Poor: 13-16; Very Poor:17-20.

2. Neoanal manometry (water perfusion four-sensor probe, connected to a pressure transducer, amplifier and chart recorder; Mui Scientific, Mississippi, Ontario, Canada), consisting of resting anal pressure (RAP), and voluntary contraction pressure (VCP) calculated as the mean value of three consecutive successful squeezes; each single value resulted from the mean of those recorded by the four sensors in the area of highest pressure.
In the presence of IPG, RAPs and VCPs were recorded in both "on" and "off" conditions. Manometric evaluations were carried out on all patients of the 1st series 1-2 months after ASC, in those who had stimulator delayed implantation also after CES training, and in all one year later. In the patients of the 2nd protocol, anomanometry was performed after CES training, just before ASC, and 1 year later in the first four.

Statistics

Scores given in the clinical assessments were reported individually, and as mean ±SD values. Manometric data (RAPs and VCPs) in both series were expressed as mean ±SD values, and whenever CES results were examined, individual examination data were also reported. Statistical comparisons were made using the Wilcoxon sum of ranks test.

RESULTS

Early and late complications

No early morbidity occurred, relating either to abdominal or perineal resective steps, or to the diverting loop colostomy. After 6 months, a minimal cysto-vaginal fistula occurred in a patient (no. 13) with T4 cancer, whose resection had involved a colpohysterectomy. After exclusion of a local recurrence, the fistula was successfully treated by Martius' procedure.

With regards to the perineal colostomy and the graciloplasty in a diabetic patient (no. 9), we reported a severe perineal infection with necrosis of the distal part of the muscles and disruption of the neosphincter. Its reconstruction, 4 months later, consisted of a peri-neorectal double sling, after longitudinal splitting of each residual gracilis muscle into two branches [73]. The abdominal stoma was closed eight months after initial surgery. A necrosis of the distal part of both muscles occurred also in patient no. 20; the extension of tissue damage and the fibrosis secondary to the perineal infection, did not permit the above reconstructive procedure. A necrosis of the colonic stump, distally to the alpha-shaped left gracilis which was probably too tight, occurred in one patient (no. 5) who, on the 5th postoperative day underwent, by perineal access only, further colonic pull-through and reconstruction of a less tight neosphincter. A mild degree of perineal infection, which was drained and/or resolved without the need for any surgical measure, occurred in 9 patients (nos. 1, 2, 3, 4, 6, 10, 12, 13 and 16). A subacute, deep perineal infection, which the patient (no. 21) revealed only 1 month after discharge, led to marked edema and secondary strangulation of the colonic stump within the tendineal wrap: the perineorectal space was opened and drained, and necrotic evolution of the stump was avoided, by detaching the tendons and loosening the neosphincter, which was reconstructed by Baeten's technique.

In two cases (no 1 and 2, respectively, at 42 and 23 months), major late complications consisted of stenosis at the level of the alpha shaped muscle, one of which (no. 1) also had an erosion of the neorectum from tendon pressure. Both cases required dissection of gracilis muscles and reconstruction of the neosphincter. Erosion of the neorectum also involved dissection of the colonic stump and its further pull-through. A more severe late complication, independent of us, consisted of a neorectal perforation by the enema nozzle, resulting in severe peritonitis and sepsis, eighteen months after prior surgery; the patient (no.18) recovered after transverse loop colostomy, which will probably be definitive, partly because the functional result had been unsatisfactory. A still asymptomatic ptosis of the pelvic floor is now developing in the patient who underwent reconstruction after necrosis of the distal part of the muscles (no. 9), and in patient no. 16.

As to major non-surgical complications, we reported a case of myocardial infarction, on the 15th postoperative day in one patient (no. 7), who recovered and was discharged on the 31st day. One patient (no. 6) died of myocardial infarction two months after discharge from hospital. One patient (no. 19) had two brainstrokes at 3 and 7 months, with full neurological recovery. A 10-month delay in CES completion and ASC was necessary.

No complications related to the stimulator implantation occurred. Although this is not a complication, two patients, up to now, have had the stimulator run down and substituted (no 2, at 43 months, and no. 9 who required high voltages, at 30 months).

Oncologic outcome.

All patients had specimen lateral margins free from tumour. Nineteen patients are evaluable from this viewpoint (minimum follow-up: 1 year, maximum: 70 months), after the exclusion of the cardiac death patient and of the last one of the series, who was operated on too recently (Tab. 1).

Withdrawn patients

In the former series, only 8 of the 13 patients underwent ASC: besides the patient who died of myocardial infarction and the one who had early metastases, three (nos. 7, 8, 13) who were poorly compliant to muscle training declined any further surgery, after good adaptation to abdominal loop colostomy.

In the 2nd protocol patients, only 6 of the 8 patients completed the CES program, since patient no. 20 had conversion into definitive abdominal colostomy and ileostomy closure eight months after prior surgery and postoperative gracilis necrosis, while the last one (no.21) is still under training.

Functional results (1st protocol)

Clinical assessments according to our 0-to-20 scoring and grading scale, showed the results reported in Table 3 in the eight patients of the first series who underwent ASC. Mean manometric values before ASC were: RAP = 30.1 ±8.6; VCP = 148.7 ±93.7. After ASC they were: RAP = 32.5 ±10.9; VCP = 171.7 ±104.4. No significant differences were found between RAP values before and after ASC, while VCPs improved significantly ($p<0.02$).

Table 3. Evaluations of functional results after TAR, according to our personal scoring and grading scale, in the eight patients of the 1st protocol who underwent ASC

Patient	AFTER ASC		IPG	EARLY AFTER CES		1 YEAR	
	scoring-grading		implant	scoring-grading		scoring-grading	
1. FF	11	(fair)	yes	7	(good)	7	(good)
2. GF	13	(poor)	yes	7	(good)	11	(fair)
3. PI	4	(very good)	no				
4. AI	6	(good)	no			7	(good)
9. IN	16	(poor)	yes	6	(good)	14	(poor)
10. SG	8	(good)	yes	4	(very good)	6	(good)
11. BM	8	(good)	yes	5	(good)	6	(good)
12. SG	4	(very good)	no			3	(very good)

Wilcoxon sum of ranks test in the five patients who had stimulator implantation.
After ASC *vs.* early after CES: not significant; early after CES *vs.* 1 year: not significant.

Selection for IPG (1st protocol)

The two patients with a "very good" result did not need the IPG support, although in one of these, only a six-month evaluation was possible after ASC. The sole survivor of these patients maintains an excellent result at a 3-year follow-up. Out of the three patients with a "good" result, the first did not receive the IPG, since it was neither strictly necessary (score = 6) nor advisable, because of an advanced tumor stage. The two others received IPG, at 2 and 7 months respectively after ASC, because of the absolute need to regain a full social life. In the three patients with a "fair" or "poor" result, a pulse generator was soon implanted, 1 to 2 months after the closure of the abdominal colostomy. Out of the three patients who did not need a stimulator, no clinical impairment over time occurred in the two (the former dead, the latter alive) who have so far completed at least one year of functional follow-up, nor was manometric worsening recorded.

Functional results after IPG (1st protocol)

In all five patients who had a stimulator implanted, continence improved, but constipation did not substantially change. In the patient who had undergone further reconstruction after necrosis of the distal part of the muscles, the improvement was also favored by a very regular intestinal habit. The score differences in these five patients showed a statistically significant improvement ($p<0.05$). One-year clinical assessments showed a worsening of the mean scores, statistically not significant. From a manometric viewpoint, comparison with the last values before stimulator implantation showed significant improvement in RAPs, only in the IPG "on" condition; the electrostimulated RAPs were also significantly higher than the unstimulated ones (Tab. 4).

Table 4. Manometric data (cm H_20) in 5 patients of the 1st protocol who underwent stimulator implantation after IES+BFB training and ASC

	LAST BEFORE CES		EARLY AFTER CES				1 YEAR LATER			
Pt. no.	(No IPG)		IPG "off"		IPG "on"		IPG "off"		IPG "on"	
	RAP	VCP	RAP	VCP	RAP	VCP	RAP	VCP	RAP	VCP
Mean	32.2	128.4	34.2	134.8	70.4	151.4	34.4	130.6	62.2	143.2
±SD	13.3	86.5	16.5	90.2	22.1	88.7	17.5	94.4	30.1	99.1
1.	23	80	21	80	50	86	20	81	45	84
2.	52	188	54	190	81	185	50	170	73	174
9.	25	25	27	30	60	68	22	26	35	40
10.	21	107	19	115	55	130	20	104	48	121
11.	40	242	50	258	106	288	55	272	110	297

Wilcoxon sum of ranks test.
RAP (IPG "on") before CES *vs.* early-after-CES: $p<0.05$.
RAP (early-after-CES): IPG "off" *vs.* "on": $p<0.05$.
All others RAP and VCP comparisons (last before CES *vs.* early after CES; early after CES *vs.* 1 year later; IPG "off" vs. "on" at any time) were not significant.

One-year manometric data demonstrated a tendentially slight decrease in three subjects, in both RAP and VCP, which did not involve amplitude increments, since a sufficient difference persisted between stimulated and unstimulated RAPs, and the clinical result did not substantially change. In the patient who had a further neosphincter reconstruction (no.9), the trend to manometric impairment was substantial, although the IPG amplitude was increased up to 5v. In the last patient, both RAP and VCP were higher at 1 year. Amplitude increments were subsequently necessary in the patients who have completed two or more years of functional follow-up.

Functional results (2nd protocol)

The clinical assessments according to our system showed the results reported in Table 5 in the five patients of the second series who had ASC. The 1-year clinical assessments, performed in only four patients, showed no significant changes, in spite of a slight score increment in two patients. Minor refinements (less than 0.5 v amplitude increments) were necessary, on clinical grounds, in all four patients. From a manometric viewpoint (Tab. 6) , the results were similar to those after CES in the 1st protocol. No significant changes occurred over time.

Table 5. Evaluations of functional results after TAR, according to our personal scoring and grading scale, in the six patients of the 2nd protocol who underwent ASC

Patient	**AFTER ASC**		**1 YEAR LATER**	
	scoring-grading		**scoring-grading**	
14. CS	5	(good)	5	(good)
15. BO	3	(very good)	3	(very good)
16. FG	10	(fair)	12	(fair)
17. CL	4	(very good)	7	(good)
18. BV	17	(very poor)		
19. PA	17	(very poor)		

Wilcoxon sum of ranks test in the fist four patients: not significant

Table 6. Manometric data (cm H_20) in 6 patients of the 2nd protocol who underwent ASC

	EARLY AFTER CES				**1 YEAR LATER**			
Pt. no.	**IPG "off"**		**IPG "on"**		**IPG "off"**		**IPG "on"**	
	RAP	**VCP**	**RAP**	**VCP**	**RAP**	**VCP**	**RAP**	**VCP**
Mean	35.3	137.5	70.6	143.6	39.5	100.5	64.7	128.2
±SD	15.7	51.4	8.2	29.8	18.7	28.6	18.8	52.4
14.	50	189	71	124	59	115	72	178
15.	18	59	61	107	17	59	50	59
16.	18	98	77	164	50	123	88	158
17.	54	136	82	123	32	105	49	118
18.	42	155	71	184				
19.	30	188	62	160				

Wilcoxon sum of ranks test.
Early-after-CES RAP: IPG "off" *vs.* IPG "on": $p<0.01$.
All others RAP and VCP comparisons (early after CES *vs.* 1 year later or IPG "off" *vs.* "on") were not significant.

DISCUSSION

In the evaluation of effectiveness, suitability and possible limitations of primary TAR, a preliminary issue is whether graciloplasty affects the oncological safety of APR. The recurrence rates reported by various authors [62, 56-57] are similar to those reported after APR without TAR. This seems to exclude any influence of graciloplasty on oncological outcome [62]. In our experience, only in the patients of the first series was a high rate of unfavourable oncological evolutions recorded. In our opinion, these can mostly be ascribed to poor selection, although stricter preoperative criteria on grounds of tumour stage would hardly have been effective: the only patient of ours who developed early metastases had a primary tumour category (T2), better than five others who did not. However, although a more selective attitude could also have been theoretically advisable in some patients of ours, we did not find practical arguments for this when the excision fulfilled correct oncological criteria, partly because a perineal colostomy favours an earlier detection of local recurrences.

Another concern regards possible surgical complication. In our patients, both early and late complications were frequent, but, apart from the cardiovascular ones which would probably have occurred independently of graciloplasty, they were never lifethreatening. The most important was necrosis of the distal part of the muscles, which occurred in two patients, one of whom was diabetic. In accordance with other authors [23, 59], we did not anticipate the ligation of the distal vascular pedicles (as suggested by Williams et al. [45] to reduce the risk of muscle ischemia. Although the blood flow in the main vascular bundle does not seem to change after clamping of the minor pedicles [74], in our opinion and experience this risk is real but unavoidable, in graciloplasty for TAR: in fact, a preliminary vascular distal pedicle ligature cannot be proposed, in patients anxious to have their tumour excised as soon as possible, who sometimes even have difficulty in accepting a delay in surgery for preoperative radiotherapy. The staged procedure as performed by Williams and co-workers might be followed, but we believe that a graciloplasty is difficult to propose, and inadvisable to carry out when the patient has just got over convalescence after a major procedure. This complication seemed the only one among the early ones, not related to learning-phase inexperience. Thus, we might expect an overall decrease in early postoperative morbidity. Unfortunately, late complications, which also seemed independent of the learning curve and had a high incidence, are likely to occur.

Since the restoration of normal defaecation is the aim of TAR, the functional outcome is the central issue regarding the suitability of the procedure. Since we used two different protocols, a specific comment on the pros and cons of both of them would be useful. Our experience with delayed, selective use of IPGs was widely discussed in our previous study [65]. In brief, we can state the following eight points, which summarise our study.

1) Manometric data in our patients suggested that IES+BFB training is very effective in developing the possibility of voluntary neosphincter contraction, while CES is effective in supporting the neosphincter basal tone.

2) Continence after IES+BFB is essentially a pseudocontinence, consisting of a sort of elastic stenosis with the added possibility of squeezing and postponing defaecation, provided that a perception of neorectal filling and impending evacuation is present, as was sometimes reported [24,25-26]. This condition involves irrigation of the colon daily or every other day, to prevent episodes of incontinence.
3) An electrically supported neosphincter permits "true" continence. However, strong peristaltic waves, whose pressure is higher than that of the neosphincter at rest, with the stimulator "on", and in the absence of normal anorectal sensitivity may cause episodes of incontinence, also in patients with a well-active IES-trained neosphincter. Thus, also in this condition, the colon has to be kept empty.
4) The CES did not necessarily involve, *per se*, better results than IES+BFB training, although whenever necessary the IPGs improved the neosphincter function, from both a clinical and a manometric viewpoint.
5) The greatest success, even in the absence of high-resting pressure values, was achieved in three patients, who had some perception of impending defaecation and did not need IPG. The reasons why neorectal sensitivity developed in these patients, and only in these, could not be explained, since the pre-IPG training was the same in all patients.
6) Although important experiences in TAR might suggest that at least in the short term functional results of static graciloplasty differ very little from those after electrodynamic support, satisfactory results in the absence of CES may be expected only in a minority of cases.
7) The possibility of satisfactory results, coupled with major postoperative complications or early cancer recurrence, may also justify a delay in IPG implantation in selected cases, thereby obviating the need for expensive devices which are unnecessary or destined to be lost.
8) Poor patient motivation or compliance with muscle-training or multiple surgical procedures, possible long-term atrophy and fibrosis of untrained muscles, and expenditure of human resources during the long and onerous outpatient IES+BFB management, were serious drawbacks to our first protocol, which induced us to try a one-stage procedure (two-stage, if we also consider ASC).

Our more recent series of patients showed both clinical and manometric data overlapping with those recorded in the patients of the 1st protocol who received IPG. In particular, it is to be noted that all patients needed enemas, though with differences regarding frequency, volume, evacuation time and efficacy. Occasional incontinence to liquid and gas were controlled by constipating or antimeteoric agents, while a mild degree of soiling was almost always present.

It is noteworthy that, except for before stimulator implantation in the first series, also in patients who had electrodynamic graciloplasty of both the 1st and

2nd protocols no relationship was noted between manometric and clinical data, thus confirming that other factors besides sphincter basal tone, contribute to continence. Thus, although manometry is useful for pathophysiological studies, for an optimal setting of the electrodynamic parameters, and for the objectivation and surveillance of the neosphincter activity, we believe that it should not be considered conclusive regarding the effectiveness of the procedure, which must be substantially evaluated on clinical grounds.

The current systems for anal incontinence were conceived for quite a different condition and not for a perineal colostomy. In particular, a factor which obviously is not included in the current methods of evaluation of faecal incontinence, but which may affect the quality of life of these patients, even after IPG implantation, is constipation, which can be very persistent. This is probably due to lack of the anorectal sampling reflex, to an altered onset of the defecation sequence, and to a possible obstacle on the part of the neosphincter, which mimics the normal sphincter activity when contracting, but does not do it enough during evacuation. We therefore devised and used a different method for functional assessment, which also considers other more specific items besides continence, in particular the necessity for enemas, which represents an indirect indicator of incontinence and a direct measure of constipation.

Psychological factors may also give rise to difficulties in the interpretation of the functional results of TAR. The presence of a neoplastic background and the absence of the native sphincter cause the disablement to be perceived differently. After TAR, the patients are fully aware that the neosphincter cannot work any more as their own anorectal apparatus did before surgery; thus they are more disposed to accept limitations and sacrifices. For example, they accept with good grace that the bowel has to be somehow re-educated, and managed not only by enemas, but also by measures such as proper diet, constipating or antimeteorism agents, or even bulk laxatives, when the tendency to constipation is predominant. Although perfect continence is barely achieved and mild soiling is always present, most of our patients were satisfied with the perineal stoma and considered themselves as being almost normal; in addition, the promise of avoiding abdominal colostomy always encouraged recovery and rehabilitation, and favoured the regaining of a full social life. After experiencing the abdominal stoma, even patients with poor functional outcome never wished to go back to the previous condition, which is viewed as a very abnormal and marginalizing condition, more so than episodic incontinence.

Our second, one-stage protocol obviated various drawbacks encountered in the first series of patients, but highlighted some other possible limitations and shortcomings. In particular, the loss of a device in the patient who had irreparable necrosis of the distal part of the muscles raises the question of health economics once again. The IPG, equipped with electrodes and hand controller, costs about $ 8,000. The risk of losing the hardware because of an early TAR complication could be obviated by implanting the stimulator two or three months after graciloplasty, as other authors did [59-60]. This delayed surgery may be easily performed under spinal anaesthesia, and involves only a further 1 or 2-day hospital-stay. Although the cost of this delayed implantation has to be multiplied by the number of patients, the staged procedure used by Baeten's group is on the whole probably more cost-effective. Other more general health economics issues in TAR are being evaluated by Williams' group: it is likely that, considering the depletion time of a stimulator the undiscounted ongoing annual cost of anorectal reconstruction and of its subsequent management, is similar to that of the ongoing cost of a permanent stoma. A still not-validated hypothesis also suggests that, in terms of improvement in the quality of life, anorectal reconstruction will offer comparable cost-effectiveness to other accepted procedures, such as cardiac surgery and renal transplantation [67].

In any case, we believe that for both clinical and economical reasons TAR involves strict patient selection, regarding tumour stage, general status, age and life expectancy, but also regarding psychological attitude, a strong motivation to avoiding abdominal stoma, and the ability to collaborate in a difficult task.

CONCLUSIONS

Patient satisfaction should be the true yardstick in evaluating the suitability of TAR. Our experience suggests that the patients are better pleased with a perineal rather than abdominal colostomy. This would be the main argument in favour of a procedure which, owing to complex related problems and to hard-to-acquire know-how, is slow to catch on.

However, if surgeons are still reluctant to adopt this procedure, we believe that their reluctance should not be based on what they see as poor functional results, but on the as yet unsolved problems, such as a still high morbidity rate, at both early and late postoperative phases, the possible drawbacks of lifelong electrostimulation, and the great drain on resources; that is, cost of the devices, prolonged hospital stay, rehabilitation and outpatient clinical care. We also believe that progression along the learning curve of both surgical and electrophysiological methodologies, coupled with further possible technical developments, and cost-effectiveness validation should reduce these problems, thereby leading to widespread acceptance of this procedure.

REFERENCES

1. Leo E, Belli F, Baldini MT, Vitellaro M, Mascheroni L, Andreola S, Bellomi M, Zucali R. New perspective in the treatment of low rectal cancer: total rectal resection and coloendoanal anstomosis. *Dis Colon Rectum* 1994; 37 (Suppl): S62-68.
2. Rullier E, Zerbib F, Laurent C, Bonnel C, Caudry M, Saric J, Parneix M. Intersphincteric resection with excision of internal anal sphincter for conservative treatment of very low rectal cancer. *Dis Colon Rectum* 1999; 42 : 1168-1175.
3. Teramoto T, Watanabe M, Katajima M. Per anum intersphincteric rectal dissection with direct coloanal anastomosis for lower rectal cancer. The ultimate sphincter-preserving operation. *Dis Colon Rectum* 1997; 40 (Suppl): S43-47.
4. Williams NS, Johnston D. The quality of life after rectal excision for low rectal cancer. *Br J Surg* 1983; 170 : 460-462.
5. Mac Donald LD, Anderson HR. The health of rectal cancer patients in the community. *Eur J Surg Oncol* 1985; 11 : 235-241.
6. Sprangers MA, Taal B, Aaronson N, Velde A. Quality of life in colorectal cancer. *Dis Colon Rectum* 1995; 38 : 361-369.
7. Chittenden AS. Reconstruction of anal sphincter by muscle slip from the glutei. *Ann Surg* 1930; 92 : 152-154.
8. Béchet M. Essai de rétablissement de la continence après amputation abdominoperineale du rectum. *Marseille Chirurgical* 1952 ; 4: 333-339.
9. Simonsen OS, Stolf NA, Aun F, Raia A, Habr-Gama A. Rectal sphincter reconstruction in perineal colostomies after abdomino-perineal resection for cancer. *Br J Surg* 1976 ; 63 : 389-391.
10. Pickrell KL, Broadbent R, Masters F, Metzger J. Construction of a rectal sphincter and restoration of anal continence by transplanting the gracilis muscle. Report of 4 cases in children. *Ann Surg* 1952; 135: 853-862.
11. Corman ML. Management of fecal incontinence by gracilis muscle transposition. *Dis Colon Rectum* 1979; 22 : 290-292.
12. Corman ML. Gracilis muscle transposition for anal incontinence: late results. *Br J Surg* 1985; 72 (suppl.) : 21-22.
13. Leguit P, Van Baal JG, Brummelkamp WH. Gracilis muscle transposition in the treatment of fecal incontinence . Long-term follow-up and evaluation of anal pressure recordings. *Dis Colon Rectum* 1985; 28 : 1-4.
14. Yoshioka K, Keighley MRB. Clinical and manometric assessment of gracilis muscle transplant for fecal incontinence. *Dis Colon Rectum* 1988; 31 : 767-769.
15. Christiansen J, Sørensen M, Rasmussen O. Gracilis muscle transposition for faecal incontinence. *Br J Surg* 1990 ; 77 : 1039-1040.
16. Morgado PJ, Alfaro R, Alfonzo R, Morgado PJ Jr. Anal incontinence: our experience with gracilis muscle transposition. *Coloproctology*1991; 13: 212-216.
17. Faucheron JL, Hannoun L, Thome C, Parc R. Is fecal continence improved by nonstimulated gracilis muscle transposition? *Dis Colon Rectum* 1994; 37 : 979-983.
18. Kumar D, Hutchinson R, Grant E. Bilateral gracilis neosphincter construction for treatment of faecal incontinence. *Br J Surg* 1995; 82 : 1645-1647.
19. Wee JT, Wong CS. Functional anal sphincter reconstruction with the gracilis muscle after abdominoperineal resection. *Lancet* 1983; ii: 1245-1246.
20. Cavina E, Seccia M, Chiarugi M, Evangelista G, Buccianti P, Chirico A, Rossi B, Sartucci F. Continenza di colostomia dopo operazione di Miles: neosfintere elettrostimolato. *Boll Soc It Chir* 1985; 6: 23-30.
21. Cavina E, Seccia M, Evangelista G, Chiarugi M, Buccianti P, Chirico A, Lenzi M, Bortolotti P, Bellomini G, Arganini M, Pieri L. Construction of a continent perineal colostomy

by using electrostimulated gracilis muscles after abdominoperineal resection: personal technique and experience with 32 cases. *It J Surg Sci* 1987; 17: 305-314.
22. Cavina E, Seccia M, Evangelista G, Buccianti P, Chiarugi M, Chirico A, Goletti O, Macaluso C, Tortora A.
Colostomia perineale continente dopo "Miles": Gracileplastica bilaterale con elettrostimolazione. Arch. e Atti 91° Congr Soc It Chir , Genova, 1989. L Pozzi, Roma, 1989, Vol. 5°: 220-255.
23. Cavina E, Seccia M, Evangelista G, Chiarugi M, Buccianti P, Tortora A, Chirico A. Perineal colostomy and electrostimulated gracilis "neosphincter" after abdominoperineal resection of the colon and anorectum: a surgical experience and follow-up study in 47 cases. *Int J Colorect Dis* 1990; 5: 6-11.
24. Seccia M, Monconi C, Banti P, Balestri R, Cavina E. Trattamento dell'incontinenza fecale mediante gracileplastica elettrostimolata. Arch. e Atti 96° Congr Soc It Chir, Roma, 1994. L Pozzi, Roma, 1994, Vol 2°: 169-182.
25. Mercati U, Trancanelli V, Castagnoli GP, Mariotti A, Ciaccarini R. Use of the gracilis muscles for sphincteric construction after abdominoperineal resection. Technique and preliminary results. *Dis Colon Rectum* 1991; 34 : 1085-1089.
26. Santoro E, Tirelli C, Scutari F, Garofano A, Silecchia G, Scaccia M, Santoro E. Continent perineal colostomy by transposition of gracilis muscles. Technical remarks and results in 14 cases. *Dis Colon Rectum* 1994; 37 (Suppl.) : 73-79.
27. Gullà N, Patriti A, Castagna V, Pucciarini LG, Bosco A, Capitanucci L, Dei Santi V, Serafini S, Giannini P, Tristaino B. Colostomia perineale con gracileplastica bilaterale elettrostimolata. *Chirurgia* 1995; 8: 432-438.
28. Mander BJ, Williams NS. The electrically stimulated gracilis neo-anal sphincter. *Eur J Gastroenterol Hepatol* 1997; 9 : 435-441.
29. Schmidt E, Bruch HP. Traitement chirurgical des incontinence sphinctériennes intestinales par autotransplant libre de musculature lisse. *J Chir* 1981 ; 118 : 315-320.
30. Lasser Ph., Dubé P, Guillot JM, Elias D. Colostomie périnéale seudo-continente. Résultats et technique. *J Chir* 1997 ; 134: 174-179.
31. Gamagami RA, Chiotasso P, Lazorthes F. Continent perineal colostomy after abdominoperineal resection: outcome after 63 cases. *Dis Colon Rectum* 1999; 42 : 626-630.
32. Salmons S, Vrbova G. The influence of activity on some contractile characteristics of mammalian fast and slow muscles. *J Physiol* 1969; 210: 535-549.
33. Hallan RI, Williams NS, Hutton MRE, Scott M, Pilot MA, Swash M, Koeze TH, Watkins ES. Electrically stimulated sartorius neosphincter: canine model of activation and skeletal muscle transformation. *Br J Surg* 1990; 77 : 208-213.
34. Pette D, Vbrovà G. Adaptation of mammalian skeletal muscle fibers to chronic electrical stimulation. *Rev Physiol Biochem Pharmacol* 1992; 120: 116-202.
35. Konsten J, Baeten C, Havenith M, Soeters P. Morphology of dynamic graciloplasty compared with the anal sphincter. *Dis Colon rectum* 1993; 36 : 559-563.
36. Shatari T, Teramoto T, Kitajima M, Minamitani H. Conversion of the rabbit gracilis muscle for transposition as a neoanal sphincter by electrical stimulation. *Surgery Today* (Jpn. J. Surg.) 1995; 25: 233-236.
37. Altomare D, Boffoli D, Scacco SC, Rinaldi M, Vicente-Prieta R, Martinelli E, Memeo V. Fast-to-slow muscle conversion by chronic electrostimulation: effects on mitochondrial respiratory chain function with possible implications for the gracilis neosphincter procedure. *Br J Surg* 1996; 83 : 1569-1573.
38. Rosen HR, Dorner G, Feil W, Zöch G, Renner K, Bittner R, Schiessel R. Muscle transformation in the sartorius muscle in a canine model. Clinical impact for electrodynamic graciloplasty as a "neosphincter". *Dis Colon Rectum* 1997; 40 : 1321-1327.
39. George BD, Williams NS, Patel J, Swash M, Watkins ES. Physiological and histochemical adaptation of the electrically stimulated gracilis muscle to neoanal sphincter function. *Br J Surg*

1993; 80 : 1342-1346.40. Williams NS, Hallan RI, Koeze TH, Watkins ES. Construction of a neorectum and neoanal sphincter following previous proctocolectomy. *Br J Surg* 1989; 76 : 1191-1194.

41. Williams NS, Hallan RI, Koeze TH, Watkins ES. Restoration of gastrointestinal continuity and continence after abdominoperineal excision of the rectum using an electrically stimulated neoanal sphincter. *Dis Colon Rectum* 1990; 33 : 561-565.

42. Baeten C, Spaans F, Fluks A. An implanted neuromuscolar stimulator for fecal continence following previously implanted gracilis muscle. Report of a case. *Dis Colon Rectum* 1988; 31 : 134-137.

43. Baeten CG, Konsten J, Spaans F, Visser R, Habets AM, Bourgeois IM, Wagenmakers AJ, Boeters PB. Dynamic graciloplasty for treatment of fecal incontinence. *Lancet* 1991; 338: 1163-1165.

44. Williams NS, Hallan RI, Koeze TH, Watkins ES. Construction of a neoanal sphincter by transposition of the gracilis muscle and prolonged neuromuscolar stimulation for the treatment of fecal incontinence. *Ann R Coll Surg* 1990; 72: 108-113.

45. Williams NS, Patel J, George BD, Hallan RI, Watkins ES. Development of an electrically stimulated neoanal sphincter. *Lancet* 1991; 1166-1169.

46. Konsten J, Baeten CG, Spaans F, Havenith MG, Soeters PB. Follow-up of anal dynamic graciloplasty for fecal incontinence. *World J Surg* 1993; 17: 404-409.

47. Baeten CG, Geerdes BP, Adang EM, Heineman E, Konsten J, Engel GL, Kester AD, Spaans F, Soeters PB. Anal dynamic graciloplasty in the treatment of intractable fecal incontinence. *N Engl J Med* 1995; 332: 1600-1605.

48. Versluis PJ, Konsten J, Geerdes B, Baeten CG, Oei KT. Defecographic evaluation of dynamic graciloplasty for fecal incontinence. *Dis Colon Rectum* 1995; 38 : 468-473.

49. Geerdes BP, Heineman E, Konsten J, Soeters PB, Baeten CG. Dynamic graciloplasty. Complications and management. *Dis Colon Rectum* 1996; 39 : 912-917.

50. Adang EM, Engel GL, Rutten FF, Geerdes BP, Baeten CG. Cost-effectiveness of dynamic graciloplasty in patients with fecal incontinence. *Dis Colon Rectum* 1998; 41 : 725-34.

51. Memeo V, Altomare DF, Boffoli D, Rinaldi M. La gracileplastica elettrostimolata sec: Williams nel trattamento chirurgico dell'incontinenza fecale. Arch Atti 96° Congr Soc It Chir, Roma, (1994). L Pozzi, Roma, Vol 2°: 206-221.

52. Seccia M, Menconi C, Balestri R, Cavina E. Study protocols and functional results in 86 electrostimulated graciloplasties. *Dis Colon Rectum* 1994; 37 : 897-904.

53. Kennedy ML, Nguyen H, Lubowski DZ, King DW. Stimulated gracilis neosphincter: a new procedure for anal incontinence. *Aust N Z J Surg* 1996; 66: 353-357.

54. Wexner SD, Gonzalez-Padron A, Rius J, Teoh TA, Cheong DM, Nogueras JJ, Billotti VL, Weiss EG, Moon HK. Stimulated gracilis neosphincter operation. Initial Experience, pitfalls, and complications. *Dis Colon Rectum* 1996; 39: 957-964.

55. Christiansen J, Rasmussen O.Ø, Lindorff-Larsen K. Dynamic graciloplasty for severe anal incontinence. *Br J Surg* 1998; 85: 88-91.

56. Altomare D, Rinaldi M, Pannarale O, Memeo V. Electrostimulated gracilis neosphincter for faecal incontinence and in total anorectal reconstruction. Still an experimental procedure? *Int J Colorect Dis* 1997; 12: 308-312.

57. Rosen HR, Novi G, Zoech G, Feil W, Urbarz C, Schiessel R. Restoration of anal sphincter function by single-stage dynamic graciloplasty with a modified (split sling) technique. *Am J Surg* 1998; 175: 187-193.

58. Sielezneff I, Malouf AJ, Bartolo DCC, Pryde A, Douglas S. Dynamic graciloplasty in the treatment of patients with faecal incontinence. *Br J Surg* 1999; 86 : 61-65.

59. Geerdes BP, Zoetmulder FAN, Baeten CGMI. Double dynamic graciloplasty and coloperineal pull-through after abdominoperineal resection. *Eur J Cancer* 1995; 31 : 1248-1252.

60. Geerdes BP, Zoetmulder FAN, Heinemann E, Vos EJ, Rongen MJ, Baeten CGMI. Total anorectal reconstruction with a double dynamic graciloplasty after abdominoperineal reconstruction for low rectal cancer. *Dis Colon Rectum* 1997 ; 40 : 698-705.
61. Mander BJ, Abercrombie JF, George BD, Williams NS. The electrically stimulated gracilis neosphincter incorporated as part of total anorectal reconstruction after abdominoperineal excision of the rectum. *Ann Surg* 1996; 224: 702-711.
62. Cavina E. Outcome of restorative perineal graciloplasty with simultaneous excision of the anus and rectum for cancer. A ten-year experience with 81 patients. *Dis Colon Rectum* 1996; 39 : 182-190.
63. Cavina E, Seccia M, Banti P, Zocco G. Anorectal reconstruction after abdominoperineal resection. Experience with double-wrap graciloplasty supported by low-frequency electrostimulation. *Dis Colon Rectum* 1998; 41 : 1010-1016.
64. Rouanet Ph, Senesse P, Bouamrirene D, Toureille E, Veyrac M, Astre C, Bacou F. Anal sphincter reconstruction by dynamic graciloplasty after abdominoperineal resection for cancer. *Dis Colon Rectum* 1999; 42 : 451-456.
65. Violi V, Roncoroni L, Boselli AS, De Cesare C, Livrini M, Peracchia A. Total anorectal reconstruction by double graciloplasty. Experience with delayed, selective use of implantable pulse generators. *Int J Colorectal Dis* 1999 ; 14: 164-171.
66. Baeten CG, Rongen MJ. Total anorectal reconstruction – Fact or fiction. *Swiss Surg* 1997; 3: 262-265.
67. Eccersley AJP, Williams NS. Anorectal reconstruction – Restoring continence after abdominoperineal excision of the anorectum. *It J Gastroenterol Hepatol* 1998; 30: 549-554.
68. Abercrombie JF, Rogers J, Williams NS. Total anorectal reconstruction results in complete anorectal sensory loss. *Br J Surg* 1996; 83: 57-59.
69. Rosen HR, Feil W, Novi G, Zöch G, Dahlberg S, Schiessel R. The electrically stimulated (dynamic) graciloplasty for faecal incontinence — first experiences with a modified muscle sling. *Int J Colorect Dis* 1994; 9: 184-186.
70. Violi V, Roncoroni L, Boselli AS, De Cesare C, Trivelli M, Peracchia A. Anorectal reconstruction after abdominoperineal excision: a state-of-the-art alternative to a conventional colostomy. *It J Gastroenterol Hepatol* 1999; 31: 267-268.
71. Rongen M-J G, Dekker FA, Geerdes B, Heineman E, Baeten CG. Secondary coloperineal pull-through and double dynamic graciloplasty after Miles resection – Feasible, but with a high morbidity. *Dis Colon Rectum* 1999; 42 : 776-781.
72. Jorge JMN, Wexner SD. Etiology and management of fecal incontinence. *Dis Colon Rectum* 1993; 36 : 77-97.
73. Violi V, Boselli AS, De Cesare C, Roncoroni L. Double-gracilis anorectal neosphincter: a technique of reconstruction after necrosis of the distal part of the muscles. *Dis Colon Rectum* 1998; 41 : 790-792.
74. Geerdes BP, Kurvers HA, Konsten J, Heineman E, Baeten CG. Assessment of ischaemia of the distal part of the gracilis muscle during transposition for anal dynamic graciloplasty. *Br J Surg* 1997; 84 : 1127-1129.

CHAPTER 17

LOCAL RECURRENCE AFTER RESECTION OF COLORECTAL CANCER

Leopoldo Sarli, Giuseppe Sgobba, Renato Costi, Luigi Roncoroni
Department of Surgery, University of Parma, Parma, Italy

Abstract
Despite therapeutical progress in the last 20 years, locoregional recurrence (LR) after a preceding colorectal resection remains a common and at the same time arduous clinical problem. The **frequency** of LR, calculated as being about a mean 16%, should be considered as underestimated. The most frequent **cause of** recurrence is neoplastic microfoci, not included in the initial exeresis; however, the implantation of exfoliated tumour cells and metachronous carcinogenesis may also be responsible. The pathological stage of the primary tumour is considered to be the most important **risk factor** for LR, although the experience of the surgeon seems also to greatly influence the risk of recurrence. The **prevention** of LR is in fact based on the correct therapeutic approach to the initial neoplasm. An intensive **follow-up** programme allows for early diagnosis of recurrence, and increases the possibilities of **therapy,** although these are somewhat limited. Initially, anastomotic LR offers greater possibilities of curative exeresis. Perianastomotic recurrences, however, prove to be in most cases inoperable; palliative surgery is possible in only a few cases.
Colo-rectal cancer is the second most frequent cause of death from cancer, and its incidence is rising throughout the western world. Despite therapeutic progress in the last 20 years, locoregional recurrence (LR), after a preceding colorectal resection, remains a common and at the same time arduous clinical problem. The onset of recurrence affects the prognosis; pelvic recurrences can also seriously compromise the quality of life of the patient.

DEFINITION

After apparently curative resection of a colorectal tumour, LR is defined as the recurrence of the disease at the primary tumour site, on the laparotomic or perineal scar, at the pericolostomy site, or along a lymphatic tree, at regional lymph nodes, or at the site of intestinal anastomosis [1-3].

A.M. Farinon (ed.), Advances in Abdominal Surgery 2002, 247-264.

The anastomosis may be the sole site of an LR, which in this case is defined as being *primarily anastomotic*. More often, however, LRs are perianastomotic and only indirectly affect endoluminal infiltration.

Isolated LRs, which are still possible to treat curatively , are distinguishable from those *associated with distant metastases*, which are indicative of a systemic disease. The concomitant presence of local and distant recurrence is more often found after resection of tumours of the colon [4-5], than after rectal ones, which are usually followed by isolated LR [6-7] (Fig. 1). A possible explanation for this phenomenon could lie in the greater possibility of diagnosing pelvic recurrences, owing to the easier accessibility of this area to simple clinical evaluations, than of identifying recurrences of colon tumours, which are often diagnosed later, and are themselves a potential cause of the spread of the disease.

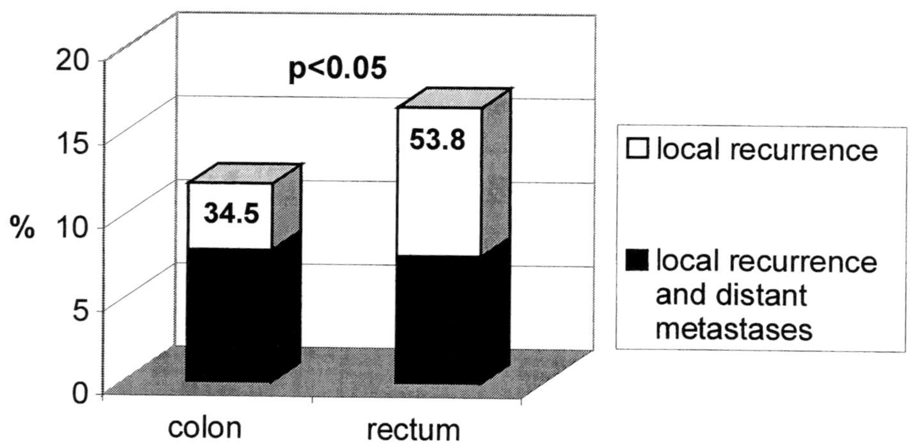

Figure 1 In the personal series of 1124 patients submitted to radical exeresis of colorectal tumours in the period 1976-1998, an LR was found in 152 cases (13.5%). The frequency of LR resulted as being higher after exeresis of rectal cancer: 65 cases (16.5%) vs 87 (11.9%) ($p<0.05$). Isolated recurrence, not associated with distant metastasis, resulted as being more frequent in patients affected by rectal cancer: 35 cases (53.8%) vs 30 (34.5%) ($p<0.05$).

Around 80% of LRs are diagnosed during the first 2 years after resection, peaking at around 12 months [8-9] (Fig. 2); in a very few cases, LR onset is diagnosed 5 years after surgery [10-11].

Recurrences of rectal neoplasms show up later than those of neoplasms of the colon [12] (Fig. 3). It is to be noted, however, that LR is diagnosed earlier after anterior resection of the rectum than after abdomino-perineal resection

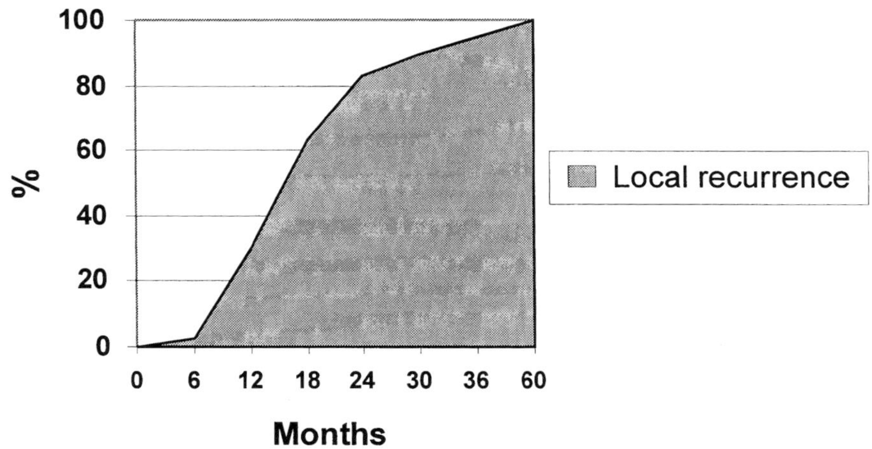

Figure 2. Interval of onset of LRs observed in 152 patients in the personal series.

[13-14], probably thanks to a greater facility of clinical detection in the presence of conserved intestinal continuity [14-15].

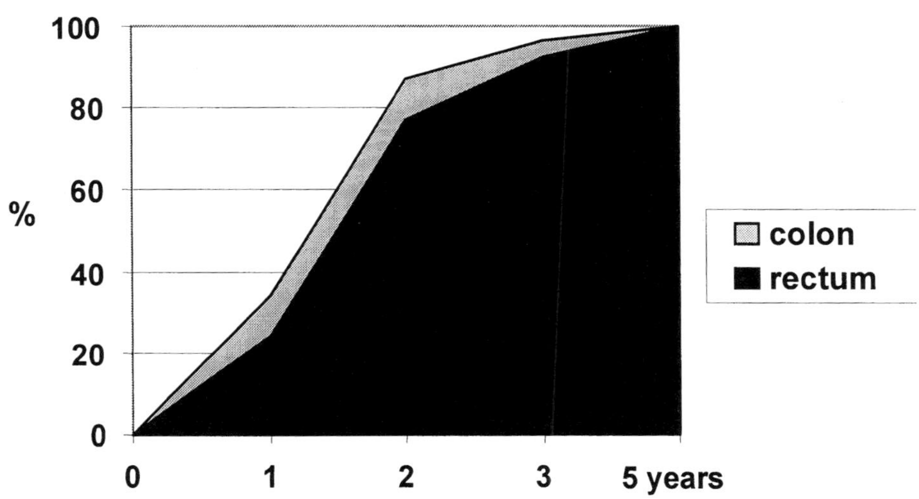

Figure 3. In the personal series the interval of onset of LRs resulted as being shorter after exeresis of colic neoplasms, although the difference is not statistically significant.

As will be seen below (Fig. 9), early onset of recurrence is considered as being an important negative prognostic value.

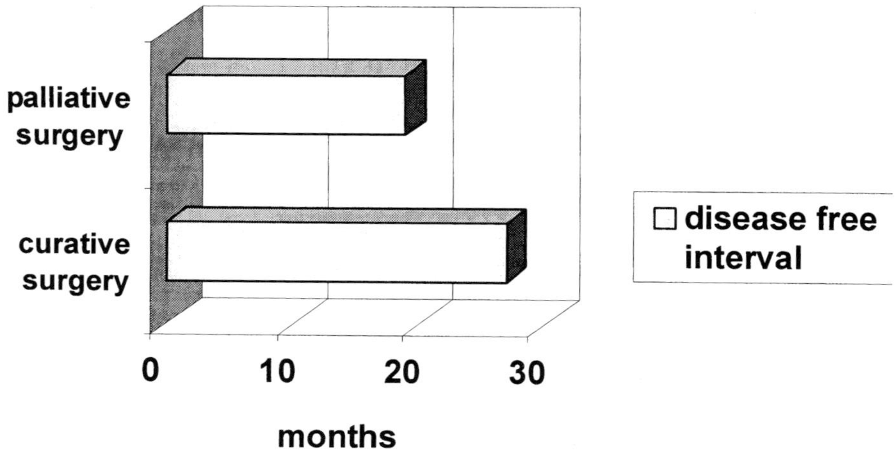

Figure 9. Correlation between disease-free interval (in months) and therapeutic possibilities in 106 cases of LR operated on in the personal series ($p<0.05$).

FREQUENCY

The frequency of LR, resulting as being around a mean 16%, differs considerably according to individual experience [12], and should in any case be considered as underestimated, since it is not supported by routine autoptic controls [16].

PATHOGENESIS

Recurrence of the disease is usually attributable to *neoplastic microfoci not included in the initial exeresis.* This hypothesis is supported by results of histopathological studies testifying to neoplastic cells in the mesocolon and in the mesorectum, corresponding with the lateral resection margins, but also in the region of lymphatic drain of a neoplasm which has been removed for the purposes of radicality [17-18]. The inadequacy of the initial exeresis, and in particular insufficient lymphadenectomy, has also been found in a high percentage of patients with LR after the resection of neoplasms of the left colon [19].

The finding, albeit less frequent, of primary anastomotic recurrences implies, however, more sophisticated alternative pathogenetic hypotheses, such as *the implantation of exfoliated tumour cells* [20-21], and *metachronous carcinogenesis* in an area of proliferative instability [22-23] .

The hypothesis of the implantation of neoplastic cells is supported by the extremely low frequency of recurrences at the level of the ileocolic anastomoses (Tab. 1), where experimental studies have demonstrated a very slight susceptibility of the ileal mucosa to the implantation of these cells [24], and could account for the 1-13% of recurrences, observed in patients who have undergone surgery for Dukes' stage A neoplasms [25].

Table. 1 Correlation beween modality of onset of LR and surgical procedures previously carried out on 106 patients under examination.

			SURGERY			
			curative		palliative	
AREA OF ONSET	N	%	N	%	N	%
Lymphatic region	70	66.3	7	10	63	90
Perianastomotic structures	24	22.6	20	83.3	4	16.7
Anastomosis*	12	11.3	12	100		

* Anastomotic recurrences regarded colo-rectal anastomosis in 5 cases and colo-colic in 2. In no case did recurrence occur from ileo-colic anastomosis.

The hypothesis of metachronous carcinogenesis is supported by studies, which show that the cellular proliferation accompanying the healing of the anastomosis leads to an instability of the intestinal mucosa, which renders it more susceptible to the effects of carcinogenic agents [23]. According to Umpleby and Williamson [26], the implantation of exfoliated cells is the mechanism for the onset of "earlier" recurrences, while metachronous carcinoge- nesis could be considered the cause of late recurrences.

RISK FACTORS

LR leads to death within 5 years from diagnosis, in 80-90% of patients affected; thus the identification of patients at high risk of LR will assist in singling out those who may benefit from adjuvant therapy and, in particular, from intensive follow-up [27]. Early diagnosis is indispensable in deciding the usefulness of further surgical treatment. It is not easy to define clearly the predictive factors of LR, as evaluations available in the literature vary considerably; however, ***pathological stage*** is considered to be the most important risk factor for LR [28] (Fig. 4).

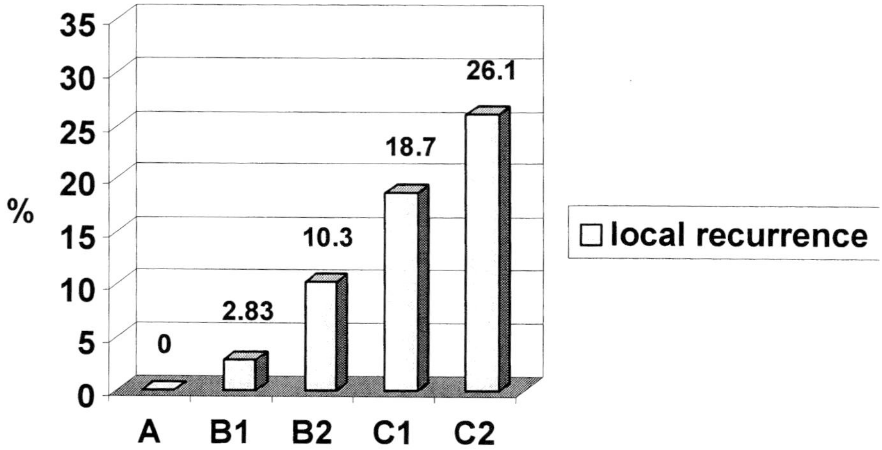

Figure 4. Stage of the primary tumour and local recurrence in the personal series. Differences are statistically significant ($p<0.001$).

In particular, the *invasion of the tumour beyond the serosa* [29], and the contemporaneous *metastatic involvement of the regional lymph nodes* [30], constitute unfavourable predictive elements. An analysis by Nicholls *et al* shows that tumours involving the perirectal cells for a depth less than 5 mm are marked by a 5% incidence of LRs, compared to 20% in those with more extensive infiltration [29].

Some contributions to the literature [30, 31] note that ***tumour size,*** the presence of ***neoplastic embolisms in the venous and lymph vessels,*** and ***perineural propagation*** also lead to a higher incidence of LR. It must be emphasised, however, that the reliability of these parameters depends on the accuracy of the histological analysis.

Tumour site seems to be a further important risk factor of LR. The frequency of LR increases progressively from locations in the right colon, in the distal direction [3]. Rectal cancer, above all extraperitoneal, proves to be at higher risk than that of all the portions of the large bowel (Fig. 5), probably because of the absence of a serous lining, and the multicentric direction of the lymphatic drain [29]. In fact, as well as the habitual centripetal direction, lymphatic trees also favor metastatis to the mesorectum at a lower level than the

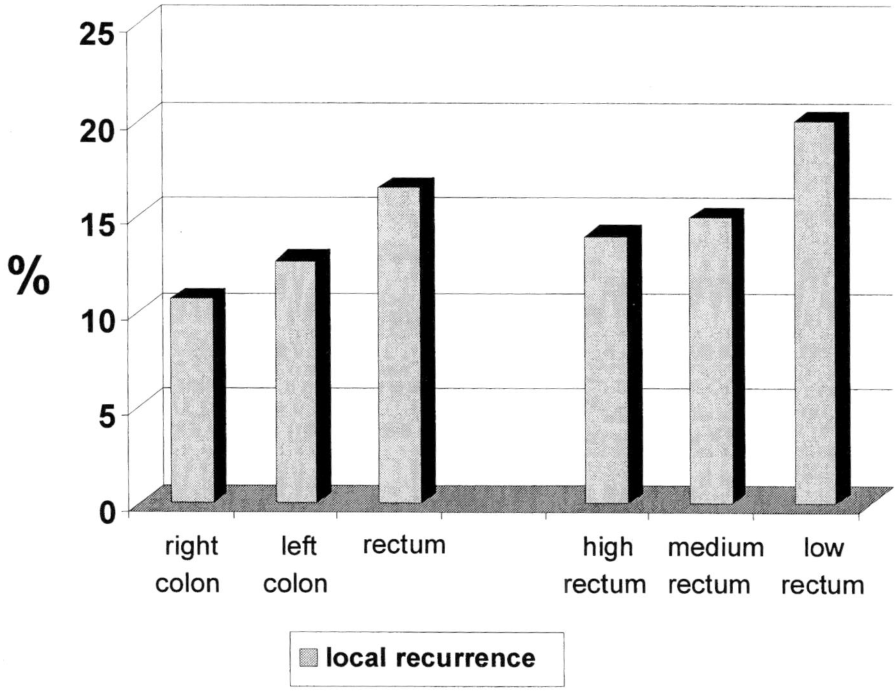

Figure 5. Tumour site and LR in the personal series.
The frequency resulted as being higher after exeresis of rectal neoplasms, and in particular those of the extraperitoneal rectum.

neoplasm, with involvement also of lateral lymph node stations (hypogastric, obturatory and common iliac). Besides anatomical factors, the risk may also be compounded by dissemination, due to manipulation of the neoplasm during surgery. Another location at risk is the left flexure [32], probably on account of the greater diagnostic difficulties, and the rapid secondary involvement of organs, around the lymphatic connections with the pancreas and spleen (the retropancreatic and splenic stations drain the lymph of the splenic flexure).

The ***complication of perforation*** of the neoplasm, or its accidental perforation during surgical manoeuvres, leads to an increase in the risk of LR [33] (Fig. 6). In a multicentric study, the 13% incidence of recurrence of the disease in the case of non-perforated neoplasms rises to 28% in perforated ones, probably because of the implantation of exfoliated tumour cells in the presence of a perforation [34].

Biological aggressivity is directly correlated to the risk of recurrence. This is demonstrated by various factors: ***macroscopic characteristics*** such as ulcerated forms [35], **histotype,** for example the variant with mucoidal aspects

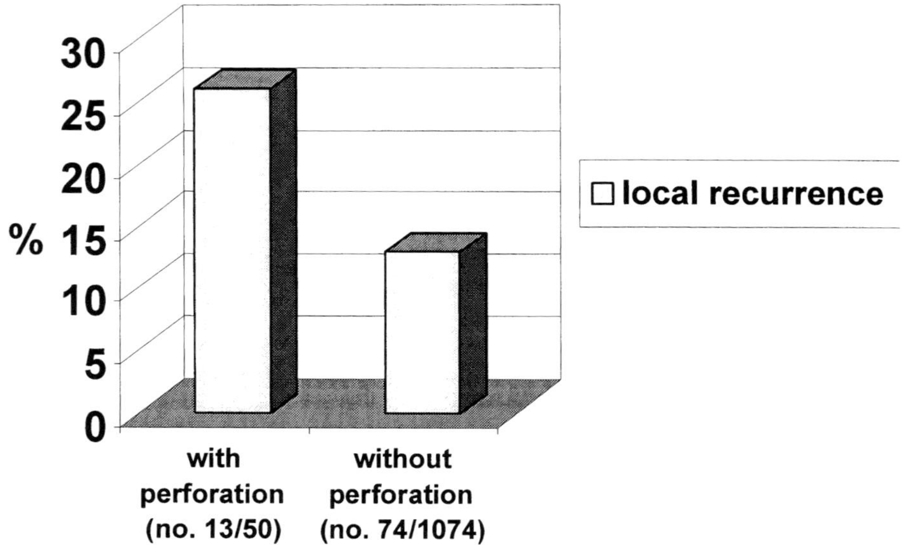

Figure 6. Influence of perforative complication of colorectal cancer on frequency of local recurrences in the personal series of 1124 patients submitted to radical exeresis of colorectal tumours.

[36], ***aneuploidy*** or a high ***DNA index*** [37-38] and an intense proliferative activity expressed by the ***labelling index*** [38], immunohistochemical properties such as the concentration of some markers in the neoplastic cells: ***CEA, Cs, TfAg*** [39], an abundance of ***sialomucin*** on the resection margins of the tumour [40], and the production of certain hormones such as ***HCG*** by the neoplasm. Although Nicholls reports an 11%, 14% and 21% incidence of LR for good, average and poor differentiation grades respectively [34], the tumour differentiation grade has lost the value attributed to it in the past, since it is now considered as being a non-independent variable, correlated to tumour stage [36]. Basically, a neoplasm that presents an unfavourable grading need not be considered at high risk of recurrence, if it is treated at an early stage.

As to LR after colo-rectal resections, some elements of ***surgical technique*** have recently been indicated as risk factors, and are thus still under discussion. The use of mechanical staplers, which has facilitated and hence rendered more frequent extra low anastomoses, in preference to resection of the rectum through an abdomino-perineal access (Tab. 2), has once again focused attention on some concepts of oncological radicality.

Table 2. Increase in time of extra low resections for cancer of the rectum (238) in the personal series.

		APR		LAR	
Years	**Number of patients**	**n.**	**%**	**n.**	**%**
1976-1985	113	66	58	47	42
1986-1998	125	54	43	71*	57*

* chi-squared with Yates' corrections: p<0.05

The distance of the resection from the tumour margin was one of the first parameters to come under question [41]. In fact, its importance has now diminished, recent studies having shown that a 2 cm. distal margin offers sufficient guarantee of radicality [42-43]. We do not consider there exists a pre-established limit to the reduction of the margin, which instead probably depends on the characteristics and stage of the neoplasm. The much-vaunted risk of increase in LR after extra low anterior resections, rather than after abdominoperineal resections, has been ruled out by recent experiences [44-45] (Fig. 7).

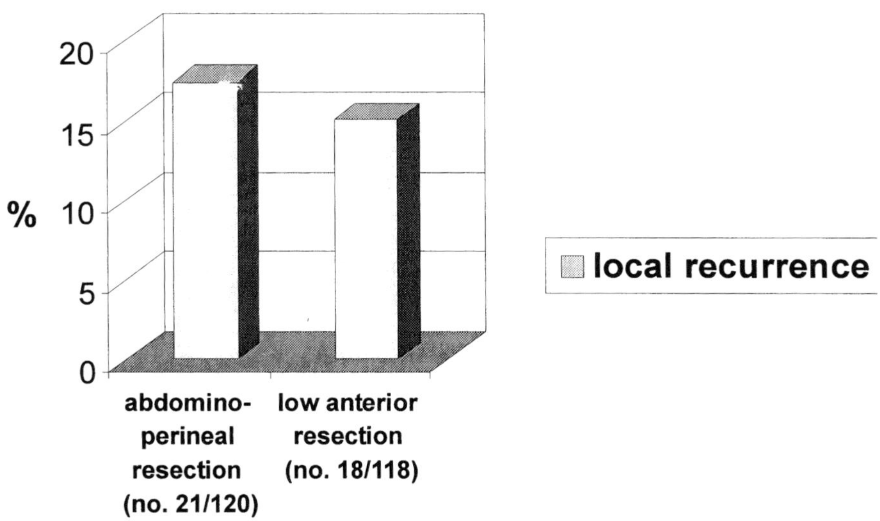

Figure 7. Frequency of LR after abdomino-perineal rectal resection (APR) and after low anterior resection (LAR) on 238 patients of the personal series.
Differences are not significant.

The experience of the surgeon seems to greatly influence the risk of recurrence [46-47]. A thorough examination of the literature has shown that the incidence of LR can range from 12% to 40%, depending on the degree of specialization available [25].

Lymphadenectomy is the fundamental technique in the prevention of recurrence of neoplasms [48].

Anastomotic dehiscence seems to give rise to a greater number of recurrences, above all after resective surgery on the left colon or the rectum [49-50] (Fig. 8). McGregor reports a 46.7% rate of recurrences after clinical and

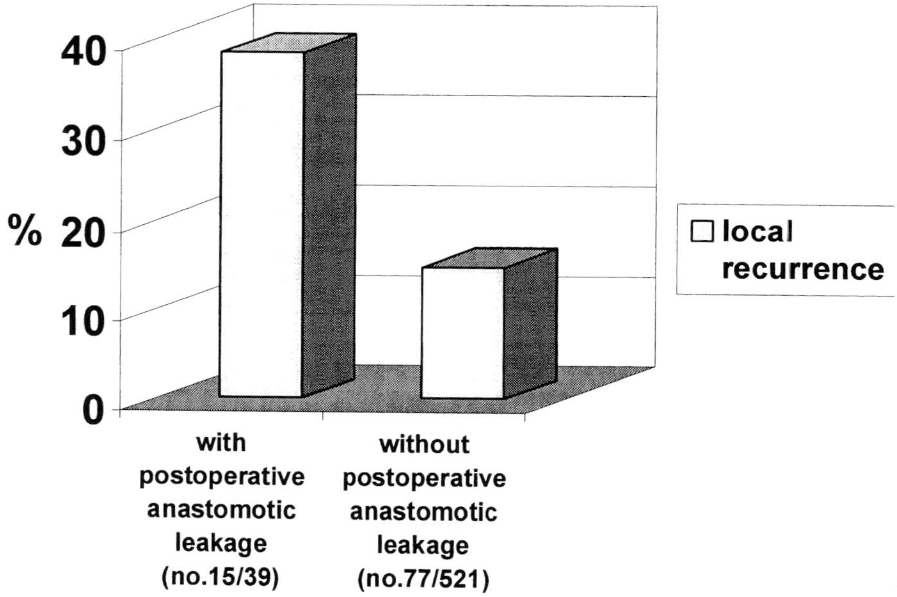

Figure 8. In the personal series the frequency of LR after 560 resections with colo-rectal anastomosis is higher if a postoperative anastomotic leak was observed ($p<0.001$).

subclinical dehiscences, a 35.3% rate after radiological dehiscences, and a rate of only 12.6% for apparently integral anastomoses [51]. A cause-effect correlation has been hypothesised, with a pathogenic mechanism comparable to that reported for the perforative complication of neoplasms of the colon: exfoliated neoplastic cells, still present in the intestinal lumen [26, 51], would seem to be able to migrate to the pericolic tissues or to the margins of the dehiscence, giving rise to recurrences [52-53]. The granulation tissue and the suture material would seem to favor the implantation of still vital neoplastic cells [54].

PREVENTION

On the basis of what has been said so far, it is evident that prevention of LR should revolve around the most correct therapeutic approach.

For this purpose, complementary therapies have been proposed.

Systemic chemotherapy seems to reduce the risk of recurrence in patients with lymph node metastasis [55].

Complementary radiotherapy, by itself or combined with systemic chemotherapy, has been proposed with a view to "sterilising" any residual neoplastic microfoci, after the resecton of rectal neoplasms [56]. While programmes of *preoperative* low-dose radiotherapy have not produced satisfactory results [57-58], and similar treatments postoperatively have yielded contradictory results [59, 60], more recent preoperative adjuvant high-dose therapy schemes have resulted in significant reductions in the frequency of LR [61, 62] after rectal resections. A clinical randomised trial, comparing the results of surgical exeresis preceded or followed by high-dose radiotherapy, revealed a significant LR reduction in the former [63]. Besides, if we consider that one of the effects of preoperative radiotherapy is that of reducing the volume of the neoplasm, thus allowing for the extension of the indication to an extra low resection, to make for easier surgery and the preservation of the sphincters [64], it is obvious that the use of this adjuvant treatment is today indispensable. Recent contributions to the literature have shown, furthermore, that the postoperative use of radiotherapy combined with systemic chemotherapy leads to better results [65]. The combined use of high-dose radiotherapy and preoperative systemic chemotherapy is the most modern therapy, yielding significantly encouraging preliminary results [66-67].

FOLLOW-UP-DIAGNOSES

When LR occurs despite preventive measures, early diagnosis is the only hope for curative treatment. The possibility of exeresis of the recurrence is greater when the latter is still asymptomatic [68]. *Intensive follow-up* schemes have thus been proposed for the first 24 months postoperatively, a period during which recurrences are most likely to show up. These schemes have led to the diagnosis of a higher number of LRs, an increase in resective surgery, and improved survival rates [27].

It is obvious that intensive follow-up procedures are more efficacious if done by specialists, able to interpret and adequately deal with the therapeutic problem of recurrence [27].

THERAPY

The optimal treatment for LR is further surgical exeresis, even though in most cases surgery is merely palliative. A longer interval between initial surgery and the diagnosis of recurrence is an orientative factor for curative exeresis (Fig. 9), probably because it is correlated to a more favourable biology of the tumour and immune status of the host [69].

Radical treatment

Radical exeresis of the local recurrence is possible in only a very small number of cases [70-71], and is the only treatment which allows for some chance of survival (Fig. 10).

The therapeutic procedure for LR must take into account not only the extension of the local infiltration, but also the possible presence of distant lesions. Single hepatic or pulmonary metastases, although not precluding the occasional possibility of exeresis, place serious doubts on the effective curative prospects of the procedure. Complementary treatments carried out previously also affect the choices of therapy for LR. We consider preoperative *high-dose irradiation* of the recurrence to be of use, although obviously only where it has not been done before surgery [72], and in any case on the basis of the principles guiding the use of radiotherapy for primary neoplasms of the rectum. However, it must be stressed that, unlike the case of primary lesions, the prognostic usefulness of this procedure for LRs has yet to be proved, although its efficacy as a palliative has already been demonstrated [73]. Adjuvant intraoperative radiotherapy, combined [74] or not [75] with preoperative radiotherapy, also seems to yield good medium term results (20 months), but does not improve the prognosis at 5 years [76]. Its combination with chemotherapy appears to be of help in the prevention, but not in the treatment, of pelvic recurrences.

Only laparotomy enables us to establish the purpose of surgery; sometimes it is not easy to distinguish the neoplastic infiltration from the marks of the preceding exeresis. The techniques cannot be schematised, but must be adapted to the individual case, since they are dependent on the location of the LR, as well as on the involvement of contiguous organs or structures.

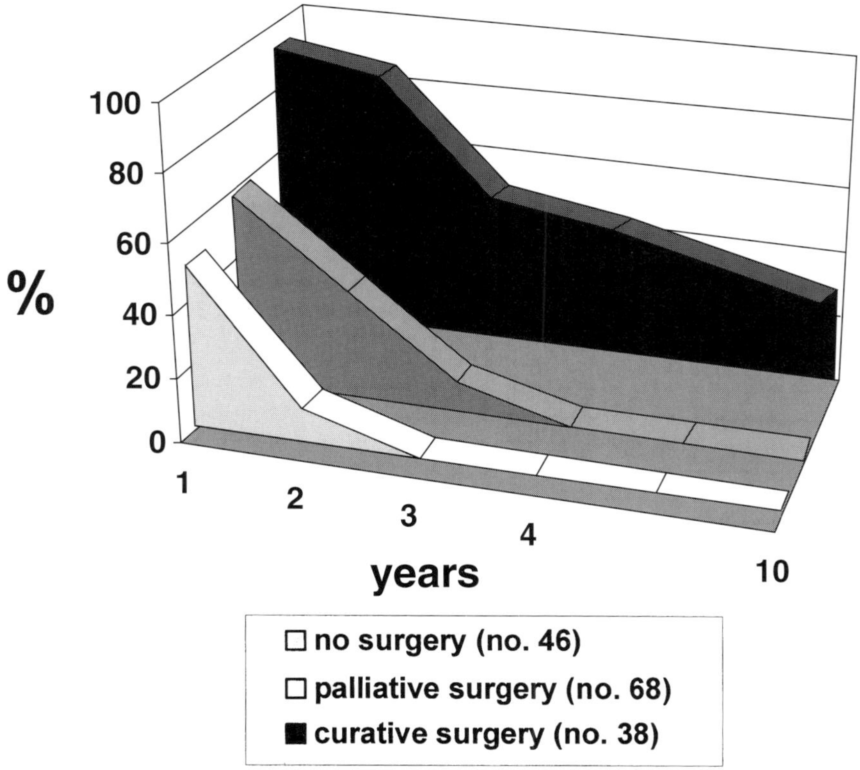

Figure 10. Possibility of treatment and actuarial survival in 152 patients in the personal series affected by LR of colorectal cancer.

Primary anastomotic LR offers the greatest possibility of curative exeresis [26, 77-78] (Tab. 1). For pelvic recurrences, abdomino-perineal resection remains the procedure of choice, although further resection is theoretically possible. In the literature, the possibility of radical exeresis of this type of recurrence varies from 5% to 28% [26, 79]. Such a wide divergence can be accounted for, by the fact that not all the authors distinguish primary anastomotic from secondary involvement, which is considerably more frequent. In particularly favourable cases of primary anastomotic LR, surgery can be repeated several times, although survival rates obviously diminish progressively [80].

Perianastomotic recurrences, however, prove to be mostly inoperable: of these, the ones affecting the elevator muscles are more frequently resectable than posterior ones, which involve the presacral fascia and the sacrum. Although in the first case abdomino-perineal resection is still possible [25, 81], with ample removal of the elevator muscles and sometimes of genito-urinary organs [82], in the second there is no possibility of cleavage [81], and radicality is impossible without drastically demolitive surgery. These are abdomino-sacral resections involving the skeletal apparatus [83], whose efficacy in terms of survival and quality of life are questionable [84]. In the experience of Wanebo et al, this type of demolition has led to a survival rate at 5 years of 12%, considering a mean duration of surgery of 18.5 hours, and an operative mortality rate of 10% [85].

In around 2% of female patients, LR is located in the ovaries [86]. Adnexectomy, when possible, is often followed by further recurrences [87] and the prognosis is particularly unfavourable [86-87].

Palliative surgery

In most cases, surgical treatment for LR is merely palliative.

Reductive exereses [88] are worthy of brief mention, since they have been credited with survival rates at times greater than those achieved with other therapeutic schemes, and have proved useful in conjunction with complementary irradiation therapy. However, a choice of this kind should be carefully considered, since the benefit of prolongation of life of an incomplete exeresis, especially if it is particularly demolitive, does not justify the operative risks.

It is for this reason that the addition of an *intestinal derivation* designed to solve problems of occlusion is usually preferable to an incomplete resection.

In the case of LR after rectal resection, techniques of *intraluminal reduction* of the tumoural mass with criotherapy [89], laser photocoagulation [90], electrocoagulation [91] or mechanical dilatations [92], as alternatives to colostomy, can solve problems of transit and bleeding, but can only partially attenuate the pain, which is the most common and most serious problem in the evolution of these recurrences.

REFERENCES

1. Goligher J C. *Surgery of the anus, rectum and colon* 1984 *(5th ed.)*; Baillière Tindall, London.
2. Sugarbaker PH. Recurrent and advanced primary colorectal cancer: therapeutic implications of new concepts of gastrointestinal tumour biology. *Clin Gastroenterol* 1989; 3: 699-712.
3. Nichelassi F, Vannucci L, Ayala JJ et al. Local recurrence after curative resection of colo-rectal adenocarcinoma. *Surgery* 1990; 108: 787-93.
4. Willett CG, Tepper JE, Cohen AM et al. Failure patterns following curative resection of colonic carcinoma. *Ann Surg* 1984 ;200: 685.
5. Russell AH, Tong D, Dawson LE, Wisbeck W. Adenocarcinoma of the proximal colon. Sites of initial dissemination and patterns of recurrence following surgery alone. *Cancer* 1984; 53: 360.
6. Rao AR, Kagan AR, Chan PM. Patterns of recurrence following curative resection alone for adenocarcinoma of the rectum and sigmoid colon. *Cancer* 1981; 48: 1492-1495.

7. Philipshen SJ, Heilweil M, Quan SH et al. Patterns of pelvic recurrence following definitive resection of rectal cancer. *Cancer* 1984; 53: 1354-1362.
8. Polk HC, Spratt JS. Recurrent cancer of the colon. *Surg Cllin North Am* 1983; 63: 151-159.
9. Schiessel R, Wunderlich M, Herbst F. Local recurrence of colorectal cancer: effect of early detection and aggressive surgery. *Br J Surg* 1986; 73: 342-344.
10. Carlsson U, Lasson A, Ekelund G. Recurrence rates after curative surgery for rectal carcinoma, with special reference to their accuracy. *Dis Colon Rectum* 1987; 30: 431-434.
11. Peracchia A, Sarli L, Carreras F et al. Recidive loco-regionali dopo chirurgia curativa per cancro del colon. *Ann It Chir* 1991; 62: 37-44.
12. Peracchia A, Sarli L, Pietra N, Giunta A. La recidiva loco-regionale, in A Peracchia, L Sarli (eds.), *Il cancro del colon e del retto operato* 1996. Minerva Medica Ed., Torino, pp. 123-151.
13. Phillips RKS, Hittinger R, Blesovsky L et al. Local recurrence following "curative" surgery for large bowel cancer: II. The rectum and rectosigmoid. *Br J Surg* 1984; 71: 17-20.
14. Williams NS. The rationale for preservation of the anal sphincter in patients with low rectal cancer. *Br J Surg* 1984; 71: 571-581.
15. Pheils MT, Chapuis PH, Newland C, Colquhoun K. Local recurrence after curative resection for rectal cancer. *Dis Colon Rectum* 1983; 26: 98-102.
16. Akyol AM, McGregor JR, Galloway DJ et al. Recurrence of colorectal cancer after sutured and stapled large bowel anastomosis. *Br J Surg* 1991; 78: 1297-1300.
17. Heald RJ, Husband EM, Ryall RD. The mesorectum in rectal cancer surgery - the clue to pelvic recurrence? *Br J Surg* 1982; 69: 613-616.
18. Durdey P, Quirke P, Dixon MF, Williams NS. Lateral spread-implication for operative management of low rectal cancer. *Br J Surg* 1987; 74: 612-627.
19. Hohenberger P, Schlag P, Kretzschmar U, Herfarth C. Regional mesenteric recurrence of colorectal cancer after anterior resection or left hemicolectomy: inadequate primary resection demostrated by angiography of the remaining arterial supply. *Int J Colorect Dis* 1991; 6: 17-23.
20. Rosemberg IL, Russel CW, Giles GR. Cell viability studies on the exfoliated colonic cancer cell. *Br J Surg* 1978; 65: 188-190.
21. Rosemberg IL. The etiology of colonic suture-line recurrence. *Ann Royal Coll Surg Eng* 1979; 61: 251-257.
22. Roe R, Fermor B, Williamson RCN. Proliferative instability and experimental carcinogenesis at colonic anastomoses. *Gut* 1987; 28: 312-315.
23. Wang Q, Gao H, Chen YL, Wang YH, He J. Transitional mucosa at anastomosis.A cause of local tumour recurrence in patients with rectal cancer after anterior resection. *Int Surg* 1992; 77: 37-40.
24. Wright HK, Thomas WH, Cleveland JC. The low recurrence rate of colonic carcinoma in ileocolic anastomoses. *Surg Ginec Obstet* 1969; 129: 960.
25. Phillips RKS, Hittinger R, Blesovsky L et al. Local recurrence following "curative" surgery for large bowel cancer: I. The overall picture. *Br J Surg* 1984 ; 71: 12.
26. Umpleby HC, Williamson RC. Anastomotic recurrence in large bowel cancer. *Br J Surg* 1987 ; 74: 873.
27. Pietra N, Sarli L, Costi R, Ouchemi C, Grattarola M, Peracchia A. Role of follow-up in management of local recurrences of colorectal cancer. A prospective randomized study. *Dis Colon Rectum* 1998; 41: 1127.
28. Peracchia A, Sarli L, Pietra N et al. La recidiva locale del carcinoma del retto: fattori prognostici extrachirurgici. *Chir Gastroenterol* 1991; 25: 637-644.
29. Nicholls RJ. Local recurrence after anterior resection. *Langenbecks Arch Chir Suppl II. Kongressbericht* 1986; 689-691.
30. Horn A, Dahl O, Morild I. Venous and neural invasion as predictors of recurrence in rectal adenocarcinoma. *Dis Colon Rectum* 1991 ; 34: 798-804.

31. Knudsen JB, Nilsson T, Sprechler M et al. Venous and nerve invasion as prognostic factors in postoperative survival of patients with resectable cancer of the rectum. *Dis Colon Rectum* 1983; 26: 613-617.
32. Aldridge MC, Phillips RKS, Hittinger R et al. Influence of tumour site on presentation, management and subsequent outcome in large bowel cancer. *Br J Surg* 1986; 73: 663.
33. Roncoroni L, Violi V, Sgobba G et al. Occlusione da carcinoma colo-rettale: esperienza personale. *Acta Chir Ital* 1987; 43: 476.
34. Nicholls RJ. La stadification preoperatoire des cancers du rectum. *Lyon Chir* 1990; 86: 689.
35. Horn A, Dahl O, Morild I. Venous and neural invasion as predictors of recurrence in rectal adenocarcinoma. *Dis Colon Rectum* 1991; 34: 798.
36. Malmberg M, Graffner H, Ling L, Olsson SA. Recurrence and survival after anterior resection of the rectum using the end to end anastomotic stapler. *Surg Ginec Obstet* 1986; 163: 231.
37. Kokal W, Sheibani K, Terz J. Tumour DNA content in the prognosis of colorectal carcinoma. *JAMA* 1986; 255: 367.
38. Pietra N, Sarli L, Carreras F et al. DNA ploidia e cinetica cellulare nel carcinoma colo-rettale. Atti XVI Congr. Naz. Soc. It. Chir. Oncol., O.C.T. Ed., Trieste 1992; p. 89.
39. Stahle E, Glimelius B, Bergstom R, Pahlman L. Preoperative prediction of late cancer specific deaths in patients with rectal and rectosigmoid carcinoma. Int J Colorect Dis 1989; 4: 182.
40. Wang Q, Wang FN, Gao H et al. Sialomucin at the resection margins and likelihood of local recurrence of carcinoma of the rectum after anterior resection. *Ann Med* 1990; 22: 31.
41. Warneke J, Petrelli NJ, Herrera L. Local recurrence after sphincter-saving resection for rectal adenocarcinoma. *Am J Surg* 1989; 158: 3-5.
42. Williams NS, Dixon MF, Johnston D. Reppraisal of the 5 cm rule of distal excision for carcinoma of the rectum: a study of distal intramural spread and of patients' survival. *Br J Surg* 1983; 70: 150-154.
43. Peracchia A, Sarli L, Pietra N et al. Recidive pelviche dopo chirurgia curativa per cancro del retto. *Ann It Chir* 1991; 62: 151-157.
44. Roncoroni L, Sgobba G, Montanari M et al. Recidive pelvi-perineali dopo chirurgia di exeresi per cancro del retto medio. Atti XII Congr. Naz. Soc. It. Ric. Chir. 1986, Monduzzi Ed., Modena; 375.
45. Wolmark N, Fisher B. An analysis of survival and treatment failure following abdomino-perineal and sphincter-saving resection in Dukes B and C rectal carcinoma. *Ann Surg* 1986; 204: 408.
46. Fielding LP. Surgeon-related variability in the outcome of cancer surgery. *J Clin Gastroenterol* 1988; 10: 130-132.
47. Mc Ardle CS, Hole D. Impact of variability among surgeons on postoperative morbidity and mortality and ultimate survival. *BMJ* 1991; 302: 1501-1505.
48. Hojo K, Koyama Y, Moriya Y. Lymphatic spread and its prognostic value in patients with rectal cancer. *Am J Surg* 1982; 144: 350-357.
49. Fujita S, Teramoto T, Watanabe M. Anastomotic leakage after colorectal cancer surgery: a risk factor for recurrence and poor prognosis. *Jpn J Clin Oncol* 1993; 23: 299-302.
50. Peracchia A, Violi V, Sarli L, Pietra N. Deiscenze anastomotiche dopo resezione del colon sinistro e del retto per cancro. Incidenza, trattamento e implicazioni a distanza. *Archivio ed Atti SIC*, Roma 1994; 58-71.
51. McGregor JR, Reinbach DH, Dahill SW, O'Dwyer PJ. Effect of fibrin sealant on perianastomotic tumour growth in an experimental model of colorectal cancer surgery. *Dis Colon Rectum* 1993; 36: 834-839.
52. Fermor B, Umpleby HC, Lever JV et al. The proliferative and metastatic potential of exfoliated colorectal carcinoma cells. *J Nat Cancer Inst* 1985;74: 1161-1168.
53. Skipper D, Cooper AJ, Marston JE, Taylor I. Exfoliated cells and in vitro growth in colorectal cancer. *Br J Surg* 1987; 74: 1049-1052.

54. Uff CR, Yiu CY, Boulos PB, Phillips RK. Influence of suture physicochemical and surface topographic structure on tumour cell adherence. *Dis Colon Rectum* 1993; 36: 850-854.
55. Sarli L, Pietra N, Longinotti E. La terapia adiuvante: ruolo della chemioterapia. In A. Peracchia, L. Sarli, *Il cancro del colon e del retto operato*. Minerva Medica Ed., Torino 1996; pp. 83-89.
56. Ibi I, Saito Y, Agnifili A et al. Biological effects of preoperative radiotherapy on metastatic lymph nodes from rectal cancer. *Am Surg* 1999; 65: 427-430.
57. Higgins GA, Humphrey EQ, Dwight RW, Roswit B, Lee LE, Keehn, RJ. Preoperative radiation and surgery for cancer of the rectum: Veterans Administration Surgical Oncology Group Trial II. *Cancer* 1986; 58: 352-359.
58. Third report of the MRC trial on behalf of The Working Party. Clinicopathological features of prognostic significance in operable rectal cancer in 17 centres in U.K. *Br J Surg* 1984; 50: 435-442.
59. Gastrointestinal Tumour Study Group. Survival after postoperative combination treatment of rectal cancer. *N Engl J Med* 1986; 315: 1294-1295.
60. Treurniet-Donker AD, Van Putten WLJ, Wereldsma JCJ et al. Postoperative radiation therapy for rectal cancer. *Cancer* 1991; 67: 2042-2048.
61. Gerard A, Buyse M, Nordlinger B. Preoperative radiotherapy as adjuvant treatment in rectal cancer- final results of a randomized study of the European Organization for Research and treatment of Cancer (EORTC). *Ann Surg* 1988; 208; 606-614.
62. Mendenhall WM, Million RR, Bland KI, Pfaff EE, Copeland EM. Preoperative radiation therapy for clinically resectable adenocarcinoma of the rectum. *Ann Surg* 1985; 202: 215-222.
63. Pahlman L, Dahlberg M, Glimelius B. Clinicopathological staging and management of colorectal cancer. Perioperative radiation therapy. *World J Surg* 1997; 21: 733-740.
64. Minsky BD. Sphincter preservation in rectal cancer. Preoperative radiation therapy followed by low anterior resection with coloanal anastomosis. *Semin Radiat Oncol* 1998; 8: 30-35.
65. Mohiuddin M, Regine WF, Marks WF, Marks JW. High-dose preoperative radiation and the challenge of sphincter-preservation surgery for cancer of the distal 2 cm of the rectum. *Int J Radiat Oncol Biol Phys* 1998; 40: 569-574.
66. Wust P, Rau B, Gellerman J et al. Radiochemotherapy and hyperthermia in the treatment of rectal cancer. Recent Results. *Cancer Res* 1998; 146: 175-191.
67. Vauthey JN, Marsh RW, Zlotecki RA et al. Recent advances in the treatment and outcome of locally advanced rectal cancer. *Ann Surg* 1999; 229: 745-754.
68. Quentmeier A, Schlag P, Smok M, Herfarth C. Reoperation for recurrent colorectal cancer: the importance of early diagnosis for resectability and survival. *Eur J Surg Oncol* 1990; 16: 319-325.
69. Peracchia A, Sarli L, Pietra N et al. Surgery of colonic suture line recurrences and of colon metachronous tumours. Atti II Corso Aggiornamento Onc Dig su stadiazione e trattamento del cancro colorettale, Verona, 1991; 60 (abstract).
70. Peracchia A, Sarli L, Pietra N et al. Chirurgia delle recidive loco-regionali del cancro del colon e del retto. *Ann It Chir* 1994; 6: 691-697.
71. Segall MM, Goldberg SM, Nivatvongs S et al. Abdomino-perineal resection for recurrent cancer following anterior resection. *Dis Colon Rectum* 1981; 24: 80-84.
72. Houry S, Vons C, Huguier M. Traitement des récidives locales des cancers coliques et rectaux traités initialement par résection-anastomose. *Gastroenterol Clin Biol* 1990; 14: 28-32.
73. Pacini P, Cionini L, Portoli L et al. Symptomatic recurrences of carcinoma of the rectum and sigmoid. The influence of radiotherapy on the quality of live. *Dis Colon Rectum* 1986; 29: 865-868.
74. Willet CG, Shellito PC, Tepper JE et al. Intraoperative electron beam radiation therapy for recurrent locally advanced rectal or rectosigmoid carcinoma. *Cancer* 1991; 67: 1504-1508.
75. Cuillière JC, Guillard Y, Mahe MA et al. Traitement des récidives pelviennes du cancer du rectum par association chirurgie-radiothérapie per-opératoire. *Lyon Chir* 1991; 87: 42-44.

76. Huguier M, Houry S. Treatment of local recurrence of rectal cancer. *Am J Surg* 1998; 175: 288-292.
77. Vassilopulos PP, Yoon JM, Ledesma EJ, Mittelman A. Treatment of recurrence of adenocarcinoma of the colon and rectum at the anastomotic site. *Surg Gynecol Obstet* 1981; 152: 777-780.
78. Liavag I. Detection and treatment of local recurrence. *Scand J Gastroenterol* 1988; 149: 163-165.
79. McDermott FT, Hughes ESR, Pihl E et al. Local recurrence after potentially curative resection for rectal cancer in a series of 1008 patients. *Br J Surg* 1985; 72: 34-37.
80. Sardi A, Minton JP, Neroda C et al. Multiple reoperation in recurrent colo-rectal carcinoma. An analysis of morbidity, mortality and survival. *Cancer* 1988; 6: 1913-1919.
81. Herfarth C, Schlag P, Hohenberger P. Surgical strategies in loco-regional recurrences of gastrointestinal carcinoma. *World J Surg* 1987; 11: 504-510.
82. Wiggers T, De Vries MR, Veeze-Kuypers B. Surgery for local recurrence of rectal carcinoma. *Dis Colon Rectum* 1996; 39: 323-328.
83. Temple WJ, Ketcham AS. Sacral resection for control of pelvic tumours. *Am J Surg* 1992; 163: 370-374.
84. Bricker EM, Butcher HR, Lawler WH, Mac Afee CA. Surgical treatment of advanced and recurrent cancer of the pelvic viscera: an evaluation of ten years experience. *Ann Surg* 1960; 150: 388-402.
85. Wanebo HJ, Koness RJ, Turk PS, Cohen SI. Composite resection of posterior pelvic malignancy. *Ann Surg* 1992; 215: 685-695.
86. Morrow M, Enker WE. Late ovarian metastases in carcinoma of the colon and rectum. *Arch Surg* 1984; 119: 1385-1388.
87. Birnkrant A, Sampson J, Sugarbaker PH. Ovarian metastasis from colorectal cancer. *Dis Colon Rectum* 1986; 29: 767-771.
88. Sugarbaker PH. Peritonectomy procedures. *Ann Surg* 1995; 221: 29-35.
89. Ftitsch A, Seidl W, Walzel C et al. Palliative and adjunctive measures in rectal cancer. *World J Surg* 1982; 6: 569-577.
90. Wodnicki H, Goldenberg R, Kaplan S et al. The laser: an alternative for palliative treatment of obstructing intraluminal lesions. *Am Surg* 1988; 54: 227-230.
91. Chistiansen J, Kirkegaard P. Treatment of recurrent rectal cancer by electroresection/coagulation after low anterior resection. *Dis Colon Rectum* 1983; 26: 656-657.
92. Kurz KR, Pitts WR, Speer D, Vaughan ED. Palliation of carcinoma of the rectum using the urologic resectoscope. *Surg Gynecol Obstet* 1988; 166: 60-62.

CHAPTER 18

MULTIMODAL TREATMENT FOR PERITONEAL CARCINOMATOSIS OF DIGESTIVE ORIGIN

Pierluigi Pilati, Simone Mocellin, Carlo Riccardo Rossi, Laura Codello, Luca Pinciroli, Mirto Foletto, Donato Nitti, Mario Lise.
Department of Surgery and Oncology, 2nd Surgical Clinic, University of Padua, Padua, Italy

Abstract
Peritoneal digestive carcinomatosis (PDC) is considered a short-term fatal condition refractory to standard treatment. Nevertheless, some authors have attempted reappraisal of the concept of incurable disease, based on the hypothesis that some of these tumors have a phase of locoregional spread during which the disease may still be curable.
Surgical treatment alone or combined with systemic chemotherapy, has yielded poor results in terms of survival and quality of life. A promising approach seems to be cytoreductive surgery (CS) combined with the intraperitoneal administration of antiblastic agents, as this sterilizes any residual tumor, following macroscopic excision, and overcomes the pharmacokinetic limits of systemic chemotherapy.
Attempts have been made to maximize the efficacy of the multimodal approach by using hyperthermic intraperitoneal intraoperative chemotherapy (HIIC). However, although results with this method of administration modality have been encouraging, no conclusions can yet be drawn, since series reported on in literature are relatively small and heterogeneous, and several clinical and technical factors (e.g. patient selection, optimal drug dosage, working temperature, evaluation of outcome) are still widely debated.

Keywords
Peritoneal carcinomatosis; intraperitoneal chemotherapy; hyperthermic antiblastic perfusion

A.M. Farinon (ed.), *Advances in Abdominal Surgery 2002*, 265-279.

INTRODUCTION

Peritoneal digestive carcinomatosis (PDC) is the most frequent cause of death in patients affected with gastrointestinal tumors [1-2]. The overall prognosis is extremely poor, the median survival ranging from 2.2 to 8.8 months [3-5].

It has not yet been demonstrated whether systemic chemotherapy, the current treatment for PDC, affects survival [6 - 8] . Surgery alone, even when macroscopically complete, is not adequate: microscopic residual disease, together with intraperitoneal surgical trauma and peritoneal seeding, cause recurrences in almost all patients [9]. Nor does this approach appear effective when combined with postoperative intraperitoneal chemotherapy [10]. An improved understanding of the biology of some of these tumors, in particular those with regional spread without evidence of systemic metastases, has prompted the search for new therapeutic approaches [4, 11]. Hyperthermic intraperitoneal intraoperative chemotherapy, potentially able to sterilize hearths of microscopic disease after CS, appears to be promising in the treatment of patients with PDC.

In the present paper, we report on the rationale behind CS combined with chemotherapy and hyperthermia, review the experience of different authors, and compare it with our own. Moreover, we deal with critical issues, including the feasibility and efficacy of, and the indications for, this multimodal treatment.

BIOLOGICAL ASPECTS OF PERITONEAL CARCINOMATOSIS

The high incidence of peritoneal seeding in patients with intra-abdominal carcinomas may be related to spontaneous intraperitoneal seeding from a primary tumor, or to iatrogenic dissemination during surgery. Cancer cells exfoliated from epithelial tumors can spread to the entire abdominal cavity [4]. On the other hand, direct manipulation of the tumor during surgical dissection may cause the leakage of malignant cells from the traumatized lymphatics, as well as malignant cell spillage from the primary tumor. However, some primary tumors with a low biological aggressiveness rarely metastasize through the lymphatic or blood vessels, whatever their size. Weiss first described this tumor behavior as “metastatic inefficiency”, since some cancers spread in the celomic cavity, but do not usually spread to distant sites through the blood stream [12]. Some investigators refer to these cancer types as “non-metastasizing” [4]. Low grade colon and appendiceal adenocarcinoma, as well as rare histological types such as pseudomixoma peritonei, often present as non-metastasizing variants, characterized by a better prognosis than other tumors. Therefore some cases of tumor spread limited to the peritoneal cavity may be amenable to a locoregional therapeutic approach.

CYTOREDUCTIVE SURGERY AND INTRAPERITONEAL CHEMOTHERAPY

Surgery appears to be inadequate and ineffective against different histological tumor types tumor, irrespective of whether it is combined with systemic chemotherapy [13]. This may be due to the presence of post-surgical residual disease, and ineffective adjuvant systemic chemotherapy, low intraperitoneal drug concentrations being achieved when drugs are administered intravenously. It is reasonable to assume that this limitation may be overcome by using intraperitoneal drug administration. In theory, the main advantage of intraperitoneal chemotherapy is that it allows the direct local delivery of high drug concentrations to the tumor site, while incurring minimal systemic exposure and toxicity. Because of low transperitoneal absorption, due to the plasma-peritoneal barrier [14], systemic drug concentrations are 18 to 620 fold lower than intraperitoneal concentrations [15], with a consequent reduction in the risk of side effects. However, results obtained so far have not met expectations, and intraperitoneal drug delivery seems no more effective than systemic drug administration [16-18]. The inefficacy of postoperative intraperitoneal drug administration may be correlated to heterogeneous drug distribution, caused by early postoperative adhesions in the peritoneal cavity, as suggested by Sugarbaker and coll. [19]. As a corollary, tumor cells may be entrapped by fibrin in surgically dissected areas, and therefore may not be exposed to the antiblastic agent in the early postoperative period.

HYPERTHERMIC INTRAOPERATIVE INTRAPERITONEAL CHEMOTHERAPY

Spratt and coll. were the first to associate heat with drugs administered intraperitoneally after CS [20], in order to enhance the antiblastic effect of intraperitoneal chemotherapy. There is experimental evidence that tumor tissue is damaged more than normal tissue, if heated to between 42 and 43 °C, because of its greater intrinsic thermosensitivity and its lower efficacy in exchanging heat through vasodilatation [21-23]. The effects of hyperthermia on tumors appear to be mediated by direct cytotoxicity, and the microcirculation peculiar to tumor tissue [24]. Hyperthermia synergically enhances the chemosensitivity of neoplastic cells to various antimitotic agents such as mitomycin-C and cisplatin [25-27].

Pharmacokinetics studies have shown that the penetration of drugs into tumor tissue is extremely limited, ranging from several cell layers to one to three millimeters from the surface. This suggests that the best possible results can only be obtained after an optimal cytoreduction.

Radiological and surgical assessment

Preoperative computed tomography (CT) scan is the only available radiological study providing useful quantitative information [30]. Some investigators sustain that CT can reliably identify patients for whom radical surgery is contraindicated, on the basis of radiological features such as mesenteric retraction [4, 31]. Nevertheless, this diagnostic tool is of limited accuracy when the tumor diameter measures less than 0.5 centimeters [32]. Alternative methods, such as CT-peritoneography (i.e. with intraperitoneal administration of contrast), positron emission tomography and magnetic resonance imaging might provide a more detailed picture of intraperitoneal spread [33-34] . However, as clinical experience with these techniques is still in its early stages, surgical exploration of the peritoneal cavity currently remains the mainstay of PDC extent assessment.

As only a few authors specify disease stage before and after surgical cytoreduction, it is difficult to compare results from different series, in terms of the indications for and the effectiveness of this multimodal therapy.

In order to obtain an accurate assessment of neoplastic distribution, Sugarbaker and coll. suggested a subdivision of the abdominal cavity into nine regions [4], each of which are given a volume score ranging from V0 to V3 (V0 = no cancer; V1 = tumors <0.5 cm; V2 = tumors 0.5 – 5 cm; V3 = tumors >5 cm). The use of the so called "peritoneal cancer index" based on these parameters was recently found to be of help in patient selection [35].

Technical features of HIIC

The ideal temperature for achieving maximum tumoricidal effect and synergistic activity with antiblastic drugs with HIIC is 43 °C [26, 36]. However, when performing HIIC, operators must bear in mind the threshold temperature for normal tissue damage. Postoperative complications are related to the mean temperature of the perfusate, particularly if it exceeds 41.5 °C [37]. Elias [38] and Yamaguchi [39] reported bowel perforation in cases in which temperatures were over 43° C. Yet no statistically significant difference has been found between the overall incidence of complications in patients who undergo HICC, and that in patients given postoperative intraperitoneal chemotherapy. Therefore a temperature within the window of 41.5 and 43° C seems to be advisable. Some teams perform HIIC using a closed circuit-system (88-92), the abdomen being closed after cytoreduction and before beginning HIIC. Fujimura [40] and Yamaguchi [39], followed by others (Tab. 1), adopted an open abdomen HIIC technique, using a peritoneal cavity expander (PCE) to facilitate the contact between bowel loops and perfusate, and to obtain a more homogeneous temperature within the abdominal cavity by mixing the perfusate manually. In our experience, the mean temperature difference between the upper and lower abdomen was higher (1.3 °C, range 0.6-1.9°C) in the first ten cases treated with the closed technique, than in the more recent cases (0.5 °C, range 0.3-0.7 °C), in which PCE was used. For an accurate evaluation of the intra-abdominal temperature, we use six thermal probes: three float freely in the abdominal cavity and three are placed immediately under the peritoneal layer. Two probes are positioned above the transverse mesocolon and two in the pelvis. We usually achieve a perfusate working temperature of 41.5 to 43 °C within 15 to 20 minutes, while the inflow temperature is around 45 to 46° C and the perfusate flow is maintained between 700 and 1000 ml/min. The perfusate volume depends on the type of circuit used and on the patient's build. Four to six liters of perfusate are usually sufficient when a closed circuit is used.

Table 1. Features of hyperthermic intraperitoneal intraoperative chemotherapy according to different authors

Author (ref.)	**PCE (*)**	**Time (minutes)**	**Temperature (° C)**
Fujimura (40)	Yes	40-60	41-43
Yonemura (45)	Yes	40-60	42
Kober (46)	No	60	42
Fujimoto (47)	No	90-180	41-43
Mansvelt (48)	No	60	> 41
Sugarbaker (49)	No	120	42
Gilly (50)	No	90	40-42
Loggie (51)	Yes	120	40.5
Elias (52)	Yes	90	41-42
Witkamp (53)	No	90	40.5
Piso (54)	yes	90	41.5
Rossi (43)	Yes	60-90	41.5

(*) PCE: peritoneal cavity expander

In view of the duration of HIIC, most authors consider that a 1 to 2 hour-period is adequate for achieving true hyperthermia and drug diffusion into tissues, and for maximizing the synergistic effect, without excessively prolonging anesthesia time. This choice is supported by findings from *in vivo* and *in vitro* studies on pharmacokinetics. Fujimoto and co-workers, who performed HIIC with mitomycin-C, found that a balance is achieved between the intraperitoneal and plasma drug concentration after one hour [41]. Moreover, Barlogie and coll. showed that cisplatin *in vitro* caused 99% of cellular death in a human colon adenocarcinoma cell line, at 42 °C after a one-hour interval, thus demonstrating that a relatively brief exposure (1–2 hours) to chemotherapy with clinically achievable hyperthermia is sufficient for achieving a significant cytotoxic effect [22].

The technical features of HIIC performed by different authors are shown in Table 1.

Drugs

As yet, few data are available on the ideal drug, or drug combination, for HIIC. The drugs most frequently used, cisplatin and mitomycin-C, have been chosen because of their activity when administered intravenously. Furthermore, the short duration of HIIC is more compatible with cell-cycle-independent drugs, such as cisplatin and mitomycin-C.

Pharmacokinetics studies on cisplatin have shown that when this drug is delivered intraperitoneally, the mean peritoneal/plasma area under the curve ratio is 6.9, indicating a higher drug concentration in the abdominal cavity than in plasma [10]. Regarding mitomycin-C, a similar pharmacokinetic advantage has been demonstrated, the peritoneal/plasma area under the curve ratio being 23 [42].

Our preliminary results with doxorubicin demonstrate both a favorable plasma/peritoneal ratio (84, range 33-115), and a good drug uptake (tumor drug concentration 5.3 μg/g; normal tissue drug concentration 2 μg/g) [43].

The types of drug and the doses used by different authors during HIIC are shown in Table 2.

New drugs now under evaluation may play a key role in improving upon results. In particular, some investigators ascertain the efficacy of biologic response modifiers such as TNFα .

Evaluation of response

One of the most important aspects of PDC management is evaluating the tumor response to treatment, also with a view to comparing different series. At present there are no standardized methods allowing a reliable quantification of tumor response, which makes it difficult to evaluate the efficacy of therapy.

Table 2 Drugs and drug associations administered during hyperthermic intraperitoneal intraoperative chemotherapy, in the treatment of peritoneal carcinomatosis of gastro-intestinal origin.

Author	MMC (*)	CDDP (*)	MMC+CDDP (*)
Fujimura	-	-	5+30
Yonemura	5	20	5+10
Kober	10	50	-
Fujimoto	10-40	30	-
Mansvelt	ns	-	-
Sugarbaker	10	-	-
Gilly	10	-	-
Loggie	10	-	-
Elias	5-10		20+200 (***)
Witkamp	10-40	-	-
Piso	-	150 (***)	-
Rossi	-	-	3.3 + 25 (**)

MMC: mitomycin-C; CDDP: cisplatin; DOXO: doxorubicin; ns: not specified; (*) mg/l (liter of perfusate); (**) $mg/m^2/l$ (liter of perfusate); (***) mg/m^2.

Second-look laparotomy has been used in young women with ovarian cancer without clinical evidence of recurrence. Most authors are reluctant to routinely undertake this invasive diagnostic procedure after CS plus HIIC, because of the risk of postoperative complications due to intraperitoneal adhesions. A thorough clinical evaluation, together with CT and ultrasound scan, allows the assessment of ascites, but cannot accurately detect small peritoneal nodules. Tumor markers, such as CA-125 for ovarian cancer, or CEA and CA-19.9 for gastrointestinal adenocarcinomas, are useful during follow-up only in cases in which preoperative levels were high. Finally, disease-free survival, when reported, refers to the clinical response, not to that found at pathology.

Clinical series

In literature, the larger series of patients with PDC who have undergone CS combined with HIIC consist of up to 200 patients (Tab. 3) [40, 45-54]. There are considerable differences between series for histology, differentiation grade and tumor stage at laparotomy.

The extent of CS differs markedly between series. The procedure was complete in all patients reported on by Spratt [20], while in other series complete cytoreduction was only achieved in some cases [39, 47], palliative surgery without debulking being performed in the others . Some authors included patients with both microscopic and macroscopic carcinomatosis [47].

Patients with early advanced gastric cancer (i.e. positive peritoneal cytology and/or tumor beyond the serosa), at a high risk of peritoneal recurrence, have been treated in an adjuvant setting with HIIC, after undergoing curative surgery for the primary tumor [56-57].

Table 3 Hyperthermic intraperitoneal intraoperative chemotherapy for the treatment of patients with peritoneal carcinomatosis of gastrointestinal origin: worldwide experience.

Authors	Year	Patients	Tumor histology (carcinoma)
Fujimura	1990	31	Gastric
Yonemura	1996	41	Gastric
Kober	1996	25	GI and others
Fujimoto	1997	141	Gastric
Mansvelt	1997	28	GI
Sugarbaker	1999	200	GI (*)
Gilly	1999	42	Gastric
Loggie	2000	84	GI
Elias	2001	27	Colorectal
Witkamp	2001	29	Colon
Piso	2001	17	Appendiceal
Rossi	2001	22	GI

(*) GI: gastrointestinal

Side effects

The postoperative mortality rate following CS combined with HIIC in the largest series reported in literature (90) was 5%. Gilly reported two deaths among 42 cases [55]. The most frequent complications are anastomotic leakage (4.5%), postoperative bleeding (4.5%) and adhesive ileus [49]. Bone marrow suppression and transitory renal failure may be related to additional side effects from mitomycin-C and cisplatin used together, in these cases [38, 49, 55]. It is widely believed that the postoperative morbidity and mortality rates are comparable to those following other major surgery approaches, in particular where patients are selected carefully; locoregional and systemic toxicity after HIIC is acceptable, rates being no higher than those reported after postoperative intraperitoneal chemotherapy.

A careful preoperative selection of patients based on their cardio-respiratory, hepato-renal and hematological status is required, in order to minimize the risk of postoperative complications.

Survival

The survivals reported by different authors after CS combined with HIIC for PDC are shown in Table 4. Since, to our knowledge, no comparative prospective studies are available, and any retrospective evaluation is unfeasible because series are heterogeneous, small, and have short follow-ups, it is difficult to reliably assess the benefits that CS with HIIC may have. However, the results so far obtained are encouraging, showing that patients treated with this approach have significantly longer survivals than those who have undergone palliative treatments. These findings should prompt formal phase III studies, in order to ascertain the actual impact on PDC of this multimodal therapeutic approach.

Results following HIIC given as adjuvant therapy to patients with early advanced gastric cancer are also promising, with a five-year overall survival ranging from 70 to 76% [56-57].

Table 4. Overall survival of patients with peritoneal carcinomatosis of gastrointestinal origin, treated with cytoreductive surgery combined with hyperthermic intraperitoneal intraoperative chemotherapy

Author	Survival
Fujimura	50% (2 years)
Yonemura	28% (3 years)
Kober	12 months (median)
Fujimoto	38% (3 years)
Mansvelt	42% (2 years)
Sugarbaker	nr
Gilly	41% (3 years) (**)
Loggie	14.3 months (median)
Elias	60.1 (2 years) (*)
Witkamp	45 (2 years)
Piso	75% (4 years)
Rossi	43% (2 years)

nr: not reported; (*) 4-year overall survival: 27.4%; (**) referred to patients subgroup with neoplastic nodules <5 mm.

Personal experience

From September 1996 through March 2001 we gave CS combined with HIIC to a total of 46 patients with peritoneal carcino-sarcomatosis. Twenty-two of these patients (15 men, 7 women; mean age, 50.3 ±11.4 years, range 21-76 years) had peritoneal carcinomatosis of gastrointestinal origin. In these cases tumor histological types were classified as adenocarcinoma of the colon (n = 7), stomach (n = 7), appendix (n = 2) and duodenum (n = 1), pseudomixoma peritonei (n = 4) and carcinoid (n = 1). The extent of peritoneal carcinomatosis was scored using the peritoneal index described by Sugarbaker. Briefly, the peritoneal cavity was divided into 13 regions, each of which was assigned a score from 0 to 3 according to the size and extent of tumor implants (total score range, 1-39). The mean number of regions with tumor spread was 8.3 ±2.7, and the mean peritoneal index was 18.5 ±7.1. CS, which was complete (disease residue < 3 mm) in all cases, included gastrointestinal resection (colon = 10, rectum = 1, stomach =5, jejunum = 4), organ resection (liver = 3, spleen = 6, ovary and uterus = 1, pancreas = 1), total peritonectomy (n = 4) and partial peritonectomy (n=19). HIIC was performed using mitomycin-C and cisplatin as reported in Table 2. The mean operating time was 8.1 ± 2 hours (range 5.4-12.2 hours).

No deaths were recorded during the postoperative period. Three patients had abdominal complications (bowel fistula, one requiring re-operation). Ten patients had pleural effusion.

According to the modified Ozol classification of locoregional toxicity , grade II (ileus > 6th < 10th postoperative day), III (ileus > 10th < 15th postoperative day) and IV (persistent ileus requiring reoperation) was observed in 13, 2 and 1 case, respectively. Hematological toxicity (grade 1-2 anemia according to the WHO classification) occurred in four cases.

After a median follow-up of 16 months (range 62-6), seven patients were alive without evidence of disease, two were alive with disease, 12 died of disease and one died of myocardial infarction. The survival analysis of patients grouped by histological grading (low vs high grade tumor) is reported in Figures 1 and 2.

CONCLUSIONS

By combining the advantages achieved from locoregional chemotherapy (high drug concentrations in abdominal cavity) with those from heat (direct cytotoxic effect and synergic effect with antiblastic agents) and surgery (tumor deposits reduction allowing drug penetration), CS associated with HIIC is an interesting proposal in the attempt to overcome the limitations of other conventional therapies.

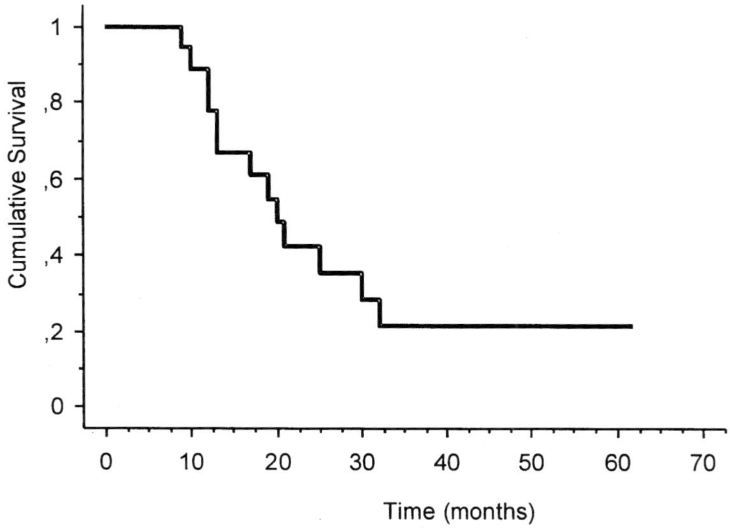

Figure 1 Kaplan-Mayer survival analysis of 22 patients affected with peritoneal carcinomatosis arising from gastrointestinal carcinomas, and treated with complete cytoreductive surgery and hyperthermic intraperitoneal intraoperative chemotherapy, at our institution.

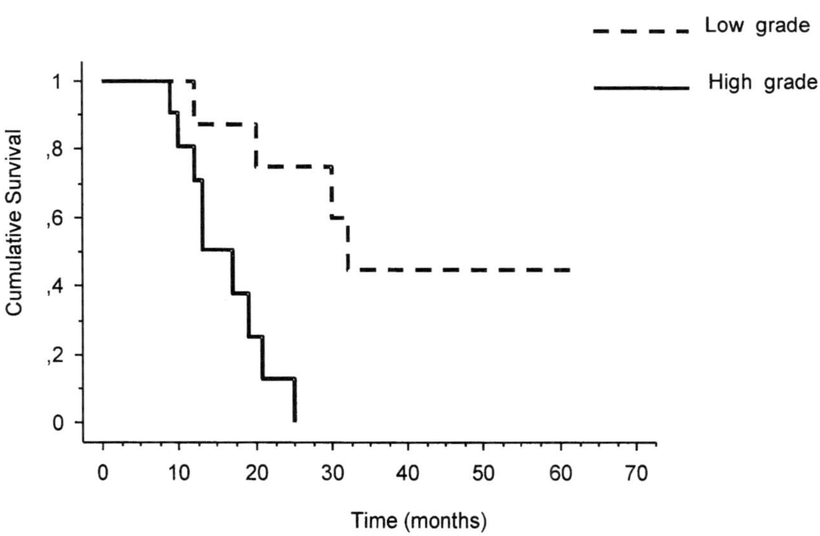

Figure 2 Survival analysis of patients with peritoneal carcinomatosis from low-grade (i.e. well-differentiated colonic adenocarcinomas, pseudomixoma peritonei and intestinal carcinoid; n=9) and high-grade (n=13) gastrointestinal carcinomas. All patients underwent complete cytoreductive surgery and hyperthermic intraperitoneal intraoperative chemotherapy, at our institution. Log-rank test: p= 0.0028.

Results from clinical series appear to confirm the activity of a multimodal approach to peritoneal carcinomatosis, based on complete CS plus intraperitoneal hyperthermic chemotherapy, according to the therapeutic principle described by Sugarbaker [49]. However, at present HIIC must be considered as an experimental treatment under investigation, and several aspects are still matter of debate. Some pilot studies have dealt with such issues, but no reliable conclusions can yet be drawn, because:

1) formal phase I/II or randomized studies have not yet been performed;

2) the severity of PDC considered in different studies is not homogeneous, ranging from minimal to advanced, with macroscopically disseminated disease even after CS;

3) the extent of CS varies greatly among series;

4) HIIC procedures are heterogeneous (differences in temperatures, drugs, doses, times, drug administration – with open or closed abdomen techniques);

5) some authors combine surgery with pre and/or postoperative chemotherapy, thereby precluding any interpretation of the effect of HIIC alone.

Survival rates are difficult to analyze because of the heterogeneity of histologic types (mostly of gastrointestinal origin), small series, and short follow-ups. However, preliminary results are encouraging, as the median survivals reported in literature are longer than those obtained with conventional therapeutic approaches.

Only through the standardization of technique, the selection of more homogeneous cases, and the use of phase I and II clinical studies, will it be possible to achieve a reliable assessment of the therapeutic value of this treatment. In particular, these results might be improved upon, through the careful selection of patients more likely to benefit from CS combined with HIIC.

We therefore believe that currently the most appropriate indication for HIIC is PDC from low grade tumors, such as well-differentiated colonic adenocarcinomas, pseudomixoma peritonei and intestinal carcinoid, provided that complete surgical cytoreduction can be achieved (residual disease macroscopically absent or < 3 mm). However, the poor results obtained so far for high-grade tumors, even in cases of limited spread of small size nodules, call for a re-appraisal of the indications for HIIC. In these cases, the administration of preoperative systemic neoadjuvant chemotherapy might be a method ex juvantibus, to test the sensitivity of these tumors to antiblastic agents to be used during HIIC.

Patients who might benefit from HIIC in an adjuvant setting are those with early advanced gastrointestinal cancer. A large-scale phase III trial should therefore be undertaken to confirm the encouraging preliminary results reported for gastric carcinoma.

REFERENCES

1. Maehara Y, Okuyama T, Kakeji Y, Baba H, Furusawa M, Sugimachi K. Postoperative immunochemotherapy including streptococcal lysate OK-432 is effective for patients with gastric cancer and serosal invasion. *Am J Surg* 1994;168:36-40.
2. Sugarbaker PH. Peritoneal carcinomatosis: natural history and rational therapeutic interventions using intraperitoneal chemotherapy. *Cancer Treat Res* 1996;81:149-68.
3. Chu DZ, Lang NP, Thompson C, Osteen PK, Westbrook KC. Peritoneal carcinomatosis in nongynecologic malignancy. A prospective study of prognostic factors. *Cancer* 1989;63:364-7.
4. Sugarbaker P. Peritoneal carcinomatosis: principles of management. Boston: Kluwer, 1996.
5. Buchholtz TW, Welch CE, Malt RA. Clinical correlates of resectability and survival in gastric carcinoma. *Ann Surg* 1978;188:711-5.
6. Machover D. A comprehensive review of 5-fluorouracil and leucovorin in patients with metastatic colorectal carcinoma. *Cancer* 1997;80:1179-87.
7. Midgley R, Kerr D. Colorectal cancer. *Lancet* 1999;353:391-9.
8. Bartlett D. Cancer Principles and practice of oncology. 6th ed: Lippincott Williams & Wilkins, 2001.
9. Benson AB, 3rd. Therapy for advanced colorectal cancer. *Semin Oncol* 1998;25:2-11.
10. Sugarbaker P. Peritoneal carcinoamtosis: drug and diseases. Boston: Kluwer, 1996.
11. Jacquet P, Vidal-Jove J, Zhu B, Sugarbaker P. Peritoneal carcinomatosis from gastrointestinal malignancy: natural history and new prospects for management. *Acta Chir Belg* 1994;94:191-7.
12. Weiss L. Cancer cell traffic from the lungs to the liver: an example of metastatic inefficiency. *Int J Cancer* 1980;25:385-92.
13. Spratt J, Edwards M, Kubota T. Peritoneal carcinomatosis: anatomy, physiology, diagnosis, management. *Curr Probl Cancer* 1986;10:558-584.
14. Jacquet P, Sugarbaker PH. Peritoneal-plasma barrier. *Cancer Treat Res* 1996;82:53-63.
15. Markman M. Intraperitoneal chemotherapy. *Semin Oncol* 1991;18:248-54.
16. Sugarbaker PH, Gianola FJ, Speyer JC, Wesley R, Barofsky I, Meyers CE. Prospective, randomized trial of intravenous versus intraperitoneal 5- fluorouracil in patients with advanced primary colon or rectal cancer. *Surgery* 1985;98:414-22.
17. Speyer JL, Collins JM, Dedrick RL, et al. Phase I and pharmacological studies of 5-fluorouracil administered intraperitoneally. *Cancer Res* 1980;40:567-72.
18. Markman M, Reichman B, Hakes T, et al. Intraperitoneal chemotherapy as treatment for ovarian carcinoma and gastrointestinal malignancies: the Memorial Sloan-Kettering Cancer Center experience). *Acta Med Austriaca* 1989;16:65-7.
19. Sugarbaker TA, Chang D, Koslowe P, Sugarbaker PH. Pathobiology of peritoneal carcinomatosis from ovarian malignancy. *Cancer Treat Res* 1996;81:63-74.
20. Spratt JS, Adcock RA, Muskovin M, Sherrill W, McKeown J. Clinical delivery system for intraperitoneal hyperthermic chemotherapy. *Cancer Res* 1980;40:256-60.
21. Giovanella BC, Stehlin JS, Jr., Morgan AC. Selective lethal effect of supranormal temperatures on human neoplastic cells. *Cancer Res* 1976;36:3944-50.
22. Barlogie B, Corry PM, Drewinko B. In vitro thermochemotherapy of human colon cancer cells with cis- dichlorodiammineplatinum(II) and mitomycin C. *Cancer Res* 1980;40:1165-8.
23. Hahn GM, Braun J, Har-Kedar I. Thermochemotherapy: synergism between hyperthermia (42-43 degrees) and adriamycin (of bleomycin) in mammalian cell inactivation. *Proc Natl Acad Sci U S A* 1975;72:937-40.
24. Dudar TE, Jain RK. Differential response of normal and tumor microcirculation to hyperthermia. *Cancer Res* 1984;44:605-12.

25. Meyn RE, Corry PM, Fletcher SE, Demetriades M. Thermal enhancement of DNA damage in mammalian cells treated with cis-diamminedichloroplatinum(II). *Cancer Res* 1980;40:1136-9.
26. Wallner KE, Banda M, Li GC. Hyperthermic enhancement of cell killing by mitomycin C in mitomycin C- resistant Chinese hamster ovary cells. *Cancer Res* 1987;47:1308-12.
27. Herman TS. Temperature dependence of adriamycin, cis-diamminedichloroplatinum, bleomycin, and 1,3-bis(2-chloroethyl)-1-nitrosourea cytotoxicity in vitro. *Cancer Res* 1983;43:517-20.
28. Kerr DJ, Kaye SB. Aspects of cytotoxic drug penetration, with particular reference to anthracyclines. *Cancer Chemother Pharmacol* 1987;19:1-5.
29. Los G, Mutsaers PH, van der Vijgh WJ, Baldew GS, de Graaf PW, McVie JG. Direct diffusion of cis-diamminedichloroplatinum(II) in intraperitoneal rat tumors after intraperitoneal chemotherapy: a comparison with systemic chemotherapy. *Cancer Res* 1989;49:3380-4.
30. Jacquet P, Sugarbaker PH. Clinical research methodologies in diagnosis and staging of patients with peritoneal carcinomatosis. *Cancer Treat Res* 1996;82:359-74.
31. Jacquet P, Jelinek JS, Chang D, Koslowe P, Sugarbaker PH. Abdominal computed tomographic scan in the selection of patients with mucinous peritoneal carcinomatosis for cytoreductive surgery. *J Am Coll Surg* 1995;181:530-8.
32. Jacquet P, Jelinek JS, Steves MA, Sugarbaker PH. Evaluation of computed tomography in patients with peritoneal carcinomatosis. *Cancer* 1993;72:1631-6.
33. Lin EC, Lear J, Quaife RA. Metastatic peritoneal seeding patterns demonstrated by FDG positron emission tomographic imaging. *Clin Nucl Med* 2001;26:249-50.
34. Kubik-Huch RA, Dorffler W, von Schulthess GK, et al. Value of (18F)-FDG positron emission tomography, computed tomography, and magnetic resonance imaging in diagnosing primary and recurrent ovarian carcinoma. *Eur Radiol* 2000;10:761-7.
35. Portilla AG, Sugarbaker PH, Chang D. Second-look surgery after cytoreduction and intraperitoneal chemotherapy for peritoneal carcinomatosis from colorectal cancer: analysis of prognostic features. *World J Surg* 1999;23:23-9.
36. Song CW, Kang MS, Rhee JG, Levitt SH. Effect of hyperthermia on vascular function in normal and neoplastic tissues. *Ann N Y Acad Sci* 1980;335:35-47.
37. Jacquet P, Stephens AD, Averbach AM, et al. Analysis of morbidity and mortality in 60 patients with peritoneal carcinomatosis treated by cytoreductive surgery and heated intraoperative intraperitoneal chemotherapy. *Cancer* 1996;77:2622-9.
38. Elias D, Detroz B, Debaene B, et al. Treatment of peritoneal carcinomatosis by intraperitoneal chemo-hyperthermia: reliable and unreliable concepts. *Hepatogastroenterology* 1994;41:207-13.
39. Yamaguchi A, Tsukioka Y, Fushida S, et al. Intraperitoneal hyperthermic treatment for peritoneal dissemination of colorectal cancers. *Dis Colon Rectum* 1992;35:964-8.
40. Fujimura T, Yonemura Y, Fushida S, et al. Continuous hyperthermic peritoneal perfusion for the treatment of peritoneal dissemination in gastric cancers and subsequent second-look operation. *Cancer* 1990;65:65-71.
41. Fujimoto S, Takahashi M, Kobayashi K, Kasanuki J, Ohkubo H. Heated intraperitoneal mitomycin C infusion treatment for patients with gastric cancer and peritoneal metastasis. *Cancer Treat Res* 1996;81:239-45.
42. Jacquet P, Averbach A, Stephens AD, Stuart OA, Chang D, Sugarbaker PH. Heated intraoperative intraperitoneal mitomycin C and early postoperative intraperitoneal 5-fluorouracil: pharmacokinetic studies. *Oncology* 1998;55:130-8.
43. Pilati P, Rossi CR, Mocellin S, et al. Multimodal treatment of peritoneal carcinomatosis and sarcomatosis. *Eur J Surg Oncol* 2001;27:125-34.
44. Bartlett DL, Buell JF, Libutti SK, et al. A phase I trial of continuous hyperthermic peritoneal perfusion with tumor necrosis factor and cisplatin in the treatment of peritoneal carcinomatosis. *Cancer* 1998;83:1251-61.

45. Yonemura Y, Fujimura T, Nishimura G, et al. Effects of intraoperative chemohyperthermia in patients with gastric cancer with peritoneal dissemination. *Surgery* 1996;119:437-44.
46. Kober F, Heiss A, Roka R. Diffuse and gross peritoneal carcinomatosis treated by intraperitoneal hyperthermic chemoperfusion. *Cancer Treat Res* 1996;82:211-9.
47. Fujimoto S, Takahashi M, Mutou T, et al. Improved mortality rate of gastric carcinoma patients with peritoneal carcinomatosis treated with intraperitoneal hyperthermic chemoperfusion combined with surgery. *Cancer* 1997;79:884-91.
48. Mansvelt B, Bertrand C, Nockerman P, et al. Study of the toxicity and results of intraperitoneal hyperthermic chemotherapy in 28 patients with peritoneal carcinomatosis. *Ann Chir* 1997;51:60-7.
49. Stephens AD, Alderman R, Chang D, et al. Morbidity and mortality analysis of 200 treatments with cytoreductive surgery and hyperthermic intraoperative intraperitoneal chemotherapy using the coliseum technique. *Ann Surg Oncol* 1999;6:790-6.
50. Gilly FN, Beaujard A, Glehen O, et al. Peritonectomy combined with intraperitoneal chemohyperthermia in abdominal cancer with peritoneal carcinomatosis: phase I-II study. *Anticancer Res* 1999;19:2317-21.
51. Loggie BW, Fleming RA, McQuellon RP, Russell GB, Geisinger KR. Cytoreductive surgery with intraperitoneal hyperthermic chemotherapy for disseminated peritoneal cancer of gastrointestinal origin. *Am Surg* 2000;66:561-8.
52. Elias D, Blot F, El Otmany A, et al. Curative treatment of peritoneal carcinomatosis arising from colorectal cancer by complete resection and intraperitoneal chemotherapy. *Cancer* 2001;92:71-6.
53. Witkamp AJ, de Bree E, Kaag MM, et al. Extensive cytoreductive surgery followed by intra-operative hyperthermic intraperitoneal chemotherapy with mitomycin-C in patients with peritoneal carcinomatosis of colorectal origin. *Eur J Cancer* 2001;37:979-84.
54. Piso P, Bektas H, Werner U, et al. Improved prognosis following peritonectomy procedures and hyperthermic intraperitoneal chemotherapy for peritoneal carcinomatosis from appendiceal carcinoma. *Eur J Surg Oncol* 2001;27:286-90.
55. Sayag-Beaujard AC, Francois Y, Glehen O, et al. Intraperitoneal chemo-hyperthermia with mitomycin C for gastric cancer patients with peritoneal carcinomatosis. *Anticancer Res* 1999;19:1375-82.
56. Kaibara N, Hamazoe R, Iitsuka Y, Maeta M, Koga S. Hyperthermic peritoneal perfusion combined with anticancer chemotherapy as prophylactic treatment of peritoneal recurrence of gastric cancer. *Hepatogastroenterology* 1989;36:75-8.
57. Fujimoto S, Takahashi M, Mutou T, Kobayashi K, Toyosawa T. Successful intraperitoneal hyperthermic chemoperfusion for the prevention of postoperative peritoneal recurrence in patients with advanced gastric carcinoma. *Cancer* 1999;85:529-34.
58. Rossi C, Foletto M, Mocellin S, et al. Hyperthermic intraoperative intraperitoneal chemotherapy with cisplatin and doxorubicin in patients undergo cytoreductive surgery for peritoneal carcinomatosis and sarcomatosis: phase I study. *Cancer* 2001.

SECTION IV

FECAL INCONTINENCE

CHAPTER 19

ANATOMICAL AND PHYSIOLOGICAL BASES OF FECAL CONTINENCE

Attilio Maria Farinon
Department of Surgery, University of Rome "Tor Vergata", Rome, Italy

Fecal incontinence, i. e. the impaired ability to control gas or stool, is a disabling and distressing condition, which, when severe, causes progressive social isolation of the patient. However, it is a common condition, especially in older individuals, where prevalence has been reported to approach 60 per cent, and in women, where incontinence as a result of childbirth reaches 54 per cent [1]. Sultan and associates [2] found that 13 per cent of primigravidae and 23 per cent of multigravidae had some degree of incontinence in the first six weeks after delivery, and Mac Arthur and colleagues [3] reported that up to two years later 4 per cent still had the symptom. Of patients surgically treated, the female-to-male ratio is 4 to 1. In a recent epidemiological study published by the University of Illinois on JAMA in 1995, fecal incontinence was determined in 2.2 per cent of the general population [4]. Data from Great Britain suggest a community prevalence of 4.2 men and 1.7 women per 1000 people who are 15 to 64 years of age, and 10.9 men and 13.3 women per 1000 people who are 65 or older [5].

Fecal incontinence is a far more common problem than is generally appreciated, and it is not confined just to elderly people. The prevalence rate among individuals aged above 15 years has been reported to be 4.3 per 1000 population, but this figure is likely to be underestimated. Congenital anorectal anomalies, an uncommon cause of fecal incontinence, occur in 1 in 5000 liveborn infants; they range in severity from an imperforate anal membrane, to total rectal agenesis. About 500 babies a year are born in the United Kingdom with anorectal agenesis, which requires surgical treatment (posterior sagittal anorectoplasty) that restores normal anatomy, but commonly leaves the child incontinent [6, 7].

* * *

A.M. *Farinon (ed.), Advances in Abdominal Surgery 2002*, 283-288.

Continence is maintained by the integrate action of the external and internal anal sphincters, the puborectalis, the levator plate, and by intact sensory pathways [8-9]. It depends on stool volume and consistency, the reservoir capacity or compliance of the rectum, the preservation of a normal sampling reflex, normal anorectum sensation, normal resting anal tone, and resistance to opening [10]. Impairment of any of the above mentioned mechanisms, alone or in combination, can lead to incontinence.

The anal canal is surrounded by a complex system of sphincters that may tightly occlude it, to prevent unwanted defecation. The muscular components consist of the internal and external anal sphincters and the puborectalis, which is a functional component of the levator ani. There are also longitudinal muscle components forming the conjoint longitudinal coat [11].

The internal sphincter lies within the ring of external sphincter muscle, and is a continuation of the inner circular layer of the smooth muscle of the rectal wall. Both under autonomic control and local innervation by an intermyenteric plexus (since activity can be blocked by circular rectal myotomy), it is maintained in a state of continuous contraction, providing for 50 to 80% of resting anal pressure (the external sphincter accounts for 25 to 30% of maximal resting tone, and the remaining 15% is attributed to expansion of anal cushions), and relaxes in response to rectal distension (rectoanal inhibitory reflex). This reflex is absent in patients with Hirschsprung's disease. With age, resting pressures progressively decrease, because of the gradual degeneration of the internal sphincter, and patients with incontinence present generally with impaired resting anal pressure [12-13].

The role of this muscle in fecal incontinence has been re-evaluated, and so have the potential role of pharmacological agents in improving sphincter function [14]. That is in contrast with the point of view of someone who concludes that although the internal sphincter must play a role in fecal continence, it does not seem to be a crucial one. Observations from general and pediatric surgeons on patients surgically treated with low anterior resection for cancer of the rectum, and with repair of high type imperforated anus seem to suggest it. In these patients, the lower part of the rectum or the most distal part of the blind rectal pouch is removed, often with a reasonably good fecal continence in spite of loss of internal sphincter.

Internal sphincter function is abolished by damage to parasympathetic nerves, as occurs in lesions affecting the sacral outflow [11, 17]. The response of the internal anal sphincter to rectal distension is the transient increase followed by decrease in the resting pressure; this constitutes the sampling reflex, or rectoanal inhibitory reflex. Its role is to initiate and control defecation; the fecal bolus enters the anal transition zone, and is recognized by the sensitive anal mucosa. The volume necessary to cause an appreciable distension is 20 to 40 ml; larger volumes in the rectum initiate a transient desire to defecate, and progressively release the feeling of a constant desire to defecate and urgency. The external sphincter and the puborectalis either relax to allow defecation or, if defecation is not desired, the pelvic floor and sphincter contract, by sending the fecal bolus back into the rectum and closing the anal canal [11]. Patients with incontinence present a higher than normal threshold of the rectoanal inhibitory reflex [18]. Although the sampling reflex may deteriorate in patients with fecal incontinence, rectal sensation does not seem to be impaired [19], except probably in diabetics with incontinence [20], and in patients with idiopathic incontinence (caused by denervation of the pelvic floor) [21]. Bilateral sacral denervation results in reduced sensory awareness to rectal distension, and to impaired discrimination between solids and liquids [22].

The voluntary sphincter is made up of the external sphincter and puborectalis muscles; these skeletal muscles behave as a functional unit, in spite of independent innervation (the external sphincter by the pudendal nerves and the puborectalis by pelvic branches of S-3 and S-4), and this enables voluntary control of continence. The external sphincter's response to stimuli (voluntary effort, rectal distension, increased intra-abdominal pressure, and anal dilatation) is contraction. Voluntary sphincter contraction normally doubles the pressure in the anal canal, though maximal voluntary contraction can be maintained only for approximately 50 seconds, after which fatigue occurs; hence, it merely provides a final control mechanism if fecal material enters the upper anal canal. This response involves different neural pathways; neurologic impairment therefore can be differentiated from muscle disorder, if the sphincter responds to any of those stimuli. Failure to respond to all stimuli is indicative either of muscle disease or of diffuse neurologic disorder [11].

The levator ani, arising from the bony pelvis and the obturator fascia, spread out to form a muscular pelvic floor. It may be divided into three parts: the puborectalis muscle formed by the inner fibers, the ischiococcygeous and iliococcygeous. The puborectalis represents the cephalad continuation of the external sphincter. It arises from the back of the symphysis and passes posteriorly around the lower part of the rectum, meeting fibers from the opposite side. The sling formed around the posterior aspect of the deep sphincter pulls the upper part of the canal forward to form the anorectal angle.

The anorectal angle, produced by the anterior pull of the puborectalis muscle, was thought to be important in maintaining continence. Parks proposed a "flap valve" mechanism, in which increased intraabdominal pressure compressed the anterior rectal wall against the pelvic floor [23]. However, this theory has been dismissed, because it cannot explain how (1) after rectopexy, although the anorectal angle is made obtuse, continence is usually maintained, and (2) how postanal repair may restore continence without necessarily changing the anorectal angle [24]. It is therefore suggested that the puborectalis acts as a sphincter, and not as a flap valve [9]. If the external anal sphincter is divided completely, satisfactory continence will theoretically be provided by the intact puborectalis. If both the external sphincter and the puborectalis muscle are divided, the patient will be incontinent. Division of the puborectalis without division of the external sphincter, which may occur for example in infants during operation for high imperforate anus, will render the patient incontinent, despite his having a normal functioning external sphincter [11].

However, adequate anorectal sensation is necessary for normal continence. Receptors in the pelvic floor, rather than the rectal wall, are thought to be important in detecting the presence of stool. Patients with fecal impaction and overflow incontinence have diminished rectal sensation, as do patients with incontinence due to diabetes mellitus or spinal disease. Patients with traumatic and idiopathic incontinence may have abnormal sensation of the anal canal. Successful repair of the anal sphincter is associated with improved sensation [25].

The anal canal is normally closed at rest and during sleep because of the constant activity of the internal sphincter; this is reinforced by the tonic activity of the external anal sphincter and puborectalis. Moreover, anal closure is assisted by the properties of the vascular anal cushions; these expand to keep the anal canal closed and prevent leakage, when anal pressures decrease. The importance of the anal cushions is obvious in patients who present with anal soiling after hemorrhoidectomy, even with normal sphincter pressures [26].

* * *

Knowledge of these anatomical and physiological data is the basis for a correct approach to fecal incontinence. However, it should be outlined that the outcome of surgical correction of anorectal anomalies depends on the adequacy of pelvic floor development, and the relation of the rectum and anus to the levator sling.

Physiological study by use of manometry, sphincter electromyography includig pudendal nerve terminal motor latency assessment, and endoanal ultrasonography will generally reveal the cause, and allow correct planning in the management of fecal incontinence. Direct sphincter repair usually gives excellent results in patients who present external sphincter defect as an isolated abnormality, even if the procedure is delayed for many years after original injury. Overlapping sphincteroplasty with internal sphincter imbrication certainly improves both the anal sphincter physiologic profile and fecal continence [27].

Whenever the external sphincter defect appears extensive, the internal anal sphincter results also as damaged, and if neuropathy is coexisting many problems are encountered, especially if a previous attempt of direct sphincter repair failed. In these patients the construction of a neosphincter may be required. There are basically two types of neoanal sphincter: one is formed by the transposition around the anal canal of the patient's own skeletal muscle, usually the electrically stimulated gracilis [28], and the other consists of a silastic cuff connected to a fluid-filled reservoir that allows the cuff to be inflated around the anal canal to occlude it [29].

REFERENCES

1. Fang DT, Nivatvongs S, Vermeulen FD, et al. Overlapping sphincteroplasty for acquired anal incontinence. *Dis Colon Rectum* 1984; 27:720-2.
2. Sultan AH, Kamm MA, Hudson CN, Bartram CI.Third degree obstetric and sphincter tears:risk factors and outcome of primary repair. *BMJ* 1994; 308:887-91.
3. Mac Arthur C, Bick DE, Keighley MRB. Faecal incontinence after childbirth. *Br J Obstet Gynaecol* 1997; 104:46-50.
4. Nelson R, Norton N, Cautley E, Furner S. Community based prevalence of anal incontinence. *JAMA* 1995; 274:559-61.
5. Cheskin LJ, Schuster MM. Fecal incontinence. In: *Hazzard WR, Andres R, Bierman EL, Blass JP, eds. Principles of geriatric medicine and gerontology.*New York: Mc Graw-Hill, 1990:1143-5.
6. Thomas TM, Egan M, Walgrave A, Meade TW. The prevalence of faecal and double incontinence. *Community Med* 1984; 6:216-20.
7. Pena A, de Vries PA. Posterior sagittal anorectoplasty: important technical considerations and new applications. *J Paed Surg* 1982; 17:796-809.
8. Bannister JJ, Gibbons C, Red NW. Preservation of faecal continence during rises in intrabdominal pressure: is there a role for the flap-valve? *Gut* 1987; 28:1242-4.
9. Bartolo DCC, Roe AM, Locke-Edwards JC, et al. Flap valve theory of anorectal incontinence. *Br J Surg* 1986; 73:1012-5.
10. Keighley MRB, Williams NS, eds. *Surgery of the anus,rectum, and colon.* Philadelphia: WB Saunders, 1993.
11. Mavrantonis C, Wexner SD. A clinical approach to fecal incontinence. *J Clin Gastroenterol* 1998; 27:108121.
12. Eckadt VF, Elmer T. Reliability of anal pressure measurements. *Dis Colon Rectum* 1991; 34:72-7.
13. Pedersen IK, Christiansen J. A study of the physiological variations in anal manometry. *Br J Surg* 1989; 76:69-71.
14. Speakman CTM, Burnett SJD, Kamm MA, Bartram CI. Sphincter injury after anal dilatation demonstrated by anal endosonography. *Br J Surg* 1991; 78:1429-30.
15. Madoff DR, Williams JG, Caushaj PF. Fecal incontinence. *N Engl J Med* 1992; 326:1002-6.
16. Williams NS. Topical issues in selected specialties: surgery of anorectal incontinence. *Lancet* 1999; 353 (suppl I):31-2.
17. Swash M, GrayA, Lubowski DZ, Nichols RJ. Ultrastructural changes in internal anal sphincter in neurologic faecal incontinence. *Gut* 1988; 29:1692-8.
18. Miller R, Bartolo DCC, Cervero F, Mortensen NJ. Anorectal sampling: a comparison of normal and incontinence patients. *Br J Surg* 1988; 75:+44-7.
19. Rogers J, Henry MM, Misiewicz JJ.Combined sensory and motor deficit in primary neuropath faecal incontinence. *Gut* 1988; 29:5-9.
20. Rogers J, Levy DM, Henry MM, Misiewicz JJ.Pelvic floor neuropathy: a comparative study of diabetes mellitus and idiopathic faecal incontinence. *Gut* 1988: 29.756-61.

21. Roe AM, Bartolo DCC, Mrtensen NJMcC. New method for assessment of anal sensation in various anorectal disorders. *Br J Surg* 1986; 73:310-2.
22. Gunterberg B, Kewenter J, Petersen I, Stener B. Anorectal function after major resections of the sacrum with bilateral or unilateral sacrifice of sacral nerves. *Br J Surg* 1976; 63:546-54.
23. Parks AG, Porter NH, Hardcastle J. The syndrome of the descending perineum. *Proc R Soc Med* 1966; 59:477-82.
24. Penninckx F, Debruyne C,, Lestar B, Kerremans RP. Observer variation in the radiological measurement of the anorectal angle. *Int J Colorectal Dis* 1990; 5:94-7.
25. Jorge JMN, Wexner SD. Etiology and management of fecal incontinence. *Dis Colon Rectum* 1993; 36:77-97.
26. Bruck CE, Lubowski DZ, King DW. Do patients with haemorrhoids have pelvic floor denervation? *Int Colorectal Dis* 1988; 3:210-4.
27. Wexner SD, Marchetti F, Jagelman DG. The role of sphincteroplasty for fecal incontinence reevaluated: a prospective physiologic and functional review. *Dis Colon Rectum* 1991;34:22-30.
28. Williams NS, Patel J, George BD, Hallan RI, Watkins ES. Development of an electrically stimulated neoanal sphincter. *Lancet* 1991; 338:1166-9.
29. Wong DW, Jensen LL, Bartolo DCC, Rothenberger DA. Artificial anal sphincter. *Dis Colon Rectum* 1996; 39:1345-51.

CHAPTER 20

ELECTROSTIMULATED GRACILOPLASTY FOR FAECAL INCONTINENCE TREATMENT

Massimo Seccia
Department of Surgery; University of Pisa, Pisa, Italy

Abstract

Treatment of severe faecal incontinence, refractory to repeated therapies or secondary to a wide anatomic loss of sphincter, remains a surgical challenge.

In these circumstances, a sphincter substitution becomes the only option available to avoid a permanent diversion or a "diapers-conditioned" quality of life.

As recently confirmed by long-term follow-up studies, a reliable surgical option is represented by the so-called dynamic graciloplasty, in which chronic elettrostimulation protocols are applied to the transposed gracilis muscles.

We present our experience based on 36 ESGPs performed since 1991 in patients affected from full faecal incontinence (N.S. Williams Scale IV and V).

Inclusion criteria, technical features and results are presented. In 21 patients (70%) continence was completely restored and due to the long follow-up length these functional results can be considered stables.

Infection remains the most severe complications, conditioning all observed failure and poorest results can be expected in some congenital diseases and in case of incontinence associated with chronic constipation.

An aggressive treatment of early postoperative complications and a correct patients selection are the crucial factors which influence early and late outcomes.

INTRODUCTION

Faecal Incontinence (FI) is a distressing, often multifactorial condition which affects patients' quality of life in various degrees.

Faecal Incontinence which arises from a focal anal sphincter defect can be primarily treated with reasonably successful rates by surgical sphincter or pelvic floor repair.

A.M. Farinon (ed.), Advances in Abdominal Surgery 2002, 289-302.

Most cases, however, require a multidisciplinary therapeutic approach (surgical, medical and/or rehabilitative).

In case of severe incontinence, refractory to repeated treatment or when there is evidence of extensive anatomic loss, a sphincter substitution becomes the only alternative to a permanent faecal diversion or to a poor "diapers-conditioned" quality of life.

Reliable solutions for this challenging problem are represented today by artificial sphincter implants and transpositions of various scheletal muscles.

Regarding the latter, the muscle which showed the most wide compliance as a sphincteric substitute is the gracilis for its anatomic properties (morphology, shape, vascularization and innervation).

Gracilis muscle transposition (graciloplasty, GP) was first described 50 years ago by Kenneth LeRoy Pickrell [1], and subsequently applied by many colorectal surgeons.

In spite of this preliminary acceptance, long term results were controversial and an overall review of long-term results following Pickrell's procedure showed that successful rates did not exceed 50% of cases. Infection, ischemia and a "passive tied sling effect" were the most observed causes of late failure [2-6].

In the 80s a significant improvement was obtained by supporting graciloplasty with electrostimulation.

Following preliminary studies in the early 80s, E. Cavina in 1987 reported his first experience with short-term electrostimulation (ES) applied to a double-wrap graciloplasty after an Abdominoperineal Resection for lower rectal cancer [7-8].

In 1988, C. Baeten first applied chronic low-frequency stimulation to support graciloplasty for FI treatment (dynamic graciloplasty) with the aim of obtain a conversion of the muscular fibers type from fast to slow in order to avoid "muscular fatigue" after a continuous stimulation [9].

Since then, a chronically electrostimulated graciloplasty was applied in various colorectal centers [10-15].

Long-term results of a prospective, multicenter trial were recently reported [16], showing significant improvement of quality of life and a decrease in incontinent events 12 and 18 month after dynamic graciloplasty GP.

Successful results were obtained in 63 and 57 percent of nonstoma patients.

In spite of these positive results, dynamic graciloplasty still must be considered as a "last option" for treatment of FI because of high cost, high postoperative complications rate and the need for an experienced team during the follow-up study.

As far as the surgical aspects are regarded, various options are described either for the muscle transposition and/or electrostimulation devices implant, showing that a uniform standard approach is still to be achieved.

We present the experience of our Unit on 36 patients treated since 1991 with electrostimulated graciloplasty for end-stage FI. All patients were submitted to chronic electrostimulation protocols, using fully implantable devices

In this experience we applied many surgical options acquired from our more consistent experience with Total Anorectal Reconstruction after A.Pe.R.

MATERIALS AND METHODS

Patient distribution

From 1991 to date, 36 patients (M: 4 - F: 35; mean age 43.8 yrs - range 16-75 yrs) were treated with chronically ESGP for end-stage incontinence (Levels IV and V of N.S. Williams' scale).

All patients except seven (extensive anal disruption following pelvic traumas) were previously submitted to medical/surgical/rehabilitative procedures and mean duration of incontinence (with the exclusion of trauma patients) was 120 months (range 12-456 months) (Tab. 2).

All patients were extensively investigated using continence scores and diaries, EMM, EMG, defecography and, more recently, with endorectal u.s. and quality of life tests ; a detailed informed consent, approved by the University-Hospital Ethical Committee was adopted in all cases.

The aetiology of incontinence is reported in Table 1.

Table 1. Etiology of faecal incontinence

CONGENITAL FI	Anal atresia	3	8%
(5 cases)	Myelomeningocele	1	4%
	Rectovaginal fistula	1	3%
ACQUIRED FI	Traumatic	7	19%
(31 cases)	Obstetric	7	19%
	Iatrogenic	8	22%
	Idiopathic	4	11%
	Rectal prolapse	3	8%
	Neurogenic	1	3%
	Verneuil's disease	1	3%

Continence was evaluated using modified N.S. Williams scale.

Preoperative evaluation was based on a continence diary in which patients referred all incontinence events for a 14 days length.

Table 2. Summary of patient history in 36 patients treated with electrostimulated graciloplasty since 1991

Patient	Sex	Age	Etiology of incontinence	Type	Previous treatment	Duration of FI
080-DME	F	71	Idiopathic	ACQ	None	5 years
081-VE	F	19	Myelomeningocele	CON	None	19 years
083-RM	F	38	Iatrogenic (rectal prolapse + hemorrhoids)	ACQ	Rectopexy	2 months
086-PD	M	16	Traumatic: traumatic hemipelvectomy	ACQ	Left colostomy	3 months
088-BN	F	73	Idiopathic	ACQ	Biofeedback	5 years
089-MG	M	23	Traumatic: pelvic crushing	ACQ	Left colostomy	8 months
091-CG	F	25	Anal atresia	CON	Pull-through	25 years
093-MW	F	55	Post-partum + constipation	ACQ	Left hemicolectomy, rectopexy	2 years
094-AG	F	19	Traumatic: gunshot wound (hunting rifle)	ACQ	Left colostomy Cannulation of anal canal with Petzer probe	2 years
095-CM	F	46	Post-partum	ACQ	Sphincteroplasty	10 years
097-CD	F	38	High congenital rectovaginal fistula	CON	None	38 years
098-IG	F	63	Iatrogenic, post-fistulectomy	ACQ	Biofeedback	18 months
102-FN	M	23	Anal atresia	CON	Pull-through, fistulectomy, fistulectomy + sphincteroplasty	6 years
111-LE	F	38	Iatrogenic, post-fistulectomy	ACQ	Multiple fistulectomies and sphincteroplasties	4 years
119-MM	F	61	Post-partum	ACQ	None	1 year
120-SA	F	72	Iatrogenic + rectocele	ACQ	Postanal repair, anterior vaginoplasty	2 years
121-TP	F	37	Post-partum	ACQ	None	17 months
124-BC	M	50	Verneuil's disease	ACQ	Colostomy	1 year
125-PM	F	52	Iatrogenic	ACQ	Biofeedback	3 years
127-SL	F	50	Iatrogenic post-fistulectomy e rectopexy	ACQ	None	20 years
128-SL	M	39	Iatrogenic post-fistulectomy	ACQ	Sphincteroplasty + colostomy	7 years
129-SL	F	58	Post-partum	ACQ	None	21 years
130-GP	M	24	Neurogenic	ACQ	Biofeedback	8 years
133-VC	F	75	Iatrogenic + descending perineum sysdrome	ACQ	Biofeedback	9 years
134-MMP	F	56	Idiopathic	ACQ	None	9 years
135-CM	F	27	Anal atresia	CON	Pull-through, anoplasty, Pickrell procedure	27 years
138-SM	F	46	Traumatic: following sexual abuse	ACQ	Hartmann procedure	2 years
139-FD	M	29	Traumatic: pelvic crushing e penetrating lesione of the rectum	ACQ	Left colostomy	2 years
144-FM	M	44	Rectal prolapse in spina bifida	ACQ	None	2 years
145-CR	F	60	Rectal prolapse	ACQ	None	1 year
146-PL	F	70	Rectal prolapse	ACQ	None	2 years
151-BE	F	65	Post-partum	ACQ	None	30 years
152-RM	F	60	Idiopathic	ACQ	Biofeedback	1 year
159-LGL	M	14	Traumatic: pelvic crushing with anorectal disinsertion + demolition of the sphincteral apparatus and pelvic floor (crushing trauma)	ACQ	Left colostomy	1 year
160-DMS	F	22	Traumatic: pelvic crushing (car accident) with penetrating lesion of the rectum + demolition of the sphincteral apparatus and of the perineum	ACQ	Left colostomy	5 years
161-BM	F	61	Post-partum	ACQ	Biofeedback	40 years

Stoma patients were evaluated by enema retention test using ortograde porridge enema and on the basis of the anatomic loss of sphincteric apparatus (Fig. 1-2)

Standard preoperative evaluation included endorectal U.S., anal manometry with VectorVolumetry evaluation, and EMG. Defecography was carried out in selected cases only.

At present, 32 patients remain at the study evaluation; two patient died during the follow up interval, two were converted to abdominal colostomy . Mean follow-up length was 49.78 months (average: 55.7, range: 6-178, S.D.: 39.4 months.).

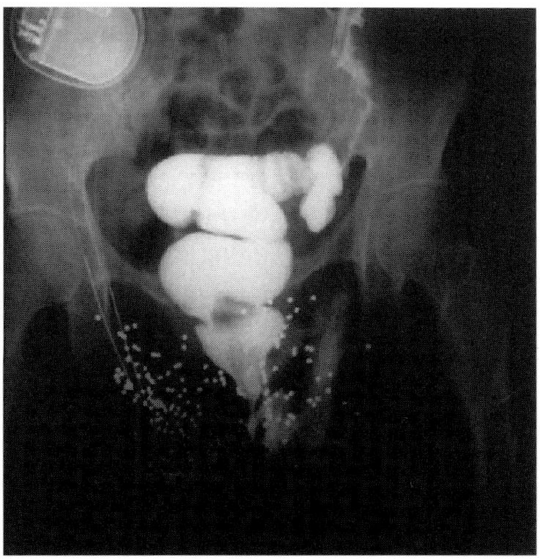

Figure 1. Gunshot wound.

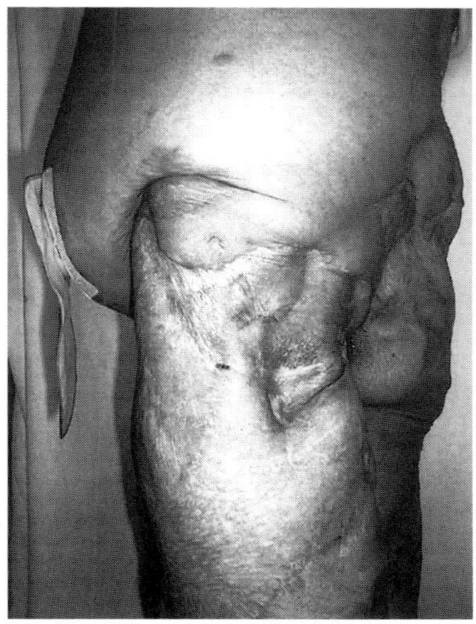

Figure 2. Pelvic trauma following automotive accident.
See color plates.

Surgical Technique

Main technical aspects of ESGP concern gracilis mobilisation and transposition, graciloplasty configuration, electrostimulation (ES) devices implant and protocols to increase fatigue resistance of transposed muscles.

As far as surgical timing is concerned, all steps (mobilisation, transposition, devices implant) are usually carried out simultaneously; if the outcome is uneventful, ES is started in the early p.o. period (3rd-4th p.o day).

Gracilis mobilization and transposition (Fig. 3, 4, 5, 6)

Long shape, superficial position and good vascularization are the anatomic properties which make the gracilis suitable for transposition. In fact, the muscle can be easily freed through three small incisions.

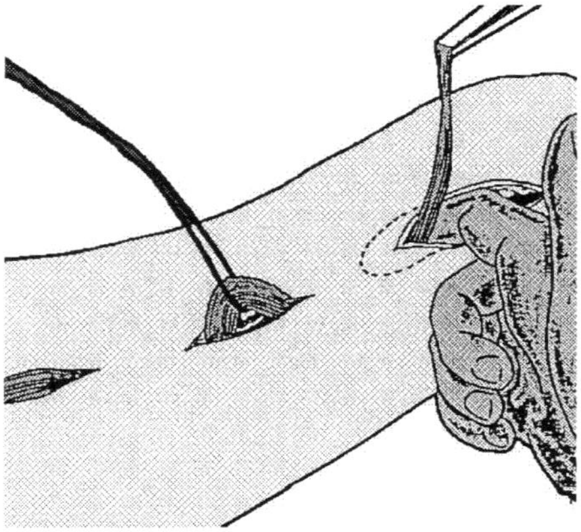

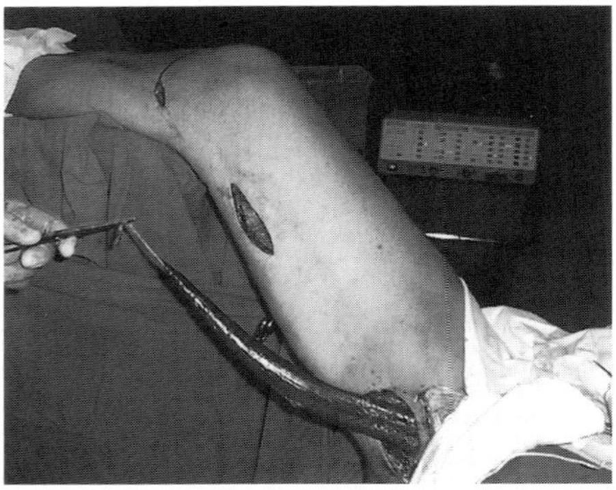

Figure 3,4. Gracilis mobilization. *See color plates.*

The patient is placed in a Lloyd's position, modified in order to obtain the widest abduction of both legs.

The first incision is usually carried out at the middle third of the thigh where the muscular belly is easily palpable during lower limb passive abduction.

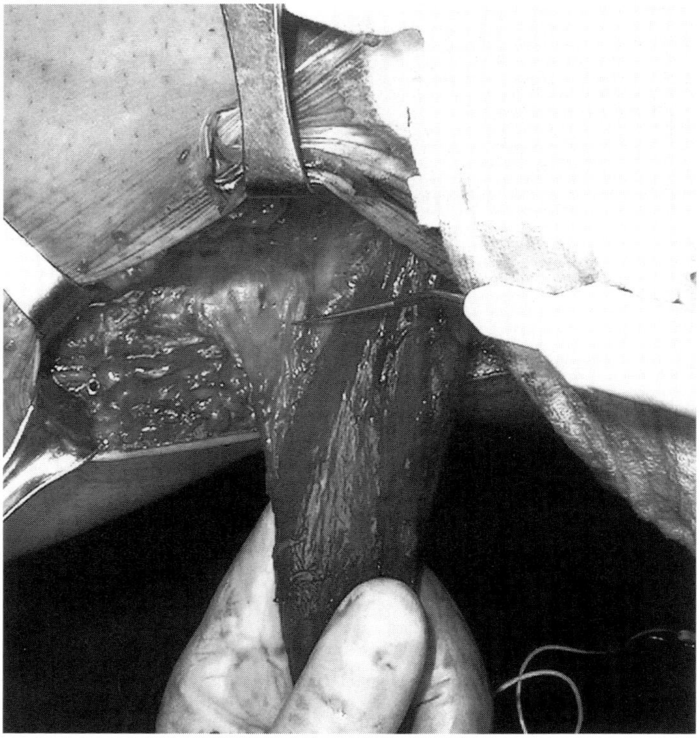

Figure 5. Nerve identification. *See color plates.*

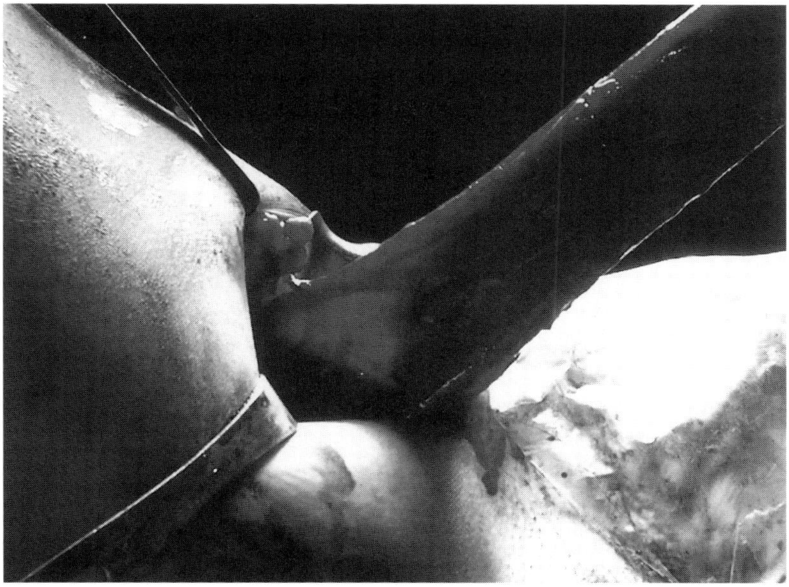

Figure 6. Nerve entry. *See color plates.*

Once the muscle is circularly freed and surrounded with a rubber band it can be proximally and distally mobilized, on the aid of a gentle traction applied to a rubber band.

At this level, one or two accessory arteries which arise from the superficial femoral artery are usuallyfound and care must be taken in their identification, legation and section.

During this surgical step a small gauze sponge and titanium clips (Ligaclip Ethicon MCA) are extremely helpful in minimizing tissue trauma.

The sacrifice of these accessory arteries is usually uneventful and no evidence of early ischemia was noted in any performed transposition.

A second incision is usually carried out at the level of the tibial shaft where the distal tendon of the muscle is inserted, being the middle part of the "pes anserinus

The distal insertion of the muscle is very easily palpable above the tibia adding a gentle traction of the already freed muscle.

Once the distal tendon is detached from its tibial insertion and the muscle is digitally freed from the adjacent structures, the gracilis is pulled out from the first incision.

The last step of gracilis mobilization is represented by the identification of its proximal insertion which is carried out through a 4-5 cms incision, made orthogonally to the inferior linea glutea.

The muscle is visible under the aponeurotic extension of the fascia lata which covers the anterior part of the muscle, joining it with the adductors muscles.

Great attention must be paid to avoid any damage to the muscle and above all to the nervous and vascular pedicle. At this level the nerve and the main artery (which emanates from the profunda femoral artery) join the muscle from the deepest and more external part of its insertion. A balance between an extensive mobilization and the preservation of a good vascular supply must be applied during this phase.

The innervation of the muscle is provided by a single main nerve which enters the muscle and gives one medial and two postero-lateral intramuscular branches. In order to guarantee a full muscular recruitment during stimulation, it is important to identify these branches before any electrode implant, using an external stimulator.

Once the gracilis is completely freed, it must be transposed to the perineum to encircle the anal canal. A circular tunnel around the anus is preliminarly performed, usually through two lateral or polar incisions.

Great attention must be paid during this phase to obtain a subcutaneous space sufficiently wide to contain the muscle and sufficiently close to the rectal wall. At the same time any rectal and/or vaginal damage must be prevented. In case of previous scars and/or fibrosis, a subcutaneous injection of saline solution (eventually added with norepinephine) can be helpful in dissociating subcutaneous tissues.

Any rectal and/or vaginal perforation-if small- must be promptly identified and carefully repaired with absorbable suture (dexon) adding a meticulous local cleansing with povidone .

The last step is represented by the transposition of the muscle, paying attention to avoid any compression exerted by the wall of the subcutaneous tunnel.

Graciloplasty configuration

Various configuration of GP are described, having the common intent to completely surround in a circular shape the anal canal.

In single-wrap GP (which is at present the preferred option) the muscle is transposed following an alfa-shaped configuration (Fig. 7-10) while the the tendon is fixed to the skin and not to a stiff structure (e.g. the ischiatic bone, as originally described by Pickrell's).

This type of tendon fixation is very useful in assessing the right tension of GP around the anus allowing also a further traction in the p.o. time, is necessary.

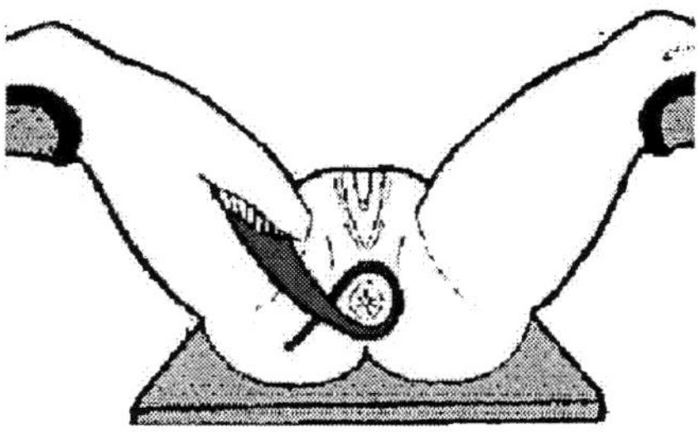

Figure 7. Alfa wrap configuration.

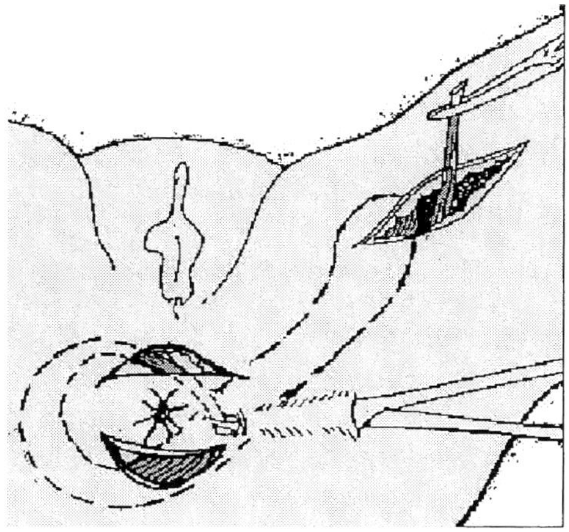

Figure 8. Alfa wrap.

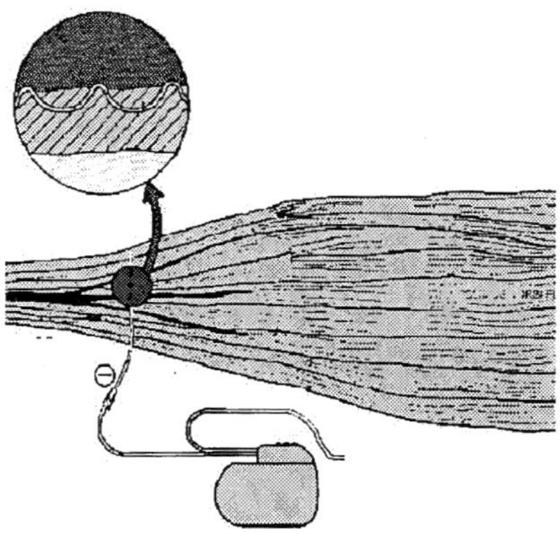

Figure 9. Electrodes implant.

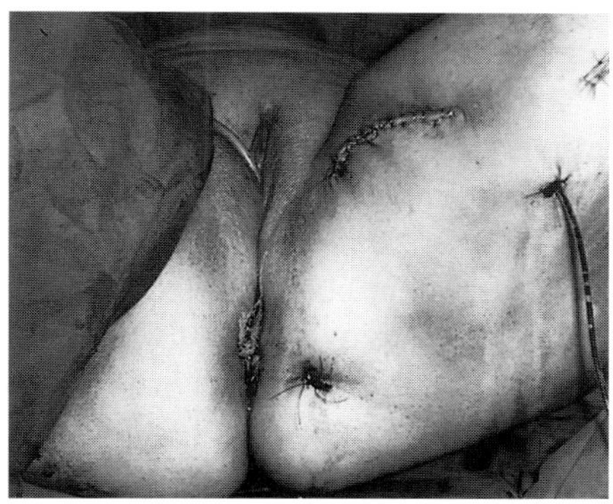

Figure 10. End of gp. *See color plates.*

In double-wrap GPs (which are rarely applied to GPs for FI) one gracilis was used to reproduce the pubo-rectalis sling function (retroanal transposition).

Electrostimulation Devices Implant

Platinum-iridium electrodes and Implantable Pulse Generators (IPG) were used in all cases to stimulate muscles. Electrodes implant must be done in such a way to allow the diffusion of electrical stimulus to the whole muscular pattern, obtaining a full recruitment of muscular fibers.

In theory, the best to way to obtain a "full stimulation" is to apply electrical stimulus directly on the main nerve. In practice, many risks contraindicate a direct electrode implant: direct or indirect nerve damage, vascular damage and electrode displacement.

In practice, the most used technique is based on an "intramuscular" placement of two electrodes, passed through the muscle, orthogonally to its main axis.

The main advantages of this method of implanting electrodes in this way are safety and effectiveness as long as the active electrode crosses the muscle completely.

Before the definitive electrodes implant, gracilis contraction can be verified with a temporary stimulation (Disposable Nerve Locator - Pulsatron N.S.-Weck Inc., Princeton, NJ) applied directly to the muscle surface and/or the nerve.

After a first experience with intramuscular implants we described a new "over-the-nerve and intramuscular" implant, obtaining a significant improvement of contraction at lower amplitudes of stimulation [17]. The first way described (intramuscular) is however to be preferred during the "learning curve" period.

After their implant, electrodes are connected to an Implantable Pulse Generator (Quadripolar IPG Itrel II model 7424, Medtronic), placed in a subcutaneous abdominal pocket in a convenient position for further activation by the patient.

Minimum amplitude necessary for some fibers contraction (just contracting threshold) and full fibers contraction (full contraction threshold) are recorded.

A correct implant with lowest contraction thresholds is crucial for further stimulation due to the fact that perineural fibrosis usually causes a progressive increase of the amplitudes necessary for the best stimulation.

I.V. cephalosporin and local flushing with gentamycin are adopted to prevent local infection, which represents the most serious postoperative complication.

Electrostimulation protocols

Electrostimulation (ES) of transposed muscles has been proved to be effective "per-se" in atrophy prevention and early vascular neogenesis; besides that, ES can offer an excellent approach for post-operative biofeedback exercises.

In addition to these properties, a long-term applied ES can induce metabolic and structural changes in scheletal muscles, allowing a conversion of the muscular pattern from fast-twitch (typical of scheletal muscles) to slow-twitch fiber conversion.

This conversion is possible when sheletal muscles are stimulated with low-frequency parameters and was applied in "dynamic graciloplasty" to increase neosphincter resistance to prolonged contraction necessary to obtain continence.

Following these principle, in our experience a chronic low-frequency (15Hz) electrostimulation was adopted in all cases.

Electrostimulation protocols were based on a first period (mean: 8 weeks) of cyclic stimulation during which off/on stimulation ratios were progressively decreased from 12:1 to 1:2.

This training period was followed by a continuous electrostimulated regimen.

Depending on muscular response , the usual amplitudes necessary to obtain a fecal continence ranged from 1.5 to 3.5 volts (mean: 3.3 volts) .

Once stimulation parameters were well assessed, and the neosphincter was able to be continuosly stimulated, patients could switch "on or off" the stimulator at their convenience using an external magnet.

Standard electrostimulation features are summarized in Table 3

Table 3. Standard electrostimulation features

Time	Features
Early postoperative period	- Stimulation is applied as soon as possible in the p.o. Period, usually for few hours/day starting from 4th/5th p.o. day - The electrostimulation is cyclic (on/off alternate periods) and the voltage is set according to parameters observed during the operation (stimulation thresholds)
Early training period	- Cyclic stimulation length is progressively increased until 24 hours/day and the voltage is set to obtain continence - The patient is discharged and the training period starts
Training period	- 8 weeks of cyclic stimulation, during which the on/off ratio is progressively increased until a resistance to a continuous stimulation is reached.
Post training period	- Continuous stimulation, activated or deactivated by the patient at his convenience

RESULTS

Early and late morbidity

No postoperative mortality (40 p.o. days) was observed. Mean hospital stay was high (36 days) due to the time necessary for treatment of coexisting diseases (as in patients with pelvic traumas) and postoperative complications.

Mean postoperative time was 20 days (min 14, max 50) and in 76% of patients the outcome was uneventful.

The overall complications rate was 19%; in 3 patients complication led to a GP failure.

The most significant complications observed were:

- local infection involving in various degrees subcutaneous tissue and/or transposed muscle, implanted electrodes and abdominal pouch;
- muscular ischemia, secondary to infection (muscular swelling-compression-ischemia);
- electrodes displacement.

Key points in complications prevention and treatment were: correct and clean technique, prompt diagnosis of any perineal fluid or blood collection, no exitation in draining these collections avoiding septic progression.

Functional results

All patients were submitted to regular clinical and physiological examination: continence scores, as well as EMM values, were recorded at 2, 4, 6, 12, 18, 24 months after ESGP and later at 6 month intervals.

Mean follow-up length was 49.78 months (average: 55.7, range: 6-130, S.D.: 39.4 months.).

To bypass logistic difficulties (70% of patients live over 300 kms away from our Unit), a ready-on-call line and facilitation for periodic audits were adopted .

At present, 30 patients are clinically evaluable (3 pts. with colostomy were excluded, 2 died, 1 is lost to the f-up) and 21 of them (70%) are continent to liquid and solid stools (I-II levels of N.S. Williams' Scale).

Preoperative and postoperative (6 months) mean EMM values rose from 34 to 59 mm.Hg (Resting Pressure) and from 53 to 112 mm.Hg (Maximum Voluntary Pressure).

In all patients mean defecation frequency passed from 4.1 times/day (max: 12/day) to 1.4 times/day (max.: 4/day) with a significant decrease in diaper use (from 4.4/day to 1.3/day).

CONCLUSIONS

Continence restoration still remain a challenge, in particular when multiple procedures failed and a permanent stoma appears to be the only alternative to a full incontinence.

Surgical substitution of an inefficient sphincter can be obtained by an electrostimulated graciloplasty in most patients suffering from direct severe trauma and sphincter disruption. In these patients the overall success rate expected is very high, ranging about 90%.

Very poor results can be expected, on the contrary, when FI is linked to congenital disorders, e.g. anal atresia.

In the remaining patients chronic constipation, postoperative complications and coexisting diseases (e.g in spina bifida) are the main causes of partial failure.

As far as the quality of life and continence are concerned, our experience confirms what has been observed in the recent Multicenter Trial with a difference of better overall results (70% vs 60%), mainly lonked to the previous experience on this field.

The procedure we adopted was based on a simultaneous muscular and electrostimulation devices implant to allow early stimulation of the transposed muscle. In comparison with other more complex procedures (two or three steps) , the surgical outcome did not appear to be affected by this choice.

Analizing failures, infection which extends to the muscular tunnels appears to play a dominant role in postoperative contractile impairment.

A further consideration must be made on the training of surgical teams in managing complications, programming correct stimulation parameters and their giving full availability to a complex follow-up study.

Reconstruction of the anal sphincter remains a surgical challenge and must be considered as the last procedure to be adopted in faecal incontinence treatment; in spite of that, in our and other Authors' experiences, gracilis transposition and chronic electrostimulation appears to be the most reliable option to restore continence.

Even considering the weight of the learning curve, it can be asserted that when adopting ESGP, continence can be fully restored in more then 60% of the patients and quality of life improved in half of the remaining.

REFERENCES

1. Pickrell KL, Broadbent TR, Masters FW, Metzger JT. Construction of a rectal sphincter and restoration of anal continence by transplanting the gracilis muscle: a report of four cases in children. *Ann Surg* 1952; 135: 853-62.
2. Corman ML. Follow-up evaluation of gracilis muscle transposition for fecal incontinence. *Dis Colon Rectum* 1980; 23: 552-5.
3. Leguit P, Van Baal JG, Brummelkamp WH. Gracilis muscle transposition in the treatment of fecal incontinence: long-term follow-up and evaluation of anal pressure recordings. *Dis Colon Rectum* 1985; 28: 1-4.
4. Yoshioka K, Keighley MRB. Clinical and manometric assessment of gracilis muscle transplant for fecal incontinence. *Dis Colon Rectum* 1988; 31: 767-9.
5. Christiansen J, Sorenson M, Rasmussen OO. Gracilis muscle transposition for fecal incontinence. *Br J Surg* 1990; 77: 1039-40.
6. Faucheron JL, Hannoun L, Thome C, Parc R. Is fecal continence improved by nonstimulated gracilis muscle transposition? *Dis Colon Rectum* 1994; 37: 979-83.
7. Cavina E, Seccia M, Evangelista G, Chiarugi M, Buccianti P, Chirico A, et al. Construction of a continent perineal colostomy by using electrostimulated gracilis muscles after abdomino-perineal resection: personal technique and experience with 32 cases. *Ital J Surg Sci* 1987; 17: 305-14.

8. Cavina E, Seccia M, Evangelista G, Chiarugi M, Buccianti P, Tortora A, et al. Perineal colostomy and electrostimulated gracilis "neosphincter" after abdomino-perineal resection of the colon and anorectum: a surgical experience and follow-up study in 47 cases. *Int J Colorectal Dis* 1990; 5: 6-11.
9. Baeten CGMI, Spaans F, Fluks A. An implanted neuromuscular stimulator for fecal continence following previously implanted gracilis muscle:report of a case. *Dis Colon Rectum* 1988;31(2):134-7.
10. Seccia M, Menconi C, Balestri R, Cavina E. Study protocols and functional results in 86 electrostimulated graciloplasties. *Dis Colon Rectum* 1994; 37: 897-904.
11. Baeten CG, Konsten J, Spaans F, Visser R, Habets AMMC, Bourgeois IM, et al. Dynamic graciloplasty for treatment of faecal incontinence. *Lancet* 1991; 338: 1163-5.
12. Williams NS, Hallan RI, Koeze TH, Pilot MA, Watkins ES. Construction of a neoanal sphincter by transposition of the gracilis muscle and prolonged neuromuscular stimulation for the treatment of faecal incontinence. *Ann R Coll Surg Eng* 1990; 72: 108-13.
13. Williams NS, Patel J, George BD, Hallan RI, Watkins ES. Development of an electrically stimulated neo-anal sphincter. *Lancet* 1991; 338: 1166-9.
14. Madoff RD, Baeten CG, Christiansen J, Rosen HR, Williams NS, Heine JA, et al. Standards for anal sphincter replacement. *Dis Colon Rectum* 2000; 43: 135-41.
15. Madoff RD, Rosen HR, Baeten CG, LaFontaine LJ, Cavina E, Devesa M, et al. Safety and efficacy of dynamic muscle plasty for anal incontinence: lessons from a prospective, multicenter trial. *Gastroenterology* 1999; 116: 549-56.
16. Baeten CG, Bailey HR, Bakka A, Belliveau P, Berg E, Buie WD, Burnstein MJ, Christiansen J, Coller JA, Galandiuk S, LaFontaine LJ, Lange J, Madoff RD, Matzel KE, Pahlman L, Parc R, Reilly JC, Seccia M, Thorson AG, Vernava AM 3rd, Wexner S.Safety and efficacy of dynamic graciloplasty for fecal incontinence: report of a prospective, multicenter trial. Dynamic Graciloplasty Therapy Study Group. *Dis. Colon Rectum* 2000; 6(43):743
17. Cavina E, Seccia M, Banti P, Zocco G. Anorectal reconstruction after abdominoperineal resection. Experience with double-wrap graciloplasty supported by low-frequency electrostimulation. *Dis Colon Rectum* 1998; 41: 1010-6.

CHAPTER 21

RESTORATION OF ANAL CONTINENCE WITH THE ARTIFICIAL BOWEL SPHINCTER (ABS ACTICON ™)

Memeo V, Altomare DF, Rinaldi M, Veglia A, Petrolino M, Guglielmi A.
Department of Emergency and Organ Transplantation, Section of General Surgery and Liver Transplantation, University of Bari, Bari, Italy

Abstract

Background A new prosthetic device, the Acticon™ artificial anal sphincter, has recently been introduced for treating severe faecal incontinence. We review the results of our experience with this procedure.

Method The data on 8 patients treated with an artificial anal sphincter for severe faecal incontinence, were reviewed after a mean follow-up of 15 months.

Results: Early complications included perineal and abdominal wound infection in 1 patient requiring removal of the device, and a haematoma in the abdominal wound in one patient. Dehiscence of the perineal wound occurred in 3 cases and cuff disconnection in one more. After activation of the device, the cuff had to be removed in 1 patient for rectal erosion. Overall, 1 patient had complete removal of the device and another removal of the cuff only. One more was reoperated for reconnection of the anal cuff. Five patients available for long term evaluation (more than 12 months follow-up) had a major improvement of faecal continence. The mean preoperative resting pressure was 18 ± 9mmHg and the mean preoperative squeezing pressure 26 ± 9 mmHg. After implantation of the anal cuff was in place deflated the mean anal pressure rose to 30 ± 12 mmHg with the cuff deflated and to 67 ± 11mmHg with the device activated ($p < 0.05$). The AMS incontinence score decreased significantly from 107 ± 12 (range 75-120) to 16 ± 4 (range 0-24) after implantation of the Acticon Neosphincter ($p<0.05$). Similar figures were observed using the CGS score: from 16.3 ± 3 (range 11-20) to 0.8 ± 1.5 (range 0-3), $p<0.05$. Three patients developed symptoms of obstructed defaecation which regressed in 2.

Conclusions Full continence was achieved after Acticon neosphincter implantation in 4 of the cases. Early infection and rectal erosion, together with difficulty in evacuating, are still the major concerns with this technique.

A.*M. Farinon (ed.), Advances in Abdominal Surgery 2002*, 303-312.

INTRODUCTION

Until the 1970s surgeons devoted most of their efforts to reducing operative mortality and morbidity but in recent years, especially in the last two decades, increasing attention has been paid improving the patients quality of life. In this perspective the treatment of faecal incontinence has posed a major challenge for surgeons. New diagnostic tools and operative strategies have been developed including very sophisticated and highly technological solutions.

The Acticon ABS neosphincter is one of the most recent prosthetic devices introduced to treat severe faecal incontinence [1] (Fig. 1).

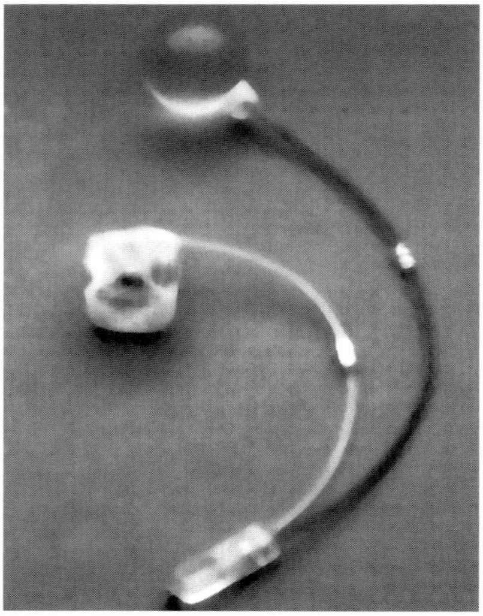

Figure 1. The Artifical Bowel Sphincter
See color plates.

It is a totally implantable silicone anal sphincter composed of an occlusive inflatable anal cuff of variable size connected to a control pump and to a pressure balloon. The system is semi-automatic and requires the patient to deflate the anal cuff by pressing the control pump located in the scrotum or the labia when he/she feels the stimulus to defaecate. The liquid shifted from the anal cuff to the pressure balloon is returned back to the neoanal sphincter within 5-10 minutes thus spontaneously restoring continence.

This kind of device was developed in the 1970s by urologists to control urinary incontinence (AMS 800™) and was first applied to treat faecal incontinence by Christiansen in 1987 [2]. Since then the device has been extensively modified and adapted to the new function.

PATIENTS AND METHODS

The current approach to patients with faecal incontinence in our Institute is summarised in the algorithm described in Figure 2 (where the role of ABS implant is also shown).

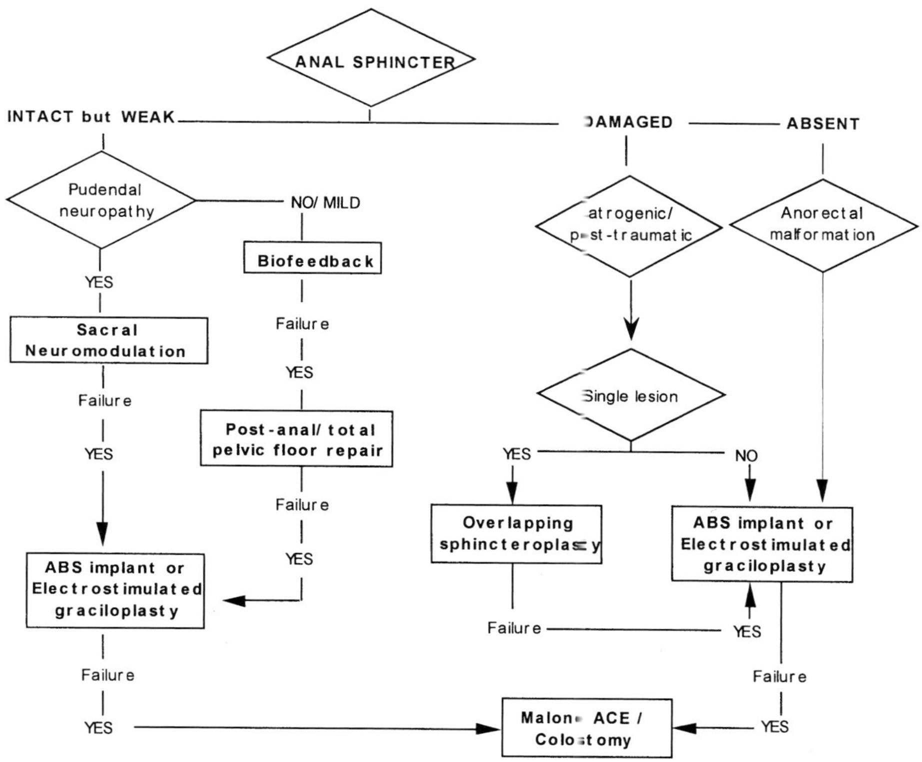

Figure 2. Therapeutic algorithm for the treatment of faecal incontinence

Eight patients (7 women and 1 man) with a mean age of 56 (range 19 - 72) years underwent implantation of the Acticon Neosphincter™ Artificial Bowel Sphincter (American Medical Systems, Minneapolis, MN, USA) over a 24-month period. The patients were affected by total faecal incontinence of idiopathic origin in all but one, in whom the cause of incontinence was imperforate anus, operated on in childhood and subsequently treated by electrostimulated graciloplasty, but with poor results. The median duration of symptoms was 8 years (range 1-25). One patient had associated urinary incontinence, previously treated with Burch's operation. One patient had undergone the Milligan and Morgan procedure for haemorroids. In 4 patients there was associated complete rectal prolapse (full thickness), treated by the Altemeier procedure (perineal rectosigmoidectomy with levatorplasty) performed six weeks before Acticon implantation in one case and by abdominal rectopexy (Wells' procedure) in two cases, performed prior to implantation in 1 case and during implantation in the other. The last patient underwent the Delorme procedure with sphincteroplasty 6 months before implantation; a Percutaneous Sacral Nerve electrostimulation test was subsequently performed to see whether this patient could benefit from a permanent sacral nerve neuromodulation, but was unsuccessful. Two patients with rectal prolapse were also affected by liver cirrhosis with a very low platelets count, while the other two suffered from diabetes.

Preoperative assessment

The severity of incontinence was evaluated with two different scoring systems, the Continence Grading Scale (CGS) and the American Medical System (AMS) score.

Anorectal manometry was performed to evaluate the mean resting and squeezing pressure and the length of the high pressure zone in the anal canal.

Electrophysiological tests including electromyography (EMG) and pudendal nerve terminal motor latency (PNTML) revealed signs of neurogenic sphincter weakness in all patients.

Trans-anal ultrasound was done to investigate sphincter integrity.

Cinedefaecography was performed in two patients, showing a large anterior rectocele in one and perineal descent in the other.

Postoperative assessment

Six months after activation of the artificial anal sphincter, all patients were reassessed by CGS [3] and AMS score [4]. At the same time anal manometry was performed to evaluate the maximal anal pressure with the cuff inflated.

Procedure

All patients gave informed consent and were apprised of the potential risks and complications.

Full mechanical preparation of the colon with osmotic solutions and enemas was performed the day before the operation. Women underwent vaginal disinfection with povidone iodate dilute solution.

Antibiotic prophylaxis with metronidazole and cephalosporins was administered in all the patients. The cirrhotic patients received fresh plasma and platelets transfusions before and during the operation. Patients were placed in the lithotomy position under general anaesthesia; in order to insert the cuff around the anal canal, a single anterior transverse perineal incision was made in 5 patients while in the other 3 a bilateral perianal incision was preferred. A tunnel was created around the anal canal by blunt dissection to allow circumferential placement of the cuff. A cuff sizer was passed around the anal canal to determine the approximate cuff length needed.

A suprapubic incision allowed placement of the pressure reservoir balloon in the laterovesical preperitoneal space, behind the rectus abdominus muscle; the tubing from the cuff was then tunnelled up towards the suprapubic incision. The balloon was filled with isosmotic radiopaque solution (Iopamiro 300) and connected to the cuff tube to enable the cuff pressurisation. The balloon was then drained and refilled. The control pump was implanted in the labia majora or in the scrotum, using blunt dissection to create a dependent pouch on the opposite side to the patient's dominant hand. Finally the pump, tubing and cuff were connected. A control X-Ray was performed postoperatively with the cuff deflated and inflated (Fig. 3-4)

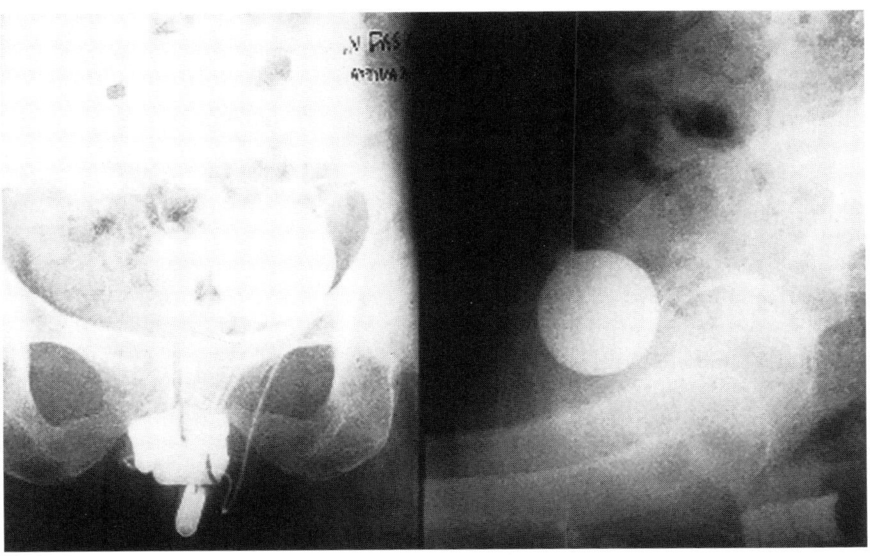

Figure 3. Pelvis X-Ray with the anal cuff inflated

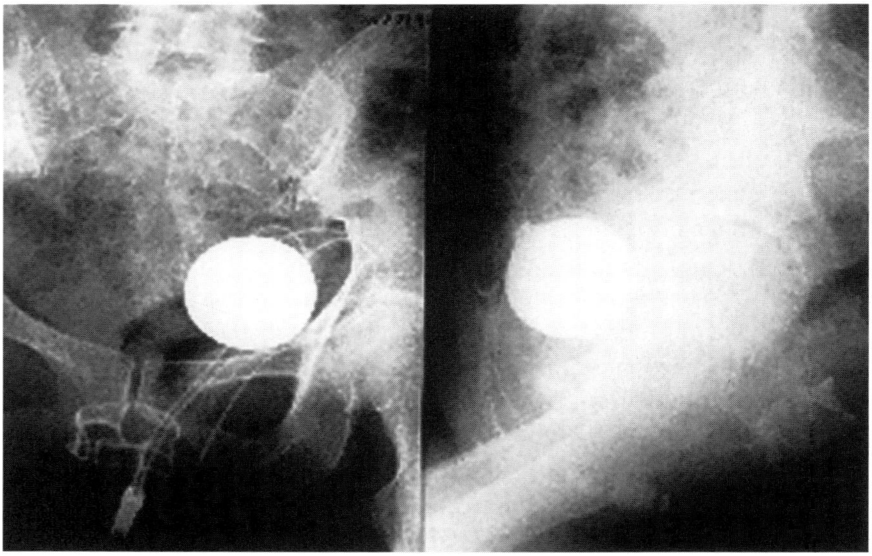

Figure 4 Pelvis X-Ray with the anal cuff deflated

Mean duration of the procedure was 80 min (range 45 - 150 min.)

The device was left deactivated (cuff deflated) for six weeks after implantation in order to allow complete wound healing and consolidation the pre-vesical space made to house the pressure balloon.

RESULTS

Mean follow-up was 15 months, with a range from 2 to 23 months.

Early complications

Infection of the perineal and abdominal wounds occurred in one diabetic patient, requiring explantation of the whole device. One haematoma occurred at the site of implantation of the balloon and required surgical drainage. Partial dehiscence of the perineal anterior wound occurred in 3 cases: in 2, surgical treatment was needed (rotating skin flap (Fig. 5) and direct wound repair, respectively). The third case healed spontaneously.

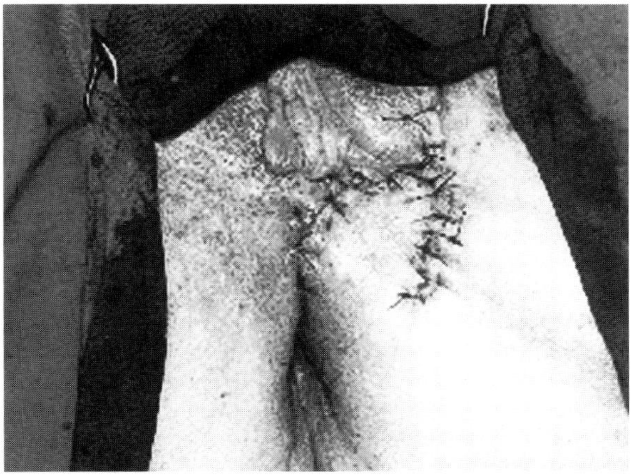

Figure 5.

Rotating skin flap for perineal repair *See color plates.*

Late complications

Three months after activation of the device, one patient, previously treated with the Altemeier operation for complete rectal prolapse, complained of anal pain. Investigation showed rectal erosion by the cuff which was removed. Accidental unhooking of the cuff required a re-operation in another patient.

Functional results

Five patients were available for long term evaluation (longer than 12 months) because 1 had had the whole device removed, one just the anal cuff, and the third is still waiting for the device to be activated. Three had some difficulty with defaecation after ABS activation; two of them improved significantly with laxatives and/or micro-enemas. The other had progressive worsening of feacal impaction due to a recto-anal intussusception, demonstrated by defaecography, that required rectopexy.

A successful outcome was obtained in the remaining 4 patients, with full continence to liquid and solid stools, confirmed by the AMS and CGS incontinence scores.

Manometric data: The mean preoperative resting pressure was 18± 9mmHg and the mean preoperative squeezing pressure 26±9 mmHg. After implantation, with the cuff deflated the mean anal pressure rose to 30 ± 12 mmHg and when the device was activated to 67± 11 ($p < 0.05$) (Fig. 6). The AMS incontinence score decreased significantly from 107±12 (range 75-120) to 16±4 (range 0-24) after Acticon Neosphincter implantation ($p<0.05$). Similar figures were observed using the CGS score: from 16.3±3 (range 11-20) to 0.8 ±1.5 (range 0-3), $p<0.05$.

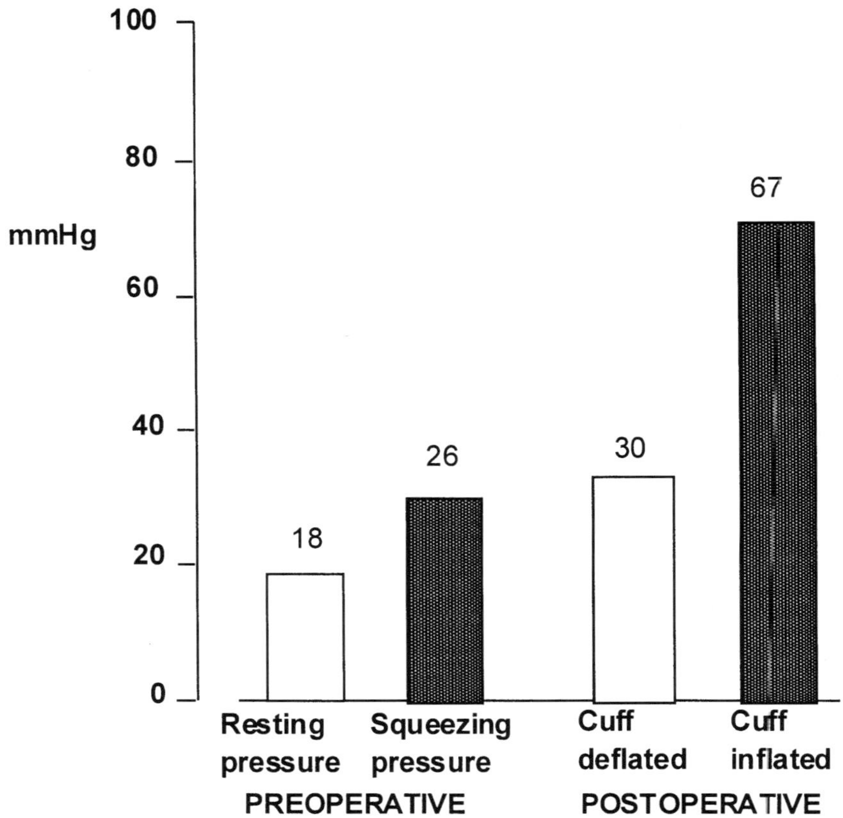

Figure 6. Anal manometry before and after artificial bowel sphincter implant

DISCUSSION

Faecal incontinence is the result of a complex integration of motor and sensory anorectal functions. The role of the artificial bowel sphincter is simply to restore a high pressure zone to the anal canal in the case of sphincter failure. Therefore, it may not be possible to restore full continence if the sensory pathway is damaged for example or if there is an associated colonic motility disorder. Moreover excessive scar tissue or infective foci around the anus following repeated surgery for complex anal fistulas or Crohn Disease are contraindication for the ABS implant. The correct indication for this procedure is idiopathic faecal incontinence (with an intact, non-functioning anal sphincter and an intact sensory pathway) or a damaged sphincter not amenable to direct repair or after failure of this approach [5].

The results of our study compare favourably with other experiences in Europe [6 - 8] and confirm that the Acticon ABS neosphincter may play an important role in the treatment of end-stage faecal incontinence.

This device is a valid alternative to the more complex electrostimulated graciloplasty which carries a similar success rate. However, comparison with this technique is not reliable because there are no randomised trials in medical literature comparing the two methods. Results from small series seems to be equivalent with a success rate ranging from 60 to 80%, although the role of the learning curve should not be underestimated. Several technical tips need to be refined. Infection of the device is certainly the most fearful complication and every effort should be made to prevent this, including accurate skin and bowel preparation, protection from the accidental passage of bowel contents through the anus by suturing a finger glove to the anal margin (this enables the surgeon to put a finger into the anus during the perianal manoeuvres without causing contamination), vaginal disinfection, frequent change of unpowdered gloves, wound irrigation with povidone-iodine solution, the use of antibiotic solution when preparing the different parts of the device and, finally, the use of two different surgical team and instruments for the perineal and abdominal phases of the procedure. The use of a protective stoma has been demonstrated to have no influence on the infection rate [9].

Some technical complications like cuff unbuttoning, and the more serious skin or rectal erosion by the cuff, are often a consequence of imperfect surgery. Too close a proximity of the device to the perianal skin should be prevented by placing it deeply within the perineum just below the pelvic floor, while mucosal erosion means that the cuff has been placed directly on the rectal wall. In one of our cases the cuff was placed on the scar of a previous colo-anal suture after an Altemeier procedure for rectal prolapse. The management of incontinent patients with an associated complete rectal prolapse should be further investigated by prospective trials as it not always clear whether the prolapse should be treated before the ABS implant or not [10].

Provided these problems are overcome, the neosphincter works well, re-establishing full continence in most patients. One of the main problems in follow-up is the onset of evacuation difficulties, which were seen in 2 of our patients and in about 20% of patients in other series [11-12]. The reason for this is not always apparent, but this inconvenience has been noted even after graciloplasty [13, 14]. Sometimes the reason is clear (rectal intussusception, rectocele), but sometimes not. Too a width an anal cuff has sometimes been blamed for this functional complication [15].

Long-term functional results are being awaited, which should establish the definitive role of this promising new procedure.

REFERENCES

1. Lehur PA, Glemain P, Bruley Des Varannes S: Artificial bowel sphincter in severe fecal incontinence. In Diagnosis and Treatment of fecal incontinence. Romano Ed, Idelson Gnocchi 2000.
2. Christiansen J, Lorentzen M. Implantation of artificial sphincter for anal incontinence. *Lancet* 1987; i:244-245
3. Jorge JMN, Wexner SD.Etiology and management of fecal incontinence. *Dis Colon Rectum* 1993; 36: 77-97.
4. American Medical Systems. Fecal incontinence scoring system. Minnetonka: American Medical Systems, 1996.
5. Madhoff RD, Baeten CGMI, Christiansen J, Rosen HR, Williams NS, Heine JA, Lehur PA, Lowry AC, Lubowski DZ, Matzel KE, Nicholls RJ, Seccia M, Thorson AG, Wexner SD, Wong WD. Standards for anal sphincter replacement.*Dis Colon Rectum* 2000;43: 135-141.
6. Lehur PA, Michot F, Denis P, Grise P, Leborgne J, Teniere P, Buzelin JM.Results of artificial sphincter in severe anal incontinence. Report of 14 consecutive implantations.*Dis Colon Rectum* 1996; 39: 1352-5.
7. Vaizey CJ, Kamm MA, Gold DM, Bartram CI, Halligan S, Nicholls RJ. Clinical, physiological, and radiological study of a new purpose-designed Artificial Bowel Sphincter. *Lancet* 1998; 351: 105-109.
8. O'Brien PE, Skinner S. Restoring control. The Acticon Neosphincter Artificial Bowel Sphincter in the treatment of anal incontinence. *Dis Colon Rectum* 2000; 43: 1213-1216.
9. Christiansen J, Sparso B. Treatment of anal incontinence by an implantable prosthetic anal sphincter. *Ann Surg* 1992; 215: 383-6
10. Dodi G, Melega A, Masin A, Infantino A, Cavallari F, Lise M. Artificial bowel sphincter (ABS) for severe faecal incontinence: a clinical and manometric study. *Colorectal Disease* 2000; 2: 207-211.
11. Devesa JM, Hervàs PL, Sanchez S. Artificial anal sphincter: functional results and complications of a large personal series. *Colorectal Dis* 2000; 2 (suppl.I), 13A.
12. Lehur PA, Roig JV, Duinslaeger M. Artificial anal sphincter. Prospective clinical and manometric evaluation. *Dis Colon Rectum* 2000; 43:1100-1106.
13. Altomare DF. Muscle transposition for fecal incontinence. Graciloplasty. In "Diagnosis and
Treatment of fecal incontinence" G. Romano Ed. Idelson-Gnocchi, Pub 2000.
14. Williams NS, Hughes SF, Stuchfield B. Continent colonic conduit for rectal evacuation in severe constipation. *Lancet* 1994; 343: 1321-4.
15. Altomare DF, Dodi G, La Torre F, Romano G, Melega E, Lise M, Montori A, Rinaldi M, Memeo V. Artificial anal sphincter (Acticon^{tm} neosphincter) for severe faecal incontinence. A multicenter retrospective analysis of 28 cases. *Br J Surg* 2001 (in press).

SECTION V

MINIMALLY-INVASIVE SURGERY

CHAPTER 22

MINI-LAPAROTOMY: A SUITABLE MINIMALLY INVASIVE TECHNIQUE FOR CHOLECYSTECTOMY

Mario Sianesi, Paolo Del Rio, Francesco Rulli*
Department of Surgery, University of Parma, Parma, Italy
** Department of Surgery, Univerisity of Rome "Tor Vergata", Rome, Italy*

Abstract
Objective To verify the effectiveness of minicholecystectomy in a short hospital stay environment.
Design Review of medical records of an on going prospective study.
Setting Surgical ward of a University Hospital.
Intervention minicholecystectomy.
Main outcome measures Complications, length of hospital stay, feasibility in a day surgery environment.
Results Of the 758 patients who underwent cholecystectomy, 702 (92.6%) were admitted for day surgery, 62.8% of whom were discharged in less than 12 hours, 28.6% in 24 hours or less, and 8.6% in more than 24 hours. Major complication rate was 0.2%; two cases required reoperation and interventional radiology drainage respectively.
Conclusions Minicholecystectomy is safe and suitable as a day-surgery procedure.

INTRODUCTION

The introduction of laparoscopic cholecystectomy progressively led to the concept of gallbladder surgery as a day-care or outpatients procedure. Minimal postoperative pain and a quick return to normal habits have been achieved. Unfortunately, women in pregnancy, and patients with severe chronic obstructive pulmonary diseases and aneurysms of the abdominal aorta, are not candidates for laparoscopic cholecystectomies. Furthermore, laparoscopic procedures are costly, and still require a longer learning curve for "traditionally trained" surgeons. Nevertheless, there have been changes in the open treatment of gallstones in the past years [1]. The incision used for "open" cholecystectomy has

A.M. Farinon (ed.), Advances in Abdominal Surgery 2002, 315-320.

become progressively smaller over the past two decades, with an attendant reduction in postoperative pain and morbidity. Several reports [2-4] indicate that minimal access is safe and allows a very short hospital stay.

This microceliotomy procedure is performed through a 3 to 6 cm transverse subcostal incision, and uses a standard operating technique with several modifications, including anterograde dissection of the gallbladder, and longer instruments [5]. It is important to note that the incision for microceliotomy cholecystectomy is located in "the minimal stress triangle" (MST) which is placed in the subxiphoid region [6] (Fig 1). In our hands, with the use of minicholecystectomy, the majority of our patients are discharged from hospital on the same day of surgery.

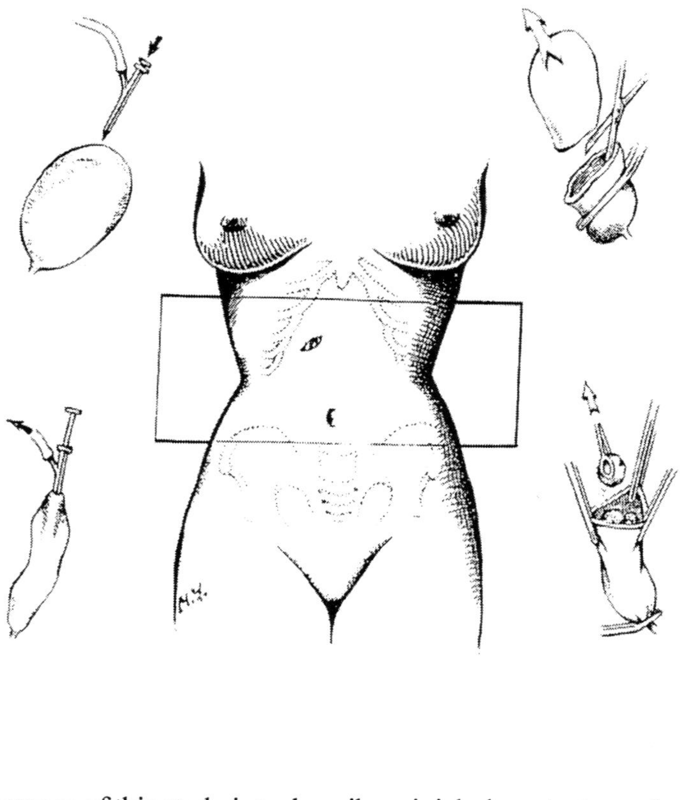

Figure 1.

The purpose of this study is to describe minicholecystectomy day-cases and assess its availability as a valid day-surgery procedure.

Our study started in December 1992 in an effort to reduce hospital-stay costs, as requested by the administration of our hospital, by including cholecystectomy in a program of ambulatory-day surgery.

We collected the records of all minicholecystectomies performed at the University Hospital of Parma. The procedure was introduced by one of us (M.S.), and performed by all the senior surgeons on the staff.

We perform minicholecystectomy as for an open one, making a small incision, preserving the rectus muscle. The operation is done through a 3 to 6 cm incision, using normal retractors. A transverse incision is used 2 to 3 cm under the costal arcade. The gallbladder is visualized and freed with laparotomy sponges. Normal retractors are then introduced, and used to elevate the liver off the Calot triangle. The gallbladder is then emptied and attached with normal Kocher forceps, in order to create traction across the common bile duct. The dissection is done with an uni- or bi-polar cautery; when necessary the gallbladder is emptied of the bigger stones or sectioned, dividing the corpus from the infundibulum (Fig 1). Then we identify the cystic artery and the cystic duct. If the gallbladder is severely inflamed and no cleavage planes are found, the anterior wall of the viscus is excised at the junction of the gallbladder bed, leaving the posterior gallbladder wall in the liver. The mucosa of the viscus is then cauterized. Cholangiography is done only when indicated and generally it does not represent a technical problem. The cystic artery and duct are then ligated or clipped and the gallbladder removed. Lidocaine and dexamethasone are introduced into the muscular layer and subcutaneous tissue. A subcuticular suture of the wound is performed.

STUDY

By the 31st of October 1999, 758 cholecystectomies had been performed on all our patients with acute or non-acute gallbladder stones: 702 by minilaparotomy and 56 by open laparotomy, because of controindications to minilaparotomy procedure (massive choledocolithiasis, choleperitoneum, a major associated surgical procedure). Patients were classified following the American Association of Anestesiology risk scale. There were 178 ASA II, 127 ASA III, and 25 ASA IV patients. Seven-hundred and two (92.6%) were patients admitted for one-day surgery . Among these 441 (62.8%) were discharged within 12 hours, 201 (28.6 %) within 24 hours, and 60 (8.6%) within more than 24 hours. One hundred and thirty-five (19.2%) patients required incisions greater than 6 cm. (to a maximum of 10 cm.) and in three cases (0.4%) a Kocher laparotomy, with rectus muscle section, was needed. These approaches were due to some acute and sclero-atrophic cholecystitis, some sclero-atrophic, and internal biliary fistulae. None of the patients required blood transfusions. Eighty-one (11.5%) patients had a common bile duct stone/s, and three a stenosing odditis (0.4%). Among these, 63 had a preoperative endoscopic sphinterotomy; 2 patients underwent a rendez-vous endoscopic sphinterotomy;

2 underwent a choledocolithotomy, and 15 a transcystic lithotomy by Dormia basket; two patients required a postoperative endoscopic sphinterotomy.

We had two complications. At the beginning of our experience (case N 21), one patient developed a choleperitoneum due to a cystic duct leakage, and she was successfully re-operated on. The second patient developed a subhepatic abscess that was treated with a percutaneous echoguided drain.

These patients experienced a poor postoperative course (pain and fever) and were kept as in-patients for more than one day.

Of the patients discharged within 24 hours, eleven were re-admitted within 30 days, but only three of these showed problems related to the surgical intervention (wound infections).

The minor complications were 15 (2,1%). All cases are reported in Table 1.

	AMBULATORY MINICHOLECYSTECTOMY 702 PATIENTS	
COMPLICATIONS		TREATMENT
	MAJOR	
BILE LEAKAGE	1	LAPAROTOMY
SUBHEPATIC ABSCESS	1	ECHOGUIDED DRAINAGE
	MINOR	
DEEP VEIN THROMBOSIS	1	MEDICAL
MYOCARDIAL ISCHEMIA	1	MEDICAL
BACK PAIN	1	MEDICAL
PNEUMONIA	1	MEDICAL
PLEURITIS	1	MEDICAL
WOUND INFECTION	2 *	INCISION AND DRAINAGE
WOUND CONTAMINATA NON INFETTA	5 *	DRAINAGE
DRAIN RETENTION IN ABDOMINAL WALL	1 *	WOUND INCISION
WOUND HAEMATOMA	2 *	DRAINAGE

* Discharged in 24 hours: postoperative ambulatory medical treatment

Post-operative pain was observed in 275 patients (39.3%), but only a few of them required more than one administration of a pain killer. Nausea was observed in 143 patients (20.5%), and vomiting in 59 (8.5 %). Urinary retention was noted in 6 cases (0.8%).

Mean hospital-stay was 1 day (min. 6 hours – max. 19 days).

Return to normal physical or intellectual activities required from 2 to 14 days for 637 patients (90.7%).

RESULTS AND CONCLUSIONS

The post-operative course of minilaparotomy without muscle sectioning was uneventful in 92.6% of the cases. Limited peritoneal exposure minimizes post-operative ileus, and patients can generally take fluids a few hours after the operation, a light meal the same evening or on the first postoperative day; normal meals thereafter. Our results confirm that the majority of minicolecystectomies can be done as out-patient surgery. Our complication-rate requiring laparotomy (one case) or interventional radiology (one case) was particularly low (0.2%).

There is a lack of data from literature about minimal invasive cholecystectomy which should be discussed. In fact, results from trials show that the learning curve of the mini-lap approach has been interrupted by the advent of laparoscopy [2, 7-11].

In conclusion, as stated by Majed and then by Bell [12, 3], we think that the advantages obtained with the laparoscopic approach still have to be compared with those of mini-laparotomy, above all considering costs and early recovery.

REFERENCES

1. Cheslin-Curtis S, Russel RCG. New trends in gallstone management. *Br J Surg* 1991; 78: 143-9.

2. Dubois F, Berthelot B. Cholecystectomie par minilaparotomie. *Nouvelle Presse Medical* 1982; 11: 1139-41.

3. Moss G. Discharge within 24 hours of elective cholecystectomy. *Arch Surg* 1986; 121:1159-61.

4. Ledet WP. Ambulatory cholecystectomy without disability. *Arch Surg* 1990;125:1434-35.

5. Sianesi M. Colecistectomia minilaparotomica ambulatoriale. *Chirurgia* 1995; 8:378-91.

6. Pelissier EP, Blum D, Meyer JM, Girard JF.Cholecystectomy by minilaparotomy without muscle section: a Short-Stay procedure. *Hepato-Gastroenterology* 1992; 39:294-95.

7. Barkun JS,Barkun AN, Sampalis JS, Fried G, Taylor B, Wexler MJ, Goresky CA, Meakins JL. Randomised controlled trial of laparoscopic versus mini cholecystectomy. *Lancet* 1992; 340:1116-119.

8. McMahon A, Russel I, Baxter J, Ross S, Anderson J, Morran C, Sunderland G, Galloway D, Ramsay G, O'Dwyer P. Laparoscopic versus minilaparotomy cholecystectomy: a randomised trial. *Lancet* 1994; 343:135-38.

9. Kent Seale A, Ledet WP. Minicholecystectomy. *Arch Surg* 1999;134:308-10.

10. Nagakawa T. Biliary surgery via minilaparotomy-A limited procedure for biliary lithiasis. *HPB Surgery* 1993; 6: 245-54.

11. Tyagi N, Meredith M, Lumb J, Cacdac R, Vanterpool C, Rayls K, Zerega D, Silbergleit A. A new minimally invasive technique for cholecystectomy. *Ann Surg* 220, 5: 617-25.

12. Majeed AW, Troy G, Nicholl JP, Smythe A, Reed MWR, Stoddard CJ, Peacock J, Johnson AG. Randomised, prospective, single-blind comparison of laparoscopic versus small-incision cholecystectomy. *Lancet* 1996; 347: 989-94.
13. Bell PRF. Surgical research and randomized trials. *Br J Surg* 1997; 84: 737-38.

CHAPTER 23

MINIMALLY INVASIVE SURGERY FOR THE TREATMENT OF FUNCTION DISEASES OF THE GASTROESOPHAGEAL JUNCTION.

Giovanni Zaninotto, Mario Costantini, Giuseppe Portale, Daniela Molena, Michela Costantino, Loredana Nicoletti, Cristian Rizzetto, Ermanno Ancona
Department of Medical and Surgical Sciences, 4th Surgical Clinic, University of Padua, Padua, Italy

INTRODUCTION

The Gastroesophageal junction (GEJ) constitutes a complex anatomical and functional entity the importance of which derives from its situation at the confines of the thorax and abdomen. The critical element in the function of the GEJ is the lower oesophageal sphincter (LES), that performs two main roles: (1) to relax during swallowing, allowing passage of food and liquid into the stomach, and (2) to maintain a resting tone that prevents free reflux of gastric contents into the lower oesophagus. Malfunction or anatomical changes in the LES lead to a variety of characteristic symptoms (heartburn, chest pain, regurgitation and dysphagia) and to different diseases. From a very schematic view, failure to relax properly at swallowing leads to oesophageal achalasia, and in other ways to epiphrenic diverticula. On the other hand, the inability to act properly as a barrier to reflux of gastric contents leads to gastroesophageal reflux disease and its complications. All these pathologies can be effectively treated by means of surgery.

The past decade has witnessed an increasingly widespread use of video-endoscopic surgery, which has also been applied in the field of gastroesophageal junction diseases. The reduction in patient discomfort and health service costs, and overall short and medium-term results potentially rendered these techniques the treatment of choice for benign oesophageal pathologies. After a number of "technical reports" in medical literature in the mid-90s, several large series of patients treated in this way have recently been published, with a

A.M. Farinon (ed.), Advances in Abdominal Surgery 2002, 321-336.

lengthy follow-up [1-6]. Objectively significant clinical conclusions can consequently now be drawn regarding the laparoscopic treatment of oesophageal function diseases, especially as far as long-term results of these techniques are concerned, as compared with the results of traditional surgery.

In this paper, we aim to review our experience of more than 400 laparoscopic procedures for gastroesophageal function diseases, focusing our discussion on the modern surgical therapy of GERD and oesophageal achalasia, that constitutes the majority of procedures performed in our institution (Tab. 1), as well as in most other dedicated centres.

Table 1. Laparoscopic treatment of gastroesophageal funtion diseases. The experience of the University of Padua Department of Medical and Surgical Sciences, Clinica Chirurgica IV, 1992-2001.

		n. of operations	**n. (%) of conversions**	**good results***
Achalasia	Heller-Dor	161	6 (3.7)	89 %
GERD	Nissen / Toupet	227	11 (4.8)	83 %
	Collis- Nissen	8	-	75 %
Epiphrenic Diverticula	Diverticulectomy + Heller-Dor	8	-	100 %
TOTAL		**404**	**17 (4.2)**	

* only patients with the operation completed laparoscopically were considered.

LAPAROSCOPIC TREATMENT OF GASTROESOPHAGEAL REFLUX DISEASE

Since 1992, 235 patients with uncomplicated and complicated (stricture, ulcers, short oesophagus) GERD have undergone laparoscopic antireflux surgery. They were 141 males and 94 females, with a median age of 48 years (5th-95th percentiles: 25-68). The indications for surgery are summarised in Table 2. A careful preoperative work-up was carried out, especially in patients with atypical symptoms, in order to confirm GERD, and avoid performing inappropriate surgery. The diagnosis was based on an accurate medical history, and a symptom score for heartburn, acid regurgitation, pain and dysphagia was obtained, based on severity (0= no symptoms, 1= mild, elicited by investigation, 2=moderate, reported but seldom requiring therapy, 3= severe, requiring continuous therapy) and frequency (1= occasional symptom, 2= once a month, 3= once a week, 4= daily) [6]. Further, given the non-specific nature of reflux symptoms [7], objective investigation was performed to confirm the disease, and rule out other causes of symptoms: a barium swallow was used to document the presence of hiatal hernia; endoscopy was performed in order to detect and classify the severity of oesophagitis, when present, and to identify complications of the disease, such as strictures or Barrett's oesophagus (the Savary-Miller classification was used for this purpose) [8]; oesophageal manometry was performed, to obtain information on LES characteristics and oesophageal body motility, following the guidelines of the "Gruppo Italiano di Studio della Motilità dell'Apparato Digerente (GISMAD)" [9]. 24-hour pH-monitoring was performed in all the patients, following standard criteria10, in order to establish the abnormal exposure of the oesophagus to gastric juice, the best objective way to define and diagnose the disease. In selected patients, 24-hour monitoring of oesophageal exposure to bilirubin, by means of Bilitec, was also performed to rule out possible associate biliary reflux [11].

Table 2. Indications for antireflux surgery in 235 patients

Indication		No. of patients	%
Uncomplicated GERD (Esophagitis 0-2)		144	61.3
Erosive esophagitis – stricture (Esophagitis 3-4)		25	10.6
Barrett's Esophagus (patients with BE and paraesophageal hernia)		28 (3)	11.9
Paraesophageal Hernia	- type II - type III-IV	3 35	1.3 14.9
TOTAL		235	100.0

Laparoscopic access to the hiatal region, for performing an antireflux procedure, is illustrated in figure 1. The division of the lesser omentum and the phrenoesophageal membrane allows exposition of the right and left hiatal crura. A "window" is then created behind the esophagus, that is isolated with a Penrose-type silastic drain, to allow safe traction without the risk of damaging the esophageal or gastric wall. The next step in the procedure involves the mobilisation of the gastric fundus, by dividing 3 to 4 short gastric vessels: the use of Ultracision (Ethicon) greatly simplifies the manoeuvre.

In order to close the hiatal defect, the crura are then approximated by using 2 to 3 non reabsorbable monofilament stitches (3.5 metric). The introduction into the esophagus, over a guide wire, of a 13 mm. bougie (Savary) avoids the risk of performing too tight a closure. In some instances, especially in the case of very large hiatal defects, the use of a double-face prosthetic mesh is necessary, in order to obtain a tension-free closure of the hiatus [12].

A fundoplication is then performed, by pulling the mobilised gastric fundus behind the esophagus through the previously created posterior window: a 360° complete posterior fundoplication, following the (floppy) Nissen technique [13], is obtained by using 2-3 non reabsorbable 3-metric stitches, of which 1 or

2 are also secured to the anterior esophageal wall, in order to prevent wrap migration. A lateral stitch between the right emivalve and the right crus can also be applied, for the same purpose. Particular care has to be paid to create a

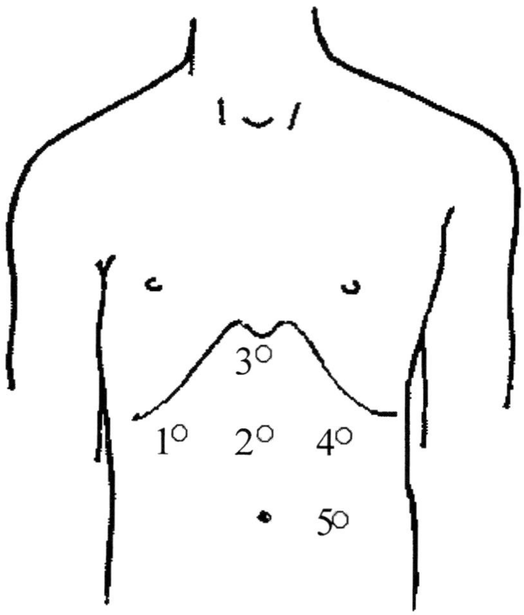

Figure 1. Schematic representation of the trocars positioning for the access to the hiatal region for the laparoscopic treatment of gastro-esophageal junction diseases. The first assistant uses port 1 for retracting the liver and port 2 for the camera. The surgeon uses ports 3 and 4 for the bimanual access to the hiatus. The second assistant, by means of a forceps introduced through port 5, maintains a gentle traction of the gastric fundus.

floppy, short (2-3 cm maximum) fundoplication, in order to prevent post-operative dysphagia.

In the case of disordered esophageal motility, a partial 270° posterior fundoplication, following the Toupet technique14, is to be preferred. Two lines of suture are made with 3-metric non reabsorbable stitches, to secure the two emivalves to both right and left lateral esophageal walls. The most proximal stitches also secure the two emivalves to the hiatal crura. In patients with a short oesophagus, even after a complete mobilization of the distal oesophagus the GEJ cannot be positioned under the diaphragm without tension, and has a tendency to return to its former position in the chest. Therefore, a lengthening procedure (Collis gastroplasty)15 needs to be performed. This procedure, usually obtained through a left thoracotomy, can now also be performed through a laparoscopic approach16. After mobilisation of the gastric fundus, with a 21-mm circular stapler inserted through an additional port in the right upper quadrant of the abdomen, a hole is created through the anterior and posterior gastric walls, 6-7 cm below the angle of His and in the proximity of a 15-mm. Savary bougie inserted into the esophagus, to avoid performing too narrow a gastric tube. A linear stapler is then passed through this gastric hole; it is fired towards the angle of His, creating a stomach tube as a continuation of the distal oesophagus. This neo-oesophagus now lies comfortably below the diaphragm without tension. A Nissen fundoplication is then performed in the usual way over the neo-oesophagus.

Results

Laparoscopic antireflux surgery was completed in 224 patients: 197 Nissen, 18 Toupet and 8 Collis-Nissen. In 13 cases of Nissen fundoplication, a large hiatal defect required the use of a double-face prosthetic mesh. The conversion rate was 4.8% (11 patients). The most common cause for conversion was a large paraesophageal hernia or adhesions from previous operations. These 11 patients were excluded from the results analysis. Mortality was nil. Intraoperative complications amounted to 3%; the most common were gastric wall perforations, occurring in 3 cases, repaired laparoscopically in 2/3 patients, and requiring conversion to laparotomy in 1 (the postoperative course was uneventful in all 3 cases). Post-operative complications were: bleeding from a trocar site in 1 case (requiring laparoscopic re-operation), cardiac arrhythmias requiring medical treatment in 3 cases, pneumonia in 5, pneumothorax in 3.

In the analysis of results, the 8 patients undergoing a Collis-Nissen fundoplication were considered separately. After a median follow-up of 21 months (5th-95th percentiles: 2-72), excellent or good results were recorded in 177 of the 216 patients undergoing a Nissen or Toupet procedure (83%). In these patients complete healing of esophagitis and the control of reflux symptoms without medications (simple antacids excluded) were obtained, without side-effects.

Thirty-nine patients continued to complain of their previous symptoms, or required continuous medication to control them, or developed new complaints (post-fundoplication symptoms): these patients were considered as failures of the laparoscopic surgical treatment. When carefully evaluating the causes of failure, postoperative dysphagia was found in 13 patients (6%), fundoplication displacement in 15 (7.3%), recurrence of reflux in 8 (6%), and gas-bloating syndrome in 4 patients (1.8%). Two additional patients (1%), both complaining of atypical symptoms, relapsed with their symptoms shortly after the operation, in spite of objective control of reflux (by 24-hour pH-monitoring). Additional endoscopic or surgical treatments were performed on 25/39 patients: 14 surgical repairs (10 laparoscopically and 4 with open surgery), 9 pneumatic dilations of the cardia and 2 pneumatic dilations of the pylorus), resulting in an improvement of symptoms in 22 patients. Therefore, the overall success rate after primary or secondary treatment rose to 92%.

As far as the patients operated with the Collis-Nissen operation are concerned, we observed an improvement in the symptom score in all patients; however, the persistence of ulcerative esophagitis was observed in one patient, and requirement for continuous medication to control his symptoms in another one. No complications or side-effect symptoms were recorded.

LAPAROSCOPIC TREATMENT OF OESOPHAGEAL ACHALASIA

Since 1993, 161 patients with primary oesophageal achalasia have undergone laparoscopic Heller myotomy. There were 90 males and 71 females, with a median age of 41.5 years (range 11-80). The median duration of their symptoms was 24 months (range 3-240). Only 32 patients (20%) had received previous treatment elsewhere: 17 had had oesophageal balloon dilations with a Rigiflex dilator (median 2 dilations, range 1-6), 10 had received up to three sessions of botulinum toxin injections at the cardia, and 5 had received both pneumatic dilations and botulinum toxin injection.

The preoperative work-up of the patients included a detailed clinical history, which was collected by using a dedicated questionnaire in which each patient's symptoms (heartburn, chest pain, food regurgitation and dysphagia) were scored according to severity and frequency [6]; a barium swallow, in order to measure the maximun diameter of the gullet; and a stationary manometry, using a low compliance pneumohydraulic perfused system, in order to assess LES pressure, length and relaxation, in addition to the oesophageal body motility [9]. Endoscopy was performed in all patients, in order to exclude malignancies.

All patients were operated using the same technique, described elsewhere in detail [17]. The access was the same as illustrated in figure 1. Briefly, only the anterior part of the oesophagus was dissected, the anterior vagus nerve was identified and a myotomy 6 to 8 cm long, extending 1-1.5 cm on the gastric side of the cardia, was performed, preferably remaining to the left of the nerve. An intra-esophageal 30 mm. balloon (Rigiflex®, Microvasive, Boston, MA) was inserted, using a guide-wire positioned endoscopically after the patient had been intubated. During the oesophageal myotomy, the balloon was gently inflated and deflated, thus facilitating the identification of the circular fibres, which were stretched and then cut or torn apart. The inflated balloon was also useful for controlling minor bleeding from the submucosal vessels, thus reducing the need for cautery. An anterior partial fundoplication (180°) according to the Dor technique completed the operation, with three stitches on each side, suturing the gastric wall to the edges of the myotomy.

A swallow test with a water-soluble contrast (Gastrografin® was routinely obtained on the 1st post-operative day, to rule out any perforation. Then the naso-gastric tube was removed and patients were allowed to drink. Patients were asked to remain on soft food for 10-15 days, and were then allowed a normal diet. They were discharged depending on the distance of their homes from the hospital (on the 2nd post-operative day, if they were within an hour's drive from the hospital; on the 4th if they came from farther away).

Patients were invited to come back to the outpatients' clinic for an interview after one month, when a barium swallow was also obtained. They were asked to repeat oesophageal manometry and undergo 24-hour pH monitoring 6 months after the operation, when they had a second interview and their symptoms were scored. Endoscopy was done after one year; thereafter, clinical check-ups were scheduled once a year. Patients who failed to report to the outpatients' clinic were interviewed over the phone.

Results

In 155 of the 161 patients the procedure was completed laparoscopically. The reasons for conversion to open surgery were 2 mucosal perforations, 1 spleen damage, and the finding of an unsuspected mass in the lower abdomen, that could not be interpreted laparoscopically, and proved to be an ectopic kidney in one patient, and adhesions from previous upper abdominal surgery in 2 patients. Mortality was nil. The most common intra-operative complication encountered was the perforation of the oesophageal mucosa while performing the myotomy: 2 mucosal tears, occurring at the beginning of our experience, were repaired by conversion to open surgery, 4 were repaired laparoscopically with 4-0 reabsorbable stitches, and one additional mucosal leak was recognised by using the water-soluble contrast swallow, routinely performed 24 hours after surgery. Other post-operative complications were: trocar site bleeding in one patient (requiring laparotomy on the 2nd postoperative day), one pneumothorax, one vocal cord palsy, one external sciatic popliteal nerve palsy, and one unexplained persistent fever. The median operating time was 150 min. (110-220). The median hospital stay was 4 days (3-11). The median time from operation to the patient's return to work was 12 days (6-21).

Only one (3.1%) of the 32 patients who had previously been treated with dilation or botulinum toxin injection, had mucosal tears during myotomy, as compared with 4.6% in the previously-untreated group (p=n.s.). The duration of the operation was similar in the patients with and without prior treatment

(135 min vs. 152 min), though all surgeons involved in the study had subjective impressions that myotomy was more difficult to perform in the previously treated patients.

After surgery, clinical follow-up was completed by all 155 patients. The median follow-up was 26 months (2-75). Excellent/good results were reported in 138 (89 %) patients. Sixteen of the 17 patients with recurrent symptoms after laparoscopic myotomy were treated with pneumatic dilations, using 3.5 and 4 cm Rigiflex balloons (median 3 dilations, range 2-6); additional pneumatic treatment was successful in 14/16 cases. One patient with severe dysphagia underwent redo open myotomy with good results. One patient, with mild dysphagia and persistent retrosternal pain, underwent thoracoscopic long oesophageal myotomy, with only minor improvements in her symptoms. The combined treatment (laparoscopic Heller myotomy plus dilations where necessary) was therefore successful in 152/155 patients (98%).

Laparoscopic treatment of epiphrenic diverticula.

Increasing experience in the laparoscopic treatment of gastroesophageal junction disease, and demonstration of the accessibility to the lower mediastinal esophagus through this access, prompted utilisation of the laparoscopic access also for the treatment of epiphrenic esophageal diverticula. With this access, all 3 steps of the traditional surgical treatment for these diverticula (diverticulectomy, myotomy, fundoplication) can be performed, giving the patient the advantage of minimally invasive access [18].

The position of the patient and location of the laparoscopic ports are the same as for Heller-Dor operation or Nissen fundoplication (Fig. 1). Also in this case, division of the Laimer membrane and exposition of the crura leads to the isolation of the abdominal esophagus, that is encircled with a Penrose-type drain, for safe traction. The mediastinal blunt dissection is then initiated, close to the esophageal wall, and the diverticulum identified. This must be completely isolated until the upper margin of its neck is clearly visible. Intraoperative endoscopy is necessary in this phase; the presence of the scope in the esophagus is also necessary to avoid excessive narrowing of the esophageal lumen, when the diverticulum is resected by means of a laparoscopic linear Endo-GIA stapler. The resected diverticulum is then removed, and the suture line protected by an interrupted oversewing suture. Hydropneumatic checking of the suture can be performed, by inflating the esophagus with air through the scope. A myotomy is then performed, on the opposite side of the esophageal wall, from the upper margin of the suture to the gastro-esophageal junction (1.0-1.5 cm on its gastric side), and an anterior (Dor's) fundoplication terminates the operation.

With this technique, in the last 3 years we have operated 8 patients with epiphrenic diverticula. At a median follow-up of 18 months (range 3-36), no recurrence of the diverticula were recorded. However, morbidity was high, with two fistulas (that required prolonged naso-gastric aspiration, PTN and antibiotics to be healed) and a post-operative pneumonia.

DISCUSSION

Laparoscopic surgery for gastro-esophageal function diseases has gained widespread diffusion, and in most centers has replaced traditional open access for the surgical treatment of such diseases. The most common field of application is in the treatment of GERD: laparoscopic fundoplication is one of the most commonly performed laparoscopic operations throughout the world [19]. Until recently, the therapy of this disease was traditionally performed with medication, in spite of the fact that, when surgery was compared to antacid and H2-blocker therapies in the long-term treatment of GERD [20-21], the overall findings suggested that antireflux surgery was consistently more effective than medical therapy. The introduction of PPIs - powerful drugs offering rapid symptom relief and curing esophagitis in the vast majority of patients – consolidated the balance already shifted towards medical treatment [22]. Until the mid '90s, antireflux surgery was consequently relegated to an ancillary role in the treatment of GERD: indications for this were relatively rare, and limited to patients failing to respond to medical therapy or developing complications. A recent report from Lundell and colleagues has shown, at last, that surgery is even more effective than omeprazole in controlling GERD [2]. Surgery has also made substantial progress: thanks to a better understanding of the mechanisms behind cardia competence, surgical technique has been refined and become more effective with fewer side effects, allowing for a more efficient selection of patients suitable for antireflux surgery. Furthermore, the introduction of laparoscopic surgery has made surgery more acceptable to gastroenterologists and patients, and the previous reluctance of physicians to refer patients for surgery has progressively decreased; the patient can now be offered two equally valid options to treat his/her disease: pills or the fiberoptic scalpel.

It has been widely reported that laparoscopic antireflux surgery is feasible, with the same low mortality and morbidity, and the same effectiveness (at least in the disease-specific short-term goal) as open surgery [23]. Several authors [1, 24, 25] reported an > 90% improvement in symptoms, and a 92-95% return to normal values in oesophageal acid exposure measured by 24-hour pH monitoring. Follow-ups of up to 7 years are now available, and they show a higher than 90% (Tab. 3) success rate in controlling GERD. However, if all the reasons for patients' dissatisfaction are considered, the overall success rate may be lower, even if this can be improved with subsequent treatment.

Table 3. Efficacy of laparoscopic fundoplication for GERD

			RESULTS			
Author	Year	Patients	% GERD control	% dysphagia	% Gas bloat	% wrap displacement
Hinder[24]	1994	198	93	6	13	n.r.
Peracchia[26]	1995	49	96	2	n.r.	n.r.
Hunter[25]	1996	252	97	4	11	3
Watson[27]	1996	253	91	11	n.r.	7
Cadière[28]	1997	224	91.6	3.9	3.9	n.r.
Anvari[29]	1998	381	96.9	2.1	n.r.	19
Landreanu[30]	1998	150	95	1	1	n.r.
Campos[31]	1999	233	87	n.r.	n.r.	n.r.
Present series	2001	216	94	6	1.8	7.3

n.r. = not reported

A prospective study has been recently carried out in Italy on behalf of the Italian Society of Endoscopic Surgery, and in two years1 more than 600 patients were collected from 20 centers all over Italy. The rate of intraoperative complications was 4.3%, and only 1% were severe complications such as esophageal or gastric perforation. The early results in more than 300 patients were very promising: symptoms were controlled in 91% of patients, and healing of severe esophagitis was achieved in 96% of patients. The patients' satisfaction after surgery, collected on a visual-analog self-testing scale from 1 to 10, was between 8 and 10 in more than 80% of patients, and less than 1% were dissatisfied with the outcome of the operation. An important side-effect of laparoscopic antireflux surgery is dysphagia. It has been shown that transient dysphagia is common after surgery, and is perhaps the sign of a well-made wrap; it generally resolves itself spontaneously in about 2 months. Persistent dysphagia has been reported in up to 11% patients, and seems to be related to the Nissen-Rossetti operation. Improved skills and certain technical modifications have resulted in a reduction of this most common side-effect of laparoscopic antireflux surgery. Complete mobilization of the gastric fundus by dividing the short gastric vessels enables a floppy, symmetrical wrap to encircle the distal esophagus. Also, by mobilizing the gastric fundus, we avoid making the mistake of encircling the esophagus not with the upper part of the fundus, but with the gastric body. In our experience, persistent post-operative dysphagia was significantly reduced after we started routinely dividing the short gastric vessels, in order to mobilize the fundus.

Gas-bloat syndrome and the inability to belch shows a reported incidence ranging between 1% and 13% (Table 3). It is necessary to assess preoperatively whether a patient already has any gastrointestinal motility disturbances. The floppy fundoplication should preserve the ability to belch, and vagal nerve injury may be responsible when these symptoms persist postoperatively. One of the most important causes of failure in antireflux surgery, which is unlikely with open surgery, is wrap displacement into the chest. A more extensive dissection of the hiatus, fewer adhesions and earlier patient mobilization may play a part in the onset of this complication. Contributing factors may include inadequate closure of the diaphragmatic crura, a short esophagus and/or insufficient esophagus mobilization; in such cases, the use of a mesh to secure the hiatal closure and a Collis-Nissen operation to adequately lengthen the esophagus should be considered. The occurrence of this complication amounted to 7.3% and was significantly more frequent in cases of paraesophageal hernia or advanced disease (Barrett, stricture) ($p<0.05$).

It is noteworthy that recurrent reflux symptoms were only recorded in 7 patients (4%); 2 of these had a Collis Nissen fundoplication repair because of esophageal stricture, 4 had a Nissen fundoplication, and 1 a Toupet. Again, the risk for GERD recurrence was higher in patients who had severe disease and shortening of the esophagus, than in patients with a normal esophageal length (2/7 vs 4/181, $p< 0.001$). Therefore, one can say that the right timing for antireflux surgery is the sooner the better!

In 1999 Campos et al. pointed out the predictive factors for a good outcome after antireflux surgery: an abnormal esophageal acid exposure, the presence of typical symptoms and a good response to medical therapy [31]. Unsatisfactory results can derive from inadequate or superficial selection of patients. A careful preoperative evaluation is therefore mandatory, especially in patients with atypical symptoms, in order to confirm GERD and avoid performing inappropriate surgery, i.e.: in order to perform the right operation for the right disease, in the right patient.

Our experience, as well as the experience of other Authors [16], showed that the Collis-Nissen operation can be performed successfully through the laparoscopic approach, giving the patient the advantages of a minimally invasive approach. However, it is a difficult operation and, given its relatively infrequent indication, it should be reserved to experienced surgeons, with both advanced laparoscopic skills and good knowledge of esophageal physiopathology. It represents, however, an additional option for the surgeon in the case of the intraoperative finding of a short esophagus, which has gone undetected by the preoperative work-up. In such a case, the alternative options are conversion to open surgery, or the performance of a fundoplication under tension or in the wrong place, with a high probability of recurrence, displacement or side-effects. The small number of patients operated with this technique cannot lead to definitive conclusions: however, the overall less favourable outcome, compared to simple fundoplication, is in line with previous experience with open surgery, where the results in these complicated patients were less satisfactory than in patients with less severe disease.

As far as esophageal achalasia is concerned, the main goal of treatment is to relieve the obstruction at LES level, that can be achieved mechanically (with a balloon or the scalpel) or using biochemical substances (botulinum toxin). In the past, open surgical myotomy produced an average 89% of good results [32]: but, for its invasiveness, this approach was commonly reserved for patients unresponsive to dilation treatment, which produced 50-65% [33] of good results after a single dilation. The advent of minimally-invasive surgery [17] may have changed this consolidated approach. With its shorter hospital stay, lower morbidity and speedier return to daily activities, it may have made surgical treatment more attractive to patients and physicians.

In previous reports [6, 34], we showed that the laparoscopic Heller-Dor operation on the basis of a 5-year follow-up in a large group of patients offers about 90% of chances to be cured from the disease, and these good results are further confirmed with the increase of the number of treated patients and the length of the follow-up. Other authors have reported very similar results (Tab. 4), that are also at least as good as previous findings with open surgery [35].

Table 4. Results of laparoscopic treatment of esophageal achalasia (1996-2001) (Only papers with more than 20 treated patients are reported)

Author	No. of patients	A/R procedure	% Good results	% reflux
Raiser, 1996[36]	35	Dor/Toupet	97	n.r.
Morino, 1997[37]	21	Dor	81	5
Boulez, 1997[38]	27	None	100	4
Graham, 1997[39]	26	Dor	90	11.1
Hunter, 1997[4]	40	Dor/Toupet	90	2.5
Vogt, 1997[40]	20	Toupet	90	10
Wang, 1998[41]	27	None	89	11
Rosati, 1998[42]	61	Dor	98.2	7
Donahue, 1999[43]	48	Dor/Toupet	83.3	n.r.
Kjellin, 1999[44]	21	None	81	21.4
Patti, 1999[5]	133	Dor*	89	17
Hunt, 2000[45]	70	Nissen#	81	4.5
Present series	155	Dor	89.4	6.9

* Including 8 patients with Toupet
# Including 13 patients with Dor
n.r. = not reported

In our study, palliation of the patients' dysphagia was achieved with no mortality and little morbidity (4.2%), and only 1 undetected mucosal tear. This low morbidity rate compares well with the outcome of endoscopic dilation, which carries a 2-6.4% perforation rate at cardia level with the currently-used new dilators [32]. The most common complication reported after Heller myotomy is post-operative, iatrogenic gastro-esophageal reflux disease (GERD). In fact, abolishing the LES barrier may lead to the abnormal presence of gastrointestinal contents in the gullet. In addition, achalasia patients have a poor peristalsis, with inadequate clearance, and GERD is potentially more harmful than in normal subjects. In most published studies on the laparoscopic approach (with or without fundoplication), post-operative reflux was reported in up to 21.4% of operated patients, with an average of 8% (Tab. 4). Our results confirmed the low incidence of pH-proven post-operative reflux, which in our hands amounted to 6.7% of patients. These data clearly show that GERD may be a problem after myotomy and that some additional measure should be adopted. Our preference for Dor's technique stems from our previous experience with open surgery [46] and from the fact that, since we do not perform any posterior dissection, the anterior fundoplication is easier to perform. Further, by covering the exposed mucosa, the anterior fundoplication protects the leakage from an undetected mucosal lesion.

In our experience, the cause of failure of laparoscopic myotomy was the persistence of uncut muscle fibres or fibrotic healing on the gastric side of the LES [47]. In most patients, the persistent or recurrent symptoms were overcome by endoscopic dilations, with no perforations or other complications. When laparoscopic surgery is not enough, the addition of endoscopic forceful dilation can ensure a 98% symptom control rate in achalasia patients.

Finally, it must be underlined that, in a previous report [6], we have shown that the so-called learning curve for performing the laparoscopic Heller-Dor operation is steep for about 20 patients, and given the rarity of the disease, this figure is probably higher than the number of achalasia patients observed during the average career of most surgeons. It is probably wise therefore to perform this operation only at designated referral centers, where experience can be gained and which can serve as "learning centers" for residents and other surgeons, in order to maintain such excellent results and avoid inappropriate complications.

The surgical treatment of epiphrenic diverticula is another promising field of application of laparoscopic techniques. This access allows the performance of all the steps necessary for the treatment of esophageal diverticula and the underlying motor disorder (diverticulectomy, myotomy, fundoplication). Alternative options have been proposed with the thoracoscopic approach, but with the omission of the myotomy (by performing a simple endoscopic pneumatic dilation of the cardia instead) and/or the fundoplication [48]. These techniques have been abandoned for the high incidence of post-operative fistulas, recurrence or reflux. The only case we treated with thoracoscopic diverticulectomy after simple ballon dilation of the cardia recurred after one year. Another advantage of the laparoscopic approach is that the stapler is parallel to the esophageal axis, thus allowing a complete diverticulectomy. Particular care has to be taken, however, when the diverticulum is large, and more than one stapling firing is necessary: the junction between the two suture lines may constitutes a "*locus minoris resistentiae*" favouring the development of post-operative fistulas, as we observed in at least one case. Our experience demonstrates that this laparoscopic approach is feasible. However, its intrinsic difficulty and the rarity of the esophageal epiphrenic diverticula lead to the same considerations already made for the Collis-Nissen and the Heller-Dor operations, on the necessity that such operations are performed in highly specialized referral centers. In spite of this, some reservations on the appropriateness of this technique are still to be maintained, especially for the high morbidity and complication rate are concerned.

CONCLUSIONS

Laparoscopic surgery has revolutionised many of the traditional concepts of surgery. Despite a decrease in the operative time with increasing experience, the average duration of laparoscopic procedures is still longer than the corresponding laparotomic techniques. The longer duration of the procedures, however, does not seem to influence the morbidity and postoperative course, in which the pain and discomfort are minimal and hospital stay and convalescence are shorter. Overall long term results are at least similar to those obtained in the past with the open access. Laparoscopic surgery has became the gold standard for the treatment of GERD and esophageal achalasia and, at present, no place should be allowed, besides particular cases, to open surgery. However, this cannot be said, yet, for other operations, such as the Collis-Nissen or the laparoscopic treatment of epiphrenic diverticula. In these fiels, other experiences are necessary to validate the appropriateness of this approach.

REFERENCES

1. Zaninotto G, Molena D, Ancona E. A prospective, multicenter study on laparoscopic treatment of gastroesophageal reflux in Italy: type of surgery, conversions, complications and early results. *Surg Endosc* 2000;14:282-288.
2. Lundell L, Miettinem P, Myrvold HE, et al. Continued (5-year) follow up of a randomised clinical study comparing antireflux surgery and omeprazole in gastrointestinal reflux disease. *J Am Coll Surg* 2001;192:172-181.

3. Bammer T, Hinder RA, Klaus A, Klinger PJ. Five- to eight-year outcome of the first laparoscopic Nissen fundoplications. *J Gastrointest Surg* 2001;5:42-48.
4. Hunter JG, Trus TL, Branum GD, Waring P. Laparoscopic Heller myotomy and fundoplication for achalasia. *Ann Surg* 1997; 225: 655-665.
5. Patti MG, Pellegrini CA, Horgan S, et al. Minimally invasive surgery for achalasia. An 8-year experience with 168 patients. *Ann Surg* 1999;230.587-594.
6. Zaninotto G, Costantini M, Molena D, et al.: Treatment of esophageal achalasia with laparoscopic Heller myotomy and Dor partial anterior fundoplication: prospective evaluation of 100 consecutive patients. *J Gastrointest Surg* 2000;4:282-289.
7. Costantini M, Crookes PF, Bremner RM, et al. Value of physiological assessment of foregut symptoms in a surgical practice. *Surgery* 114:780-87, 1993.
8. Savary M, Miller G. The esophagus. In: Gassmann SA (Ed.), Handbook and atlas of endoscopy. Verlag 1978, Solothurn, Switzerland, pp. 135-142.
9. Passaretti S, Zaninotto G, DiMartino N, Leo P, Costantini M, Baldi F. Standards of oesophageal manometry. A position statement from the Gruppo Italiano di Studio per la Motilità dell'Apparato Digerente. *Dig Liv Dis* 2000;32:46-55.
10. Zaninotto G, DiMario F, Costantini M, et al.. Oesophagitis and pH of the refluxate: experimental and clinical study. *Br J Surg* 79:161-164, 1992.
11. Bechi P, Pucciani F, Baldini F, et al. Long-term ambulatory enterogastric reflux monitoring: validation of a new fiberoptic technique. *Dig Dis Sci* 38:1297-1306, 1993.
12. Basso N, De Leo A, Genco A, et al. 360° laparoscopic fundoplication with tension-free hiatoplasty in the treatment of symptomatic gastroesophageal reflux disease. *Surg Endosc* 2000; 14:164-169.
13. Nissen R: Gastropexy and fundoplication in surgical treatment of hiatal hernia. *Am J Dig Dis* 1961; 6:954-961.
14. Toupet A. Technique d'oesophago-gastroplastie avec phrenogastropexie appliquée dans la cure radicale des hernies hiatales et comme complement de l'operation de Heller dans les cardiospasmes. *Mem Acad Chir* 1963; 89:386-389.
15. Collis JL. An operation for hiatus hernia with short esophagus. *J Thorac Cardiovasc Surg* 1957; 34:768-771.
16. Johnson AB, Oddsdottir M, Hunter JG. Laparoscopic Collis gastroplasty and Nissen fundoplication. *Surg Endosc* 1998; 12:1055-1060.
17. Ancona E, Anselmino M, Zaninotto G, et al. Esophageal achalasia: laparoscopic versus conventional open Heller-Dor operation. *Am. J Surg* 1995; 170: 265-270
18. Rosati R, Fumagalli U, Bona S, Bonavina L, Peracchia A. Diverticulectomy, myotomy and fundoplication through laparoscopy: a new option to treat epiphrenic esophageal diverticula? *Ann Surg* 1998; 227:174-178.
19. Perdikis G, Hinder RA, Lund RJ, Raiser F, Katada N. Laparoscopic Nissen fundoplication: where do we stand? *Surg Laparoscopy & Endosc* 1997;7:17-21.
20. Behar J, Sheahan DG, Biancani P, et al. Medical and surgical management of reflux esophagistis. A 38-month report on a prospective clinical trial. *N Engl J Med* 1975;293:263-268.
21. Spechler SJ, and the Department of Veterans Affairs Gastroesophageal Reflux Disease Study Group: Comparison of medical and surgical therapy for complicated gastroesophageal reflux disease in veterans. *N Engl J Med* 1992; 326:786-92.
22. Vigneri S, Termini R, Leandro G, et al. A comparison of maintainance therapies for reflux esophagitis. *N Engl J Med* 1995;333:1106-1110.
23. Peters JH, De Meester TR, Crookes P, et al. The treatment of gastroesophageal reflux disease with laparoscopic Nissen fundoplication. *Ann Surg* 1998; 228:40-50.
24. Hinder RA, et al. Laparoscopic Nissen fundoplication is an effective treatment for gastroesophageal reflux disease. *Ann Surg* 1994; 220:472-483.
25. HunterJG, Trus TL, Branum GD, Waring JP, Wood WC. A physiologic approach to laparoscopic fundoplication for gastroesophageal reflux disease. *Ann Surg* 1996; 223:673-687.

26. Peracchia A, Bancewicz J, Bonavina L, et al. Fundoplication is an effective treatment for gastro-oesophageal reflux disease. *Gastroenterology Intern* 1995; 8:1-9.
27. Watson DI, et al. Changing strategies in the performance of laparoscopic Nissen fundoplication as a result of experience with 230 operations. *Surg Endosc* 1995; 9:961-966.
28. Cadière GB, Himpens J, Rajan A, et al. Laparoscopic Nissen fundoplication: laparoscopic dissection technique and results. *Hepatogastroenterology* 1997; 44:4-10.
29. Anvari M, Allen C. Laparoscopic Nissen fundoplication: two-year comprehensive follow-up of a technique of minimal paraesophageal dissection. *Ann Surg* 1998; 227:25-32.
30. Landreanu RJ, Wiechmann RJ, Hazelrigg SR, et al.: Success of laparoscopic fundoplication for gastroesophageal reflux disease. *Ann Thorac Surg* 1998; 66:1886-93.
31. Campos GMR, Peters JH, DeMeester TR, et al. Multivariate analysis of factors predicting outcome after Nissen fundoplication. *J Gastrointest Surg* 1999; 3:292-300.
32. Vaezi MF and Richter JE. Current therapies for Achalasia: Comparison and efficay. *J Clin Gastroenterol* 1998;27:21-354.
33. Bruley des Varannes S and Scarpignato C. Current trends in the management of achalasia. *Digest Liver Dis* 2001;33:266-277.
34. Anselmino M, Zaninotto G, Costantini M, et al. One-year laparoscopic Heller-Dor operation for esophageal achalasia. *Surg Endosc* 1997; 11: 3-7.
35. Andreollo NA, Earlam RJ. Heller's myotomy for achalasia: is an added anti-reflux procedure necessary? *Br J Surg* 1987;74:765-769.
36. Raiser F, Perdikis G, Hinder RA, et al. Heller myotomy via minimal-access surgery. An evaluation of antireflux procedures. *Arch Surg* 1996; 131:593-598.
37. Morino M, Rebecchi F, Festa V, Garrone C. Preoperative pneumatic dilation represents a risk factor for laparoscopic Heller myotomy. *Surg Endosc* 1997;11:359-361.
38. Boulez J, Meeus P, Espalieu Ph. Oesocardiomyotomie de Heller sans anti-reflux par voie laparoscopique. *Ann Chir* 1997;51:232-236.
39. Graham AJ, Finley RJ, Worsley DF, Dong SR, Clifton JC, Storseth C. Laparoscopic esophageal myotomy and anterior partial fundoplication for the treatment of achalasia. *Ann Thorac Surg* 1997;64:785-789.
40. Vogt D, Curet M, Pitcher D, Josloff R, Milne RL, Zucker K. Successful treatment of esophageal achalasia with laparoscopic Heller myotomy and Toupet fundoplication. *Am J Surg* 1997;174:709-714.
41. Wang PC, Sharp KW, Holzman MD, Clements RH, Holcomb GW, Richards WO. The outcome of laparoscopic Heller myotomy without antireflux procedure in patients with achalasia. *Am Surg* 1998;64:515-521.
42. Rosati R, Fumagalli U, Bona S, Bonavina L, Pagani M, Peracchia A. Evaluating results of laparoscopic surgery for esophageal achalasia. *Surg Endosc* 1998;12:270-273.
43. Donahue PE, Teresi M, Patel S, Schlesinger PK. Laparoscopic myotomy in achalasia: intraoperative evidence for myotomy of the gastric cardia. *Dis Esoph* 1999;12:30-36.
44. Kjellin AP, Granqvist S, Ramel S, Thor KBÅ. Laparoscopic myotomy without fundoplication in patients with achalasia. *Eur J Surg* 1999;165:1162-1166.
45. Hunt DR and Willis VL. Laparoscopic Heller myotomy for achalasia. *Austr N Z J Surg* 2000;70:582-586.
46. Zaninotto G, Costantini M, Anselmino M, Boccù C, Ancona E. Onset of oesophageal peristalsis after surgery for idiopathic achalasia. *Br J Surg* 1995;82:1532-1534.
47. Zaninotto G, Costantini M, Portale G, et al. Etiology, diagnosis and treatment of failures after laparoscopic Heller myotomy for achalasia. *Ann Surg* 2002 (in press).
48. Rosati R, Fumagalli U, Bona S, Bonavina L, Chella B, Peracchia A. Chirurgia mini-invasiva dei diverticoli epifrenici dell'esofago, in: Zaninotto G, Ancona E (Eds.) La Chirurgia Toraco-Laparoscopica, Stato dell'Arte e Prospettive Future, Cortina, Verona 1997, pp. 119-24.

CHAPTER 24

LAPAROSCOPIC MANAGEMENT OF PANCREATIC TUMORS

Andrea Pietrabissa, Ugo Boggi, Carlo Moretto, Franco Mosca
Department of Surgery and Organ Transplantation, University of Pisa, Pisa, Italy

Abstract
Laparoscopic distal pancreatectomy and splenectomy for cystic tumors of the pancreas is feasible, and appears to correlate with accelerated recovery. The procedure can be accomplished in the lateral position with a three-trocar technique, provided the stomach is suspended to the abdominal wall, and the spleen attachments to the diaphragm are divided last. The hand-assisted technique can be useful in complicated cases, or when tactile feed-back is required to identify occult lesions. Robotic assistance can improve the ergonomics of the procedure and facilitate the more difficult steps of laparoscopic distal pancreatectomy.
Unilateral thoracoscopic truncal splanchnicectomy (TS) is safe and effective for pain relief in patients with unresectable pancreatic cancer. This procedure offers substantial relief of pain in the short term, in patients with unresectable pancreatic cancer, and significantly ameliorates the quality of their residual life.

Keywords
Laparoscopic pancreatectomy, hand-assisted surgery, pain relief.

INTRODUCTION

Laparoscopic resective surgery of the pancreas has witnessed an extraordinary evolution, which is still going on and, although initially restricted to a few pioneer centers, it is currently practised at a growing number of institutions. The first report of a laparoscopic pancreatoduodenectomy dates back to 1992 [1]. This particular procedure was later abandoned by its own proponents,

A.M. Farinon (ed.), *Advances in Abdominal Surgery 2002*, 337-346.

mainly because patients derived no appreciable benefit from this approach, which implies considerable technical skill and prolonged operating times [2]. In contrast, several reports from different authors, have shown how laparoscopic distal pancreatectomy can provide, in selected instances, significant benefit to the patient [3-5] and, with the aid of the latest technology, the procedure seems reproducible with relative ease by most surgeons, particularly if they are already familiar with the advanced laparoscopic techniques of splenectomy and left adrenalectomy. Indeed, several steps of the procedure are common to these two operations. In the following paragraphs the indications and technical points adopted at *ENDODOC* - the Regional Center of Tuscany for Minimally Invasive Surgery and Advanced Technology at the University of Pisa – Italy – in the performance of distal pancreatectomy are presented and discussed.

Disabling pain for many patients with unresectable pancreatic cancer is poorly managed, and can remain a significant problem up until their death. Results and effectiveness of percutaneous celiac plexus block have been controversial, and addiction to opiates often becomes the most prominent feature of these patients. Video-assisted TS has recently emerged as an efficient alternative to the chemical blocks, and to the more invasive open approaches. Our more recent experience with this procedure is also presented and discussed in the following pages.

INDICATIONS TO DISTAL PANCREATECTOMY

Oncological reservations have been expressed concerning the use of laparoscopic surgery in malignant diseases. Moreover, cancer of the pancreatic body and tail is often discovered at an advanced stage, when surgery is no longer useful or requires the combined resection of adjiacent organs for palliative intent. For these reasons, laparoscopic surgery is best indicated for removal of cystic lesions of the pancreas, often benign in nature or with a low malignant potential, and also in the management of islet cell tumors.

Cystic lesions of the pancreatic body or tail include inflammatory pseudocysts (which account for 70% of all lesions), true cysts, serous cystadenomas, mucinous cystadenomas (10% malignant) and cystadenocarcinomas [6]. Preoperative differential diagnosis is based on clinical presentation, imaging techniques and percutaneous biopsy, but remains challenging for the surgeon, with a potential for diagnostic errors that approaches 20%. In absence of symptoms or of a clear demonstration of malignancy, observational management and resection have both been recommended. Today, the availability of the minimally invasive approach can offer the surgeon an attractive alternative, providing the patient with less discomfort and faster recovery, in comparison to the open technique. Considering laparoscopic distal pancreatectomy earlier in the management of cystic lesions of the pancreas will reduce the risk of mistreatment of possible malignancies.

Islet cell tumors represent in our experience another good indication for laparoscopic surgery. These tumors are benign and solitary in over 90% of cases and can easily be enucleated (when in a favourable position) or resected by laparoscopy [7]. Correct intraoperative localisation can occasionally be problematic, and is greatly facilitated by the use of laparoscopic contact ultrasonography , [8] and in selected instances with the digital palpation of the gland (Hand-Assisted Laparoscopic Surgery).

OPERATIVE TECHNIQUE OF LAPAROSCOPIC DISTAL PANCREATECTOMY

Patient position and operative setting

The patient is placed in the right semi-lateral position, and both surgeon and camera-person stand to the patient's right side. Three-trocars are usually enough to complete the procedure.

Pneumoperitoneum is created just above the umbilicus, where the first trocar (10 mm) is positioned. The 30° telescope is advanced through this port for initial exploration. Two additional trocars are then inserted under laparoscopic view: one 10 mm in the subxifoid region, mainly used for exposure and retraction , and one 12 mm in the left flank, used for the placement of scissor, harmonic scalpel, clip applier and stapling device

Exposure of the pancreatic body and tail

By use of the harmonic scalpel and hemoclips the gastrocolic ligament and the short gastric vessels are divided, to allow access to the lesser sac and expose the pancreatic body and tail. The position of the patient on the right flank greatly facilitates these maneuvers as stomach, omentum and left transverse colon fall apart by gravity. To improve access to the pancreatic neck and to the origin of the splenic artery, the stomach is then suspended to the anterior abdominal wall by two interrupted stitches. Sutures mounted on a 5-cm straight needle are used for this purpose. The straight needle is hand-driven percutaneously through the abdominal wall in the left hypocondrium, until a sufficient length emerges from the peritoneal surface. The needle is then grasped internally by a needle holder, is passed through the gastric wall along the greater curvature, and then reversed and guided inside-out through the abdominal wall, in the vicinity of the entrance point. The two ends of the suture are grasped with a Kelly clamp and put in traction, to maximize exposure of the pancreatic body and tail.

Vascular control, pancreatic transection and extraction of the specimen

In the open technique for distal pancreatectomy the spleen is usually first detatched from the diaphragm, and lifted as a handle for quick mobilization of the body and tail of the pancreas. In laparoscopy, on the contrary, the patient being in the flank position, the spleen attachments to the diaphragm should be divided last, to avoid the collapse of the spleno-pancreatic block towards the right hypocondrium. The first passage is therefore the isolation and division of the splenic artery between hemoclips, to reduce the vascular inflow and minimize bleeding during the following dissection. Next, the inferior edge of the pancreas to the left of the superior mesenteric vein is gently lifted, further directing the dissection to the creation of a retroperitoneal tunnel posterior to the pancreatic tail, until the left crus of the diaphragm comes into view. The splenic vein is then dissected off the posterior aspect of the pancreatic neck and encircled with right-angle forceps, to free a sufficient lenght of this vessel for the safe placement of the stapler loaded with a vascular cartridge (Fig. 1). After division of the splenic vein, the pancreatic neck is transected with repeated application of the stapling device. It is preferable to chose a 45 mm stapler which allows a wide opening of the jaws, as the thickness of the pancreas at the transection line is unpredictable, and problems can be encountered in positioning and firing a device of inferior length. Bleeding from the pancreas at the staple line can effectively be controlled with the application of an argon beamer. Then, the pancreas and the spleen can easily be freed from their posterior and superior attatchments.

Once the specimen is ready for extraction, the surgeon can choose any site within the abdomen for the delivery incision. It is our practice in this as in many other circumstances (laparoscopic nephrectomies, splenectomies, etc.), to make a suprapubic transverse skin incision, which is then deepened by longitudinal division of the linea alba and lateral muscles splitting. A purse-string suture is made on the intact peritoneum around the passage of the shaft of a large-size endoscopic retrieval bag, to prevent loss of pneumoperitoneum. The bag is opened in the left hypocondrium, the specimen caught and delivered through the suprapubic incision, after digital dilatation of the small peritoneal defect. A small size drain is usually left close to the pancreatic stump, and both trocar sites and main wound are closed after careful checking of hemostasis in the surgical field.

SPECIAL CONSIDERATIONS

Hand-Assisted pancreatic resection

In Hand-Assisted Laparoscopic Surgery (HALS) of the pancreas, the non-dominant hand of the surgeon is inserted into the abdomen, via special devices that allow maintenance of pneumoperitoneum throughout the procedure [9-10]. The assisting hand is used for display, exposure and blunt dissection. Furthermore, with HALS the surgeon retains tactile feedback which is particularly useful, with the combined adoption of laparoscopic ultrasonography, to detect small occult insulinomas.

Another advantage of having a hand inside the surgical field relates to the immediate control of hemorrhage that can be achieved, a fact not to be disregarded in approaching pancreatic resection. A sub-xiphoidal 7 cm midline incision is our preferred access for HALS in distal pancreatectomy (Fig. 1).

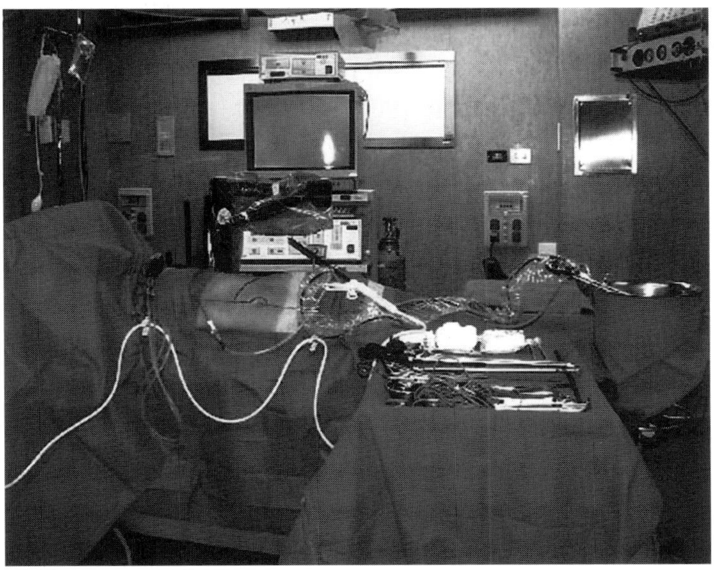

Figure 1. Operative setting for Hand-Assisted distal pancreatectomy using the Omniport device and a robotic visualization system *See color plates.*

It is preferrable to wear brown gloves, as conventional white gloves create a shining effect that interferes with good endoscopic vision. Until new sets of mini-intruments specially designed for HALS become available, one has to realize that the helping hand has limited assisting potential. Particularly for technically demanding dissections, such as dissecting the splenic artery or encircling the splenic vein, it is preferable in our view to have an assisting non-dominant instrument rather than the naked hand. Therefore, during HALS distal pancreatectomy, either the left hand is inserted at a later stage of the procedure, or at times it is withdrawn and replaced by an instrument advanced inside a trocar, placed through those HALS devices that allow a gas-proof regulation of the entrance point, such as the Omniport Hand-Access Device (Advanced Surgical Concepts, Bray, Ireland) or the Lap Disk (Hospital Services Srl, Rome, Italy).

Robotics and solo-surgery

At ENDODOC the AESOP 3000 robotic visualization system (Computer Motion, Santa Barbara, CA, USA) is routinely employed for laparoscopic surgery of the adrenal, spleen, kidney and distal pancreas (Fig. 2).

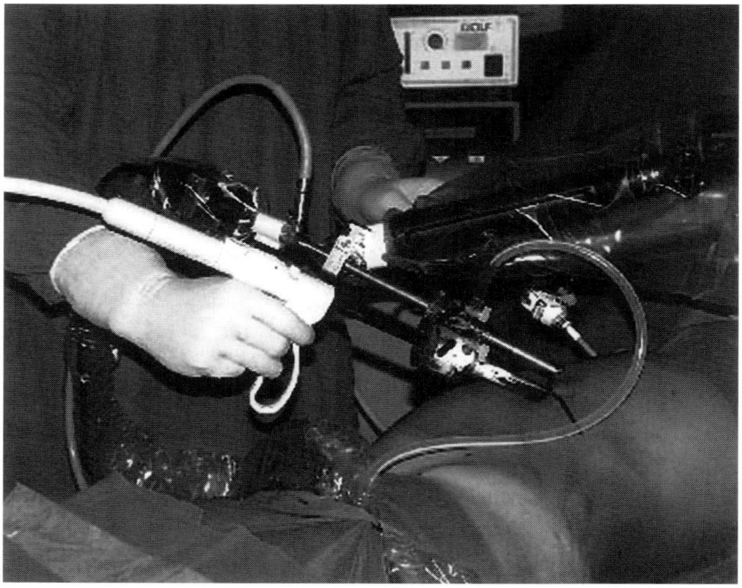

Figure 2 The robotic visualization system AESOP 3000 allows the performance of laparoscopic distal pancreatectomy in "solo-surgery". *See color plates.*

The robotic system imitates the form and function of a human arm, and eliminates the need for an assistant to manually control the camera. The first advantage of using robotic assistance during distal pancreatectomy relates to the ergonomics of the procedure. In fact, the preferred position for the endoscope is in between the two operating instruments, a setting that, when using a camera-person, produces a conflict of ergonomics with the operating surgeon. As a consequence, the surgeon that holds the camera tires very quickly with negative effects on steadiness of images and concentration. Moreover, AESOP provides the surgeon with direct control of a steady operative field of view. The surgeon can in fact maneuver the camera using the speech recognition technology. An established set of voice commands are previously recordered by the operating surgeon onto a voice card, which is inserted into the system controller before surgery. The availability of a motionless operative field is of great benefit for the surgeon who is about to perform a difficult and delicate task such as looping a major vessel. The only movements on the monitor will then be caused by operating instruments and by respiratory excursions. This makes it easier to focus on anatomical details, and contributes towards limiting the occurrence of dissection mistakes.

THORACOSCOPIC SPLANCHNICECTOMY

Severe pain is the single most distressing and debilitating feature of pancreatic cancer. The majority of patients have pain at some time during the course of their disease, and failure to control this symptom often results in major behavioural changes or depression. Thoracoscopic splanchnicectomy (TS), which obviates the morbidity of thoracotomy and of the laparotomic transhiatal approach to the splanchnic nerves, has recently been proposed by a number of authors as an attractive alternative, in the management of upper abdominal pain syndromes secondary to chronic pancreatitis, or supramesocolic malignancies, including unresectable pancreatic cancer. This procedure has the potential to achieve, through a minimally invasive approach, an interruption of pain fibres which is similar to the percutaneous block, with a higher degree of precision, also avoiding the side effects associated with the local diffusion of neurolytic solutions.

Operative technique

Right splanchnicectomy is performed for right-sided pain, while centralised, bilateral and left-sided pain are managed by left splanchnicectomy. Under general anesthesia, with conventional endotracheal double-lung ventilation, the patient is placed in the flank thoracotomy position. Partial pulmonary collapse and down-displacement of the diaphragm are induced by CO^2 insufflation delivered via a Veress needle and maintained at 8 mm Hg throughout the procedure. A 5 mm port for the 30-degree telescope is placed in the sixth intercostal space along the mid-axillary line. One operative 5 mm port is subsequently inserted under visual control, in the eighth intercostal space at the posterior axillary line (Fig. 3).

A three cm horizontal incision is made on the pleura along the costophrenic reflection, just lateral to the descending aorta as it leaves the thorax on the left,

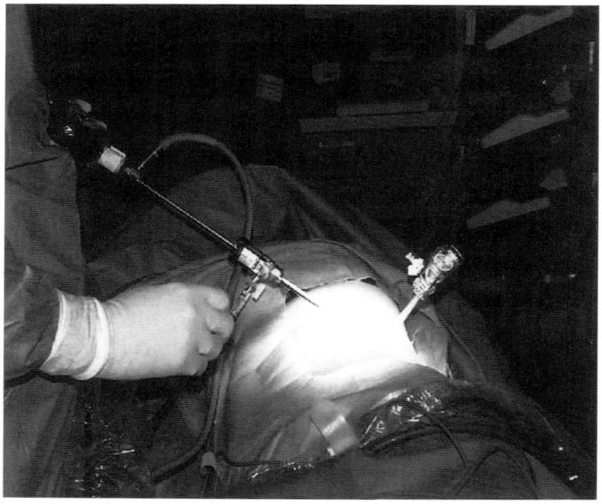

Figure 3. Positioning of trocars for thoracoscopic splanchnicectomy.
See color plates.

and lateral to the azygos vein on the right side. The main trunk of the greater splanchnic nerve is isolated by blunt dissection as distally as possible, and sectioned between hemoclips (Fig. 4). Also, the lesser nerve is always looked for and, if identified, transected. The lung is then completely reinflated under visual control, and no chest tube is usually left in place.

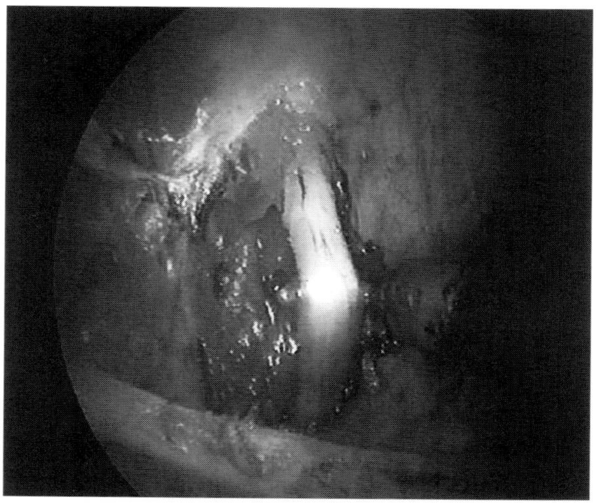

Figure 4. The greater splanchnic nerve is identifyed and then sectioned
See color plates.

Four patients were classified as technical failures, due to dense and diffuse pleural adhesions which made it impossible to reach and section the splanchnic nerves. In the other cases, the main trunk of the greater splanchnic nerve was always identified and transected, while the lesser nerve was seen and divided in only 10 instances. There were 39 left and 11 right splanchnicectomies. Three patients required a contralateral procedure for right back pain recurrence, 8 to 12 weeks after a left splanchnicectomy. The mean duration of the procedure was 23 ± 9 minutes. No death or complication occurred during TS. One patient required postoperative insertion of a chest tube for 24 hours to drain a residual pneumotorax. No orthostatic change of blood pressure was observed after the procedure. Patients were always discharged on the third postoperative day. Transient intercostal pain, at the site of insertion of the 10 mm trocar was common during the first two weeks after TS, but always resolved spontaneously. No patient was lost to follow-up which ranged from 3 to 8 months. At the time of this report follow-up was completed until death in 42 patients. Mean postoperative survival in this group was of 3.6 months. Eight patients are still alive, and their mean postoperative follow-up is 4.6 months. The Nottingham Health Profile questionnaire was used in our patients, to measure perceived health problems secondary to chronic pain before and after TS. The high preoperative scores in each of the five areas considered by this test, which encompass social, psychological, behavioural and physical functioning, reflected the relevant number of problems experienced by patients with severe pain.

At one month after TS, NHP scores were significantly reduced, approximating the estimated scores of a "normal" population, [11]. NHP was confirmed to be a sensitive marker to changes in perceived health, concomitant with sudden relief from severe pain.

Our data indicate that thoracoscopic unilateral truncal splanchnicectomy is safe and effective. The use of CO^2 insufflation makes TS a simple procedure that can usually be performed in less than 30 minutes. It results in significant reduction of pain and consequent improvement of quality of life in patients with unresectable pancreatic cancer. Possibly this technique should be indicated earlier in the course of pancreatic cancer, before the onset of drug-seeking behaviour, rather than as a savage procedure in patients already refractory to narcotics.

REFERENCES

1. Gagner M, Pomp A. Laparoscopic pylorus-preserving pancreatoduodenectomy (Abstract). 2nd Annual Congress, Canadian Society for Endoscopic and Laparoscopic Surgery, Ottawa, Ont., Canada, Sept. 1992; 10(11):26-29.

2. Gagner M, Pomp A. Laparoscopic pancreatic resection: is it worthwhile? *J Gastrointest Surg* 1997; 1(1): 20-26.

3. Cuschieri A, Jakimovicz J. Laparoscopic distal 70% pancreatectomy and splenectomy for chronic pancreatitis. *Ann Surg* 1996; 223(3):280-285.

4. Cuschieri A. Minimally invasive surgery: hepatobiliary-pancreatic and foregut. *Endoscopy* 2000; 32(3): 331-344.

5. Park A, Schwartz R, Tardan V, Anvari M. Laparoscopic pancreatic surgery. *Am J Surg* 1999; 177: 158-163.

6. Shachter PP, Anvi Y, Gvirz G, Rosen A, Czerniak A. The impact of laparoscopy and laparoscopic ultrasound on the management of pancreatic cystic lesions. *Arch Surg* 2000; 135: 260-264.

7. Gagner M, Pomp A, Herrera MF. Early experience with laparoscopic resection of islet cell tumors. *Surgery* 1996; 120: 1051-1054.

8. Berends FJ, Cuesta AM, Kazemier G, van Eijck CHJ, de Herder WW, van Muiswinkel JM, Bruining HA, Bonjer HA. Laparoscopic detection and resection of insulinomas. *Surgery* 2000; 128: 386-391.

9. Klingler PJ, Hinder RA, Menke DM, Smith LS. Hand-Assisted laparoscopic distal pancreatectomy for pancreatic cystadenoma. *Surg Laparosc Endosc* 1998; 8 (3): 180-184.

10. Cuschieri A. Laparoscopic hand-assisted surgery for hepatic and pancreatic disease. *Surg Endosc* 2000; 14: 991-996.

11. Pietrabissa A, Vistoli, F, Carobbi A, Boggi U, Bisà M, Mosca F. Thoracoscopic splanchnicectomy for pain relief in unresectable pancreatic cancer. *Arch Surg* 2000; 135(3): 332-335.

CHAPTER 25

MINIMALLY INVASIVE SURGERY FOR THE TREATMENT OF RECTAL TUMORS: 10 YEARS EXPERIENCE.

Mario Guerrieri, Andrea Tamburini, Francesco Feliciotti, Alessandro Maria Paganini, Angelo De Sanctis, Francesca Crosta, Emanuele Lezoche*.
Institute of Surgical Sciences, University of Ancona, Ancona, Italy
**2nd Surgical Clinic, University of Rome "La Sapienza", Rome, Italy*

INTRODUCTION

Traditional surgery has been used side by side with minimally invasive surgical techniques, which have been widely utilized in the field of benign diseases, as is demonstrated by the use of laparoscopy in cholecystectomy, appendectomy, fundoplication, hernioplasty, splenectomy and adrenalectomy etc. Such procedures are safe and have in common favorable postoperative course with minimal stress for the patient, as demonstrated by several reports (1-5). For this reason, also in malignant diseases, the concept of minimally invasive surgery that utilizes a laparoscopic or transanal endoluminal technique has been introduced. These techniques, associated with preoperative neoadjuvant radiotherapy, could guarantee the same oncological radicality, with minimal surgical stress for the patient. The aim of this study was to evaluate short and long-term results in 169 patients with rectal cancer, who underwent radiotherapy and laparoscopic surgery, or trans-anal endoscopic microsurgery (TEM).

PATIENTS AND METHODS

All operations performed in emergency have been excluded from our series. Indications for a laparoscopic approach have been T2 (ø > 3 cm) and T3 carcinomas. T1 cancers have been treated by TEM as well as T2 carcinomas in patients older than 75, associated with preoperative radiotherapy, and in T2 and T3 high risk patients, or a minimal percentage of patients who refused an ab-

A.M. Farinon (ed.), Advances in Abdominal Surgery 2002, 347-355.

dominal perineal rectal resection (Miles technique). The following parameters were assessed in our protocol: conversion rate, duration of operation, return to normal bowel function, request of drugs for postoperative pain control, duration of hospital stay, clearance of the margins of the specimen, morbidity, mortality, local recurrences rate, metastases and survival. In the laparoscopic approach also the specimen's length and the lymph nodes number have been assessed. After operation the patients were followed-up prospectively by clinical examination, blood exams including tumor markers, colonoscopy, hepatic ultrasound and CT scan every six months.

Relative contraindications to laparoscopic approach were the following: patients who had undergone previous multiple abdominal operations and patients with severe preoperative respiratory insufficiency.

Contraindications to TEM were considered: tumors located into the intra-peritoneal portion of the rectum, lesions larger than 4 cm, N+ lesions and recurrent neoplasm.

Technical steps.

In patients who underwent preoperative radiotherapy, the health margins of the lesion were marked before the treatment with Indian ink.

In the laparoscopic approach four 10-12 mm trocars and a 45° angled scope with a 3CCD camera werer utilized. In all patients a high legation of the inferior mesenteric vessels with vascular staplers (endo-GIA) was performed. All the main oncological concepts of traditional surgery were followed, such as extensive limphadenectomy, a total meso-rectal excision en-bloc with the rectum and a correct clearance of the specimen's margins. The operative specimens were removed through a 5-6 cm sovra-pubic or sub-umbilical mini-laparotomy. After the first 10 operations a wound protector sleeve was used to prevent the possible implant of cancer cells. In the case of abdominal-perineal amputation the specimens were removed through the perineal access. When an anastomosis was required, it was performed intracorporeally with visceral stapler according to the Knight-Griffen technique. If the hydro-pneumatic test results as being positive, a reinforce laparoscopic intracorporeal suture is placed.

At the end of the operation a left para-colic and para-anastomotic drains were placed with the successive extra-peritonealization, when possible, of the anastomosis and drain. Then the operative specimens were measured and fixed in a 10% solution of formaline for 24 hours; the lymph nodes were counted and isolated with standard methods.

TEM technique requires general anesthesia, even if in some selected high-risk patients regional anesthesia was used. The surgeon approaches the operative field through a modified rectoscope connected to sealing elements to prevent gas loss, and introduces the microsurgical instruments. The rectal cavity is inflated with CO2, monitoring continually the internal pressure. The dissection is carried out using a multifunctional cutting-suction-coagulation instrument [9, 41]. A full-thickness resection is performed, including the peri-rectal fat and regional lymph nodes. At the end an abundant washing of the residual cavity is performed using a solution of saline and Mitomicine C (10 mg in 200cc of saline). The specimen is then washed and arranged on a cork sole where it is fixed by needles and sent to the pathologist. The wound is closed using a PDS 3-0 semi-continual suture with a silver clip at both end of the wire, in order to avoid intracorporeal knots.

Sixty-two patients (34 males, 28 females, with a mean age of 64.2 years, ranging from 32-86 years) underwent laparoscopic resection of rectal tumors, whereas 107 patients (66 males, 41 females, with a mean age 65.6 years, ranging from 31-95 years) underwent TEM approach to rectal tumors.

All patients of both groups, excluding the pT1 cases, underwent preoperative radiotherapy (5.040 cGy in 5 weeks) and were operated after 40 days.

In 45 cases the operations done by laparoscopy were sub-mesorectal resections, and 17 abdominal-perineal amputations. In 3 patients with preoperative Duke's D staging, synchronous hepatic metastases were treated with open cryotherapy, after the laparoscopic resection of the primary tumor. A sub-costal bilateral incision was used in order to obtain a better exposition of the liver.

RESULTS

Among the patients treated by radiotherapy combined with minimally invasive techniques, an excellent response was observed in 50% of the patients, moderate in 35%, and absent in 14.8%.

No operative mortality was observed in either group.

Nine out of 62 patients (8 anterior rectal resection and 1 abdominal-perineal resection) were converted to open surgery for the following reasons: in 7 cases difficulty in dissection of the rectum, and in 2 cases for bleeding. The global conversion rate in the first 31 patients was 23.3% and the one of the last 31 cases was of 6.6%, as a result of a learning curve. No conversions were needed in patients treated by TEM approach.

The mean operative time for the laparoscopic operations was 270 minutes (ranging from 150-470 minutes). In the series of patients treated by TEM the mean operative time was 116 minutes (ranging from 45-200 minutes). The NG tube was removed routinely at the end of the operation in both groups. Sixty-four per cent of patients of the laparoscopic group and 86% of patients of the TEM group reached normal bowel function on the second postoperative day. The most marked advantage of minimally invasive approaches was the significant reduction of postoperative discomfort, compared with patients operated by open traditional approach; in fact both in the TEM group and in the laparoscopic group postoperative pain and pain killer drugs were minimal.

Mean postoperative hospital stay in patient operated by laparoscopic technique was 10.2 days (ranging from 6-35 days), for the group operated by TEM technique the mean postoperative hospital stay was 5 days (ranging from 3-12 days) with mobilization on the first postoperative day and also resuming a solid diet on the third postoperative day.

Two postoperative minor complications (5.9%) were present in the laparoscopic group and were represented as follow: 1 patient showed a mild stenosis of the anastomosis requiring dilatation; 1 patient showed urinary retention.

Major complications were observed in 4 patients (7.5%) treated laparoscopically: 3 patients presented an anastomotic leak, in 1 case requiring reoperation with derivative colostomy, and the two other cases were treated by conservative therapy. In one case a postoperative ileus was observed, and was solved by NG tube and medical therapy.

Minor complications in patients who underwent TEM were observed in 11 cases (10.3%): in 7 patients a partial dehiscence of the suture, concerning 1/3 of the circumference, was observed between the third and seventh postoperative day, and was treated by conservative therapy. Three cases of fecal incontinence were observed, and were treated by physiotherapy and biofeedback after 2 months. A single case of hemorrhage requiring blood transfusion occurred.

Major complications in the TEM group were observed in 2 cases (1.9%), and were represented by: a recto-ureteral fistula treated conservatively by urinary catheter, and a recto-vaginal fistula in a patient who had refused preoperative radiotherapy. This patient, who was preoperatively staged as pT2 and postoperatively resulted as pT3, underwent successively abdominal-perineal rectal amputation.

The definitive histology of patient who underwent laparoscopic resection resulted as follow: 15 pT1 (29%), 19 pT2 (37%), 13 pT3 (25%) e 5 pT4 (9%). The mean length of specimens' length was 24.7 cm; the mean length of the free tumor margin was 3.0 cm, the mean number of lymph nodes' identified in the specimens was 10.3.

The mean number of lymph nodes number identified in the specimens of TEM cases was one. The definitive postoperative staging of rectal tumors treated by TEM was as follow: 15 cases with no cancer cells identified in the specimen (pT0) (14%), 24 pT1 (22,4%), 52 pT2 (48,6%) e 16 pT3 (15%).

The mean follow-up in the laparoscopic group was 39.7 months (ranging from 12-76 months). No trocars tumor cells implantation was observed on the trocars site or on the wound of laparotomies. Local recurrences were observed in 10.6% of patients, which required reoperation.

A single patient who had previously undergone abdominal-perineal resection was reoperated 3 months later, and died a few days later of peritoneal diffusion. A patient who underwent anterior rectal resection stage pT3, N1 and was reoperated 2 months later by Hartman procedure, is alive at 45 months from the reoperation (specimen's margin is disease free). A third patient who underwent sub-mesorectal resection, presented a massive local recurrence 9 months later, and died two months after a palliative colostomy. The last patient returning 37 months after having been operated for abdominal-perineal amputation, presented a local massive recurrence requiring a pelvic exenteratio, and is alive 6 months after this operation.

In the TEM group local recurrences were observed in 6.5% of patients at a mean follow-up of 44 months (range 6-108). Five recurrences were observed in the pT2 stage and 2 in pT3 stage. Among the five pT2 patients, three did not undergo preoperative radiotherapy. One patient underwent radiotherapy followed by video-assisted abdominal perineal rectal amputation, and died 46 months later of esophageal cancer, free from rectal disease.

Another old high-risk patient was treated with radiotherapy and TEM, and is alive and disease free 60 months after the reoperation. A cirrhotic patient underwent open resection after 12 months. Two pT2 patients, who had previously undergone radiotherapy, developed a recurrence respectively at the 30th and 6th months of follow-up, and were treated with abdominal-perineal amputation. In two cases, being high-risk pT3 patients, a radiotherapy cycle was repeated, and these patients are alive at 20 and 15 months respectively of follow-up.

Metachronous metastases were observed in 14.9% of cases in the laparoscopic group and in 1.9% in the TEM group. Among the last group a patient has underwent hepatic resection 14 months after the previous operation and is alive at 30 months from the second operation.

A second patient operated for hepatic resection 26 months after the TEM operation died 13 months later.

At follow up, the survival rate (excluding unrelated mortality) was 100% for T0 and T1 patients in both groups. In laparoscopic series the survival for T2, T3, and T4 patients was 78,8%, 61,6% and 20%, respectively. In TEM group it was 81% and 62,5% for T2 and T3 patients, respectively.

DISCUSSION

Our study started in 1992, with the aim of analyzing the feasibility and short and long-term results of rectal resections carried out by laparoscopic approach and TEM. The majority of recent reports demonstrate that laparoscopic rectal surgery is safe and feasible, with an acceptable percentage of conversions to open surgery (12-18%), low morbidity (5-20%) and low mortality (0-5%) [12-16]. In our series the conversion rate is 17% and is similar to the one reported by other authors. The most frequent cause of conversion resulted as being the difficulty in isolation of the rectum, which is in part being overcome by progress of experience [17-18]. The general belief is anyway that the times of return to bowel functions and the hospital stay, are shorter in laparoscopic surgery (3,5 and 6 days, respectively) [10-11, 14]. Some authors did not observe a significant difference in terms of hospital stay, as compared with open surgery (7-14 day) [5, 21-22]. All the authors underlined a significant reduction of post-operative pain and discomfort, as documented by clinical observation and a lower request for painkiller drugs. In our series, the majority of patients recovered bowel function and resumed a liquid diet rapidly in both groups. As described in several reports, postoperative pain reduction in colo-rectal minimally invasive surgery has been the most relevant aspect as compared with the open procedure.

The feasibility of a colorectal oncologically correct laparoscopic resection has been demonstrated in previous reports [8, 11, 19-21]. Jacobs (3), who first described the first 20 cases treated laparoscopically, observed that the extension of bowel and mesenteric resection was comparable with that usually obtained with open surgery. Other authors [12, 15-16, 22-23], who reported that the number of lymph node included in the operative specimen is not different from the one obtained with open procedures, confirmed these conclusions.

Oncological concerns are related to the risk of implantation in the trocars or specimen extraction sites, and the effect of CO_2 on malignant cell growth; there are several studies regarding this topic [26-28]. In any case, the real incidence of trocars site recurrences is not well known. Several measures are suggested in order to prevent them: avoid direct manipulation of the tumor; limit the instruments' insertion; protect the minilaparotomy with a plastic sleeve; avoid squeezing the specimen, but extend the incision; peritoneal cavity washing and aspiration; washing of the trocars site and minilaparotomy, with saline or heparin or povidone solution (dilution tumor cells), and complete aspiration of the solution; complete disinflation of the pneumoperitoneum before instrument removal and suture. Recent advances in minimally invasive techniques have rendered possible treatment with curative intention of the initial rectal cancer, by local excision associated to preoperative radiotherapy [30-32]. TEM can also be applied in more invasive tumours (pT2, pT3), in high-risk patients or in patient who, informed about their pathology, refused an abdominal perineal rectal amputation. The advantages, compared to traditional transanal resection, consist in a better exposition given by the distension obtained with gas, and three-dimensional magnification that allows precise dissection and lower incidence of recurrences (10-24% transanal resection). We consider mandatory an accurate preoperative staging of the lesions: for this reason we utilize a specific protocol, which includes clinical examination, endoscopy with multiple macro biopsies, transanal ultrasound CT scan and MRI. In our TEM series 12 lesions were preoperatively understaged: 4 were adenomas preoperatively considered pT1, which however underwent curative TEM, because full thickness excisions were conducted. In other 8 adenomas, in which preoperative transanal ultrasound was not performed, because their location was more than 12 cm from the anal verge, a clinically relevant understating was observed (7 pT2 and 1 pT3). These patients underwent radiotherapy and were reoperated by anterior rectal resection. Lastly, in a patient preoperatively considered pT2, a pT3 tumor resulted at the definitive histology, and he was reoperated.

Preoperative radiotherapy did not determine increased difficulty in tissues dissection, or in the suture, and did not increase the dehiscence risk, either in cases operated by open surgery or laparoscopically. The 7 cases of dehiscence after TEM procedure were observed in wide full-thickness recections, with consequent tension of the suture. Undoubtedly, a more favorable clinical result was observed in a patient with a suture dehiscence after TEM than in a patient with dehiscence after submesorectal laparoscopic resection. In fact, in TEM technique the perirectal fat dissection is limited, and this facilitate the healing of the cavity. However, almost all dehiscences, except in a case reoperated after laparoscopy, have been treated conservatively. The major complication rate after TEM (1 dehiscence and 1 recto-vaginal fistula) was low (1.9%).

At follow up the recurrence rate was low in both techniques and cancer related mortality was comparable with the literature data.

CONCLUSIONS

The results reported by our study confirm that laparoscopic surgery shows a better postoperative course in terms of minimal pain, rapid resuming of bowel functions and mobilization. In patients treated with preoperative radiotherapy, the advantage is extended to a lower rate of local recurrences.

Minimally invasive surgery has gained therefore a primary role in the treatment of all colo-rectal pathologies, but a definitive judgment on its application in the oncological field is not at the moment decisive. Conclusions of our study need to be confirmed: oncological long-term results are not completely known, and further prospective randomized protocols have to be carried out before these procedures can be widely approved.

REFERENCES

1. Cooperman AM, Katz V, Zimmon D, Botero G. Laparoscopic colon resection a case report. *J Laparosc Endosc Surg* 1991; 1: 221.
2. Fowler DL, Sharon AW. Laparoscopy-assisted sigmoid resection. *Surg Laparosc Endosc* 1991; 1: 3.
3. Jacobs M, Verdeja JC, Goldestein HS. Minimally invasive colon resection (laparoscopic colectomy). *Surg Laparosc Endosc* 1991; 1: 144.
4. Corbitt JD. Preliminary experience with laparoscopic guided colectomy. *Surg Laparosc Endosc* 1992; 2: 791.
5. Monson JRT, Darzi A, Corey PD, Guillon PS. Prospective evaluation of laparoscopic-assisted colectomy in unselected group of patients. *Lancet* 1992; 340: 831-833.
6. Musser PJ, Boorse RC, Madera F, Reed FJ III. Laparoscopic colectomy: at what cost? *Surg Laparosc Endosc* 1994; 4: 1-5.
7. Peters WR, Bartels TL. Minimally invasive colectomy: are the potential benefits realized? *Dis Colon Rectum* 1993; 36: 751-756.
8. Feliciotti F, Paganini AM, Guerrieri M, Lezoche E. Gasless laparoscopy for greater respect of oncological criteria during laparoscopic colon resection. Abstract Atti 4th Int. Congr. of European Ass. for Endosc. Surg. (E.A.E.S.) , June 1996, Trondheim, n. 79.
9. Guerrieri M, Paganini AM, Feliciotti F, Zenobi P, Proietti A, Lezoche E. Trattamento locale del carcinoma del retto mediante microchirurgia endoscopica transanale (TEM) associata a radioterapia: risultati a cinque anni di follow-up. *Chir Gastroent* 1997; 31: 1.
10. Phillips EH, Franklin M, Carrol BJ, Fallas MJ, Ramos R Rosenthal. Laparoscopic colectomy. *Ann Surg* 1992; 216: 6.
11. Franklin ME, Rosenthal D, Norem RF. Prospective evaluation of laparoscopic colon resection vs open colon resection for adenocarcinoma. *Surg Endosc* 1995; 9: 811-816.
12. Fielding GA, Lumley J, Nathanson L, Hewitt P, Rhodes M, Stitz R. Laparoscopic colectomy. *Surg Endosc* 1997; 11: 745.
13. Fine AP, Lanasa S, Gannon MP, Cline CW, James R. Laparoscopic colon surgery: report of a series. *Ann Surg* 1995; 61: 5.
14. Lacy AM, Garcia-Valdecasas JC, Delgado S, Grande S, Fuster J, Tabet J, Ramos C, Pique JM, Cfuentes A, Visa J. Postoperative complications of laparoscopic assisted colectomy. *Surg Endosc* 1997; 11: 119-22.
15. Tucker JG, Ambroze WL, Orangio GR, Duncan TD, Mason EM, Lucas GW. Laparoscopic assisted bowel surgery. *Surg Endosc* 1995; 9: 297-300.
16. Fingerhut A. Laparoscopic colectomy. The French experience. Laparoscopic Colorectal Surgery Churchill Livingstone, New York 1995; 253-257.
17. Larach SW, Salomon MC, Williamson PR, Goldstein E. Laparoscopic assisted colectomy: experience during the learning curve. *Coloproctology* 1993; 1: 38-41.
18. Falk PM, Beart RW, Wewner SD, Thorson AG, Jagelman DG, Lavery IC, Johanses OB, Fizgibbons RJ Jr. Laparoscopic colectomy: a critical appraisal. *Dis Colon Rectum* 1993; 36: 28-34.
19. Wilson JP, Hoffman GC, Baker JW, Fitchett CW, Vansant JH. Laparoscopic assisted colectomy. Initial experience. *Ann Surg* 1994; 219, 732-743.
20. Senagore AJ, Luchtefeld MA, Mackeigan JM, Mazier WP. Open colectomy versus laparoscopic colectomy: are there differences. *Am Surg* 1993; 59, 549-554.
21. Wexner SD, Cohen SM, Johansen OB, et al. Laparoscopic colorectal surgery: a prospectie assessment and current perspective. *Br J Surg* 1993; 80, 1602-1605.
22. Wexner SD, Cohen SM, Ulrich A, Reissman P. Laparoscopic colorectal surgery: are we being honest with out patients? *Dis Colon Rectum* 1995; 38, 1-5.

23. Van Ye TM, Cattery RP, Henry LG. Laparoscopic assisted colon resections compare favorably with open technique. *Surg Lap Endosc* 1994; 4 (1): 25-31.
24. Bohm B, Milsom JW, Kitago K, Brand M, Fazio VW. Laparoscopic oncologic total abdominal colectomy with intraperitoneal stapled anastomosis in a canine model. *J Laparoendosc Surg* 1994; 4, 23-30.
25. Milsom JW, Bohm B, Deconini C, Fazio VW. Laparoscopic oncologic proctosigmoidectomy with low colorectal anastomosis in a cadaver model. *Surg Endosc* 1994; 8, 1117-1123.
26. Nduka CC, Monson JRT, Menzies-Gow N, Darzi A. Abdominal wall metastases following laparoscopy. *Br J Surg* 1994; 81, 648-652.
27. Alexander RJ, Jacques BC, Mitchell KG. Laparoscopically assisted colectomy and wound recurrences. *Lancet* 1994; 249-250.
28. Fusco MA, Paluzzi MW. Abdominal wall recurrence after laparoscopic assisted colectomy for adenocarcinoma of the colon. *Colon Rectum* 1993; 36, 858-861.
29. Lezoche E, Paganini AM, Cuschieri A. Minimally invasive colorectal surgery. Documento Editoriale S.R.L., Milano 1994.
30. Frazee RC, Patel R, Belew M, Roberts JW, Hendricks R. Transanal excision of rectal carcinoma. *Am Surg* 1995; 61, 714-717.
31. Read DR, Sokil S, Ruiz-Salas G. Transanal local excision of rectal cancer. *Int J Colorectal Dis* 1995; 10, 73-76.
32. Said S, Stippel D, Zieren J. Minimal invasive surgery in the local treatment of rectal cancer. *Ann Chir Gynaecol* 1994; 83, 167-173.
33. Hartley JE, Mehigan BJ, Mac Donald AW, Lee AW, Monson JR. Patterns of recurrence and survival after laparoscopic and conventional resections for colorectal carcinoma. *Ann Surg* 2000; 2: 181-186.
34. Khalili TM, Fleshner PR, Hiatt JR, Sokol TP, Manookian M, Tsushima G, Phillips EH. Colorectal cancer: comparison of laparoscopic with open approach. *Dis Colon Rectum* 1998; 41: 832-838.
35. Kockerling F. Prospective multicenter study of the quality of oncologic resections in patients undergoing laparoscpic colorectal surgery for cancer. *Col Rect* 1998; 8: 963-970.
36. Lezoche E, Feliciotti F, Paganini AM, Guerrieri M, Campagnacci R, De Sanctis A. Laparoscopic colonic resections versus open surgery: a prospective non-randomized study on 310 unselected cases. *Hep Gastroent* 2000; 47: 697-710.
37. Lezoche E, Feliciotti F, Paganini AM, Guerrieri M, Campagnacci R, De Sanctis A. Colonic cancer by elective laparoscopy versus open procedures. EAES expert' s opinion conference on colonic cancer by elective laparoscopy.8th Int Cong EAES, Nice, France, 2000.
38. Lord SA, Larach SW, Ferrara A, Williamson PR, Lago CP, Lube MW.Laparoscopic resection for colorectal carcinoma: a three-years experience. *Dis Colon Rectum* 1996; 39: 148-154.
39. Milsom JW, Bohm B, Hammerhofer KA, Fazio V, Steiger E, Elson P. A prospective, randomized trial comparing laparoscopic versus conventional techniques in colorectal surgery: a preliminary report. *J Am Coll Surg* 1998; 187: 46-57.
40. Puolin EC, Mamazza J, Schlachta CM, Gregoire R, Roy N. Laparoscopic resection does not adversely affect early survival curves in patients undergoing surgery for colorectal adenocarcinoma. *Ann Surg* 1999; 4: 487-492.
41. Lezoche E, Guerrieri M, Paganini AM, Feliciotti F. Transanal Endoscopic Microsurgical excision of irradiated and nonirradiated rectal cancer. A 5 year experience. *Surg Lap & Endosc* 1998; 8: 249-256.

SECTION VI

TRANSPLANTATION

CHAPTER 26

PANCREAS PROCUREMENT FROM CADAVERIC DONORS OF MULTIPLE GRAFTS

Ugo Boggi, Fabio Vistoli, Marco Del Chiaro, Andrea Pietrabissa, Gabriele Catalano, Piero Marchetti, Stefano Del Prato*, Franco Mosca
*Department of Surgery and Organ Transplantation, *Endocrinology and Metabolism, Section of Metabolism, University of Pisa, Pisa, Italy*

Abstract
Background This paper describes a modified technique for concurrent procurement of pancreas, liver, kidneys and isolated small bowel. The main distinctive features of this procedure are avoidance of direct portal perfusion and simplification of in vivo and bench-work dissection.
Methods Between December 1997 and December 2001, 893 grafts were retrieved in 223 multiorgan procurements.
Results All procurements progressed expeditiously and no graft sustained injuries precluding transplant. Vascular variations were identified in 82 donors (36.7%). A total of 64 pancreata were transplanted by our team, including 48 simultaneous pancreas-kidney transplants, 6 simultaneous cadaveric pancreas living kidney transplants and 10 pancreas transplants alone. One additional pancreas was procured and shipped to another center for isolated grafting. Three pancreata were employed for islet cell transplantation and 96 for islet cell isolation and in vitro viability and secretion studies. The remaining 59 pancreata were discarded. A total of 181 livers (174 full size grafts, 6 split grafts and 1 reduced size graft), 419 kidneys and 2 isolated small bowels were also procured and transplanted at 17 different institutions. In 20 instances the liver was not allocated to our center. Nineteen liver teams (95%), from 9 different institutions, agreed to procure their grafts according to our method. Seven procurements were done entirely by our team, and 12 by a surgeon from the liver transplant team assisted by one of us.
Conclusions This procurement technique is quick, simple, safe, standardized, flexible and at least as effective as other "conventional" procedures. Since one team can procure all abdominal organs, this technique may facilitate organization and reduce costs of multiorgan procurement.

A.M. *Farinon (ed.), Advances in Abdominal Surgery 2002*, 359-383.

INTRODUCTION

Multiple organ procurement is a unique surgical operation: it takes place almost constantly overnight, often after a busy working day, and involves multiple surgical teams, each devoted to the retrieval of a specific organ and therefore mostly concerned with their own needs. Time for organization is usually limited, and the procedure can rarely be delayed significantly without the risk of losing the donor [1], or compromising the quality of the organs [2]. Hemodynamic instability of the donor may boost the above factors, and contribute towards creating an atmosphere of competition among surgical teams [3]. Moreover, the operating room staff of hospitals not actively involved in recipient operations is usually not accustomed to procurement procedures and techniques. Consequently, while someone may be interested in the novelty of the procedure and become strongly cooperative, others may regard organ procurement merely as an additional working load, and may be indifferent, or even overtly hostile [4]. Under these circumstances, meticulous in situ dissections, the necessity for close intraoperative monitoring or support and, more generally any necessity that complicates or prolongs the procedure, may lead to suboptimal procurement because of unfavorable operative conditions.

The ideal technique for abdominal organ procurement, capable of overcoming these difficulties, should be quick, simple, safe, standardized, flexible and effective, and should involve as few teams as possible. Speed is required to avoid destabilization of a frail donor [5, 6], improve collaboration among different procurement teams [7], reduce intraoperative hemorrhage [8], and to prevent warm ischemic injury occurring after prolonged normothermic dissections, as a consequence of vasospasm, unintentional vascular occlusion and hemodynamic instability [2-3, 6-7, 9-10]. Simplicity and safety are required to allow the procurement of anatomically intact grafts [11]. Effectiveness is required to ensure the procurement of grafts of good quality with high rates of immediate functional recovery [6]. Flexibility is required to assure quick, simple, safe and effective procurement of all organs, including those not usually procured, such as the intestines, under any logistic, anatomic or hemodynamic conditions. Standardization is required to enhance cooperation among procurement teams, and to facilitate shipping of grafts among transplant centers [4]. The limited number of the teams, ideally one for the chest and another for the abdomen, would greatly facilitate organization, reduce costs, and, hopefully, improve cooperation [4, 11-13].

We describe the results of a quick en bloc technique of subtotal abdominal evisceration, employed for the combined procurement of pancreas, liver, kidneys, and small bowel. This technique, developed to expand the donor pool for pancreas transplant, is an evolution of the one described in 1992 by Nakazato and co-workers [13]. The main improvements of the modified procedure are avoidance of direct portal perfusion and simplification of in vivo dissection, achieved by keeping organs not planned for procurement out of the operative field. Other changes have been made to both in vivo dissection and benchwork preparation of the grafts.

MATERIALS AND METHODS

In the period between December 1997 and December 2001, 223 multiple-organ procurements were done with the technique described below. A total of 893 organs were retrieved including 223 livers, 223 pancreata, 445 kidneys (1 donor donated a single kidney) and 2 small bowels (Tab. 1). The grafts were perfused with UW solution (Viaspan, Dupont Pharmaceuticals, Stevenage, Herts, UK) in 195 procurements (87.5%) and with Celsior® (Celsior, Imtix Sangstat Lyon, France) in the remaining 28.

Thirteen donors (5.8%) were found to harbour an occult tumor in the prostate (n= 6), in the kidneys (n=4), in the uterus (n= 1), in the adrenal gland (n=1), and in the liver (n=1). None of the organs retrieved from these donors was transplanted.

Eight pancreata procured from the first 8 consecutive donors of this series were also discarded. They were not suitable for transplant, and were used to verify the technique of in-vivo dissection and bench work preparation of the grafts. Subsequently, a total of 65 pancreata were procured and transplanted alone (n= 11), or simultaneously with a kidney procured from either the same cadaveric donor (n=48) or a living donor (n=6). Four (5.8%) out of 68 grafts allocated to whole pancreas transplant, on the basis of the selection criteria set up by local transplant agencies, were procured and subsequently discarded, because of severe fibro-fatty infiltration (n=1), kidney tumor (n=1) and poor histologic score of kidney biopsy (n=1). All the organs procured from a donor with severe and prolonged hemodynamic instability were discarded, after histologic documentation of liver necrosis and severe tubular necrosis of the kidneys. The remaining 134 pancreata were allocated to our research and clinical program of islet cell transplant. Thirty-five grafts were found not suitable for islet cell isolation, because of a donor age above 80 years (n=7), chronic pancreatitis (n=11), and donor infection with hepatitis B and C viruses (n=17). The remaining 99 pancreata were used for either insulin secretion studies under different conditions (n=96), or transplant (n=3).

The procurement team consisted of one licensed surgeon and two residents. Once the grafts were separated on the back table, one additional surgeon was called in to complete the preparation of the liver.

Data are presented as mean (± standard deviation)

Table 1. Donor characteristic

Characteristics	**With whole pancreas transplantation (n=65)**		**Without pancreas transplantation (n=158)**	
	mean or n°	SD or %	mean or n°	SD or %
Age (yr)	30.3	± 10.9	53.5	± 17.6
Sex				
Male	42	64.6%	91	57.6%
Female	23	35.4%	67	42.4%
Donor diagnosis				
Closed head trauma	36	55.4%	54	34.2%
Intracranial hemorrhage	29	44.6%	104	65.8%
Mechanical ventilation (hr)	57.2	± 49.3	76.8	± 54.6
Body mass index	24.2	± 3.2	28.3	± 5.2
Vasopressors				
Use	60	92.3%	144	91.1%
Dopamine				
Use	41	63%	142	89.9%
Dose (mg/kg/min)	7.1	± 3.5	5.2	± 4.2
Dobutamine				
Use	7	10.7%	22	13.9%
Dose (mg/kg/min)	4.3	± 1.3	2.5	± 4.2
Norepinephrine				
Use	34	52.3%	62	39.2%
Dose (mg/kg/min)	0.5	± 0.3	0.6	± 0.1
Systolic blood pressure				
Low (< 100 mmHg)	6	9.2%	12	7.6%
High (> 100 mm Hg)	59	90.7%	146	92.4%
Hypotensive events (<60 mmHg)	25	38.5%	68	43%
Cardiac arrest	3	4.6%	11	7%
Heart beating during retrieval	64	98.5%	158	100%
Transfusions (units)	3.3	± 4.5	4.6	± 5.8
Serum amlyase level (U/L)	163.4	± 58.3	172.8	± 51.8
Blood glucose level (mg/dl)	143.2	± 42.2	153.6	± 44.8
Serum creatinine level (mg/dl)	1.02	± 0.39	1.4	± 0.89
Admission Cokroft-Gault (mg/dl)	112.7	± 18.2	101.6	± 38.2

SELECTION CRITERIA FOR PANCREAS DONATION

All donors aged less than 55 years without history of diabetes, pancreatic disease, or pancreatic trauma were considered eligible for pancreas donation. Donor hyperglycemia or hyperamylasemia, hemodynamic instability (including short-lived episodes of cardiac arrest) requiring either low or high doses of vasopressors, and long periods of intensive care unit stay, were not considered as absolute contraindications. The final decision to accept a graft was based on the gross appearance of the pancreas (i.e. presence of calcifications, fibrosis or extent of fatty infiltration), and on the quality of the vessels (i.e. evidence of severe atherosclerotic disease). Quality of perfusion was also considered, and it was thought to be adequate if the liver blanched homogeneously and quickly with easy drainage of clear venous effluent.

PROCUREMENT TECHNIQUE

In vivo normothermic dissection

Donors were prepped from the chin to the pubis and a long midline incision was made from the sternal notch to the symphysis pubis. After division of liver ligaments (round, falciform, left triangular and left coronary) the abdomen was quickly checked to verify the quality of the organs to be retrieved, and the presence of anatomic variations in arterial liver supply. Attention was also paid to identify any occult disease. Next, the infrarenal aorta was encircled just above the bifurcation. The inferior mesenteric artery was not ligated. The supraceliac aorta was exposed by transcrural dissection from the right side of the abdominal esophagus or, in case of anomalous left hepatic arteries, from the left side. A nasogastric tube, placed prior to laparotomy, was advanced into the duodenum and 500 ml of 20% povidone-iodine solution instilled.

In case of combined procurement of the bowel, the right colon was mobilized towards the left, the colo-epiploic ligament was dissected and the middle colic vein and artery were divided and tied. The superior mesenteric vessels were then isolated at the level of the uncinate process of the pancreas, while paying particular attention to spare the ileocolic vein (Fig. 1). After sectioning the mesenteric root as close to the pancreas as possible the small bowel graft remained connected to the donor only through the skeletonized mesenteric vessels. Any bleeding point was identified at this stage, in order to prevent post-reperfusion hemorrhage in the recipient.

When the liver was to be shared by 2 recipients, the split was be performed either with the intact donor circulation or entirely as a bench work procedure, depending on the degree of hemodynamic stability of the donor and the preference of the liver procurement team.

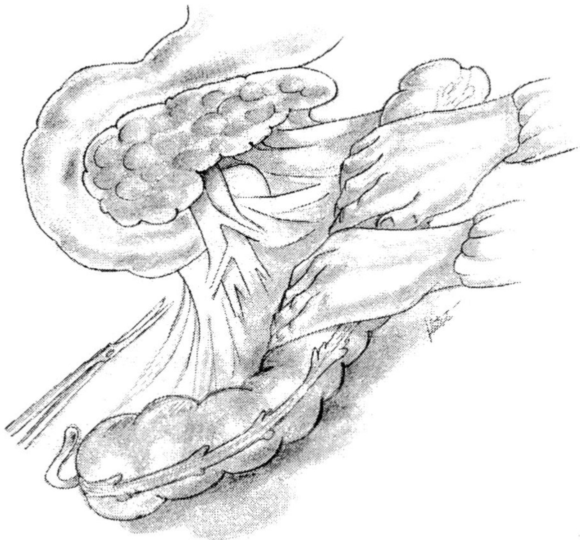

Figure 1. Complete mobilization of the right colon allows identification of the superior mesenteric vein and artery

As soon as the thoracic teams were ready, the donor was fully heparinized and the distal aorta was cannulated with a large bore cannula (12 to 18 F, Medtronic, DLP, Grand Rapids, MI, USA) connected to a gravity flush system primed with chilled preservation solution.

In vivo hypothermic dissection

As the cardiac surgeon induced the heart arrest, and incised the inferior vena cava at its junction with the right atrium, the abdominal team crossclamped the supraceliac aorta, began the perfusion of abdominal organs and filled the abdomen with ice slush saline solution. The preservation solution was then allowed to flow freely during the procurement of thoracic organs, or until it was deemed necessary. In the meantime, the gallbladder was opened and washed with chilled saline solution, the supraceliac aorta was tied and the vascular clamp withdrawn. In case of combined procurement of the intestine, the small bowel was removed first: the superior mesenteric vessels were divided, leaving a proximal stump of about 0.5 cm including the pancreaticoduodenal artery and vein. The small bowel was procured en bloc with the right colon, in order to facilitate proper graft positioning at the time of transplant. The colon was readily removed after reperfusion.

In all the other cases, removal of abdominal organs began with a complete mobilization of the stomach. The gastrocolic ligament and the short gastric vessels were sectioned, the first portion of the duodenum was closed and divided with the GIA stapler, the lesser curvature was dissected up to the cardia (thus leaving the intact hepato-gastric ligament with the liver), and the stomach was swept up into the pericardium (Fig. 2). The colon was mobilized next and swept down onto the donor's legs (Fig. 3). The diaphragm was widely incised

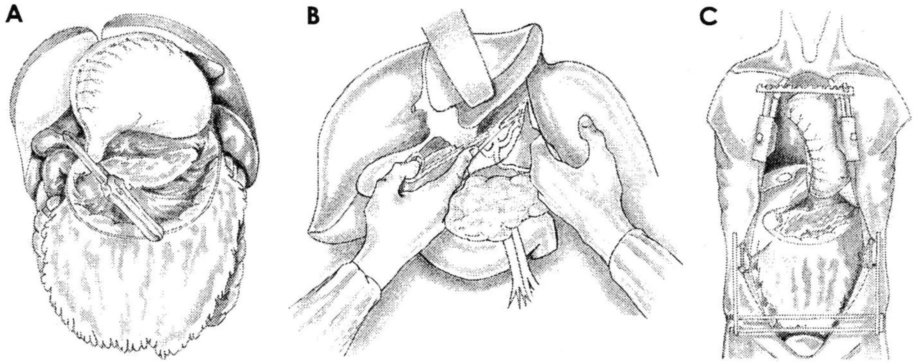

Figure 2. A: Mobilization of the greater curvature of the stomach and closure of the duodenum; B: With an assistant gentling lifting and retracting the stomach to the left, the surgeon dissects the hepato-gastric ligament as close to the lesser curvature as possible; C: The stomach is swept up into the chest

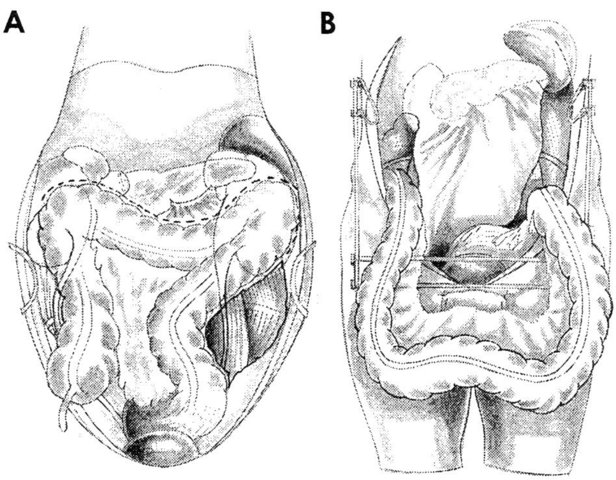

Figure 3. A: The colon is fully mobilized; B: The mesentery is transected and the colon is swept onto donor's legs

close to the thoracic walls (Fig. 4). The ureters were transected near the bladder, tagged and dissected up to the iliac vessels with the surrounding adipose

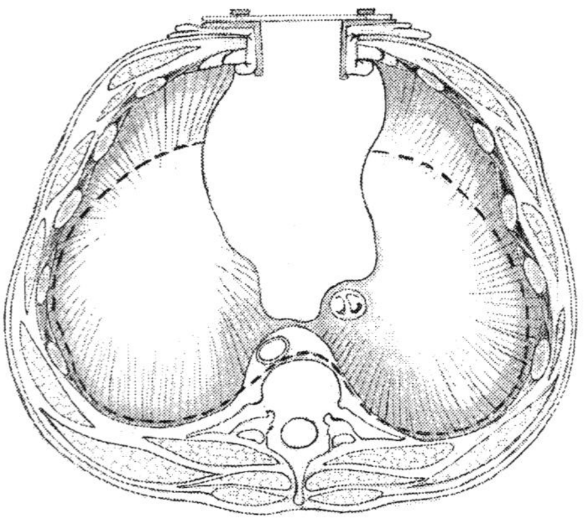

Figure 4. The diaphragm is incised close to the chest wall

tissue and vasculature (Fig. 5). The superior rectal artery was isolated between forefinger and thumb of the left hand and sectioned just in front of aortic bifurcation, thus completely releasing the specimen from the pelvis.

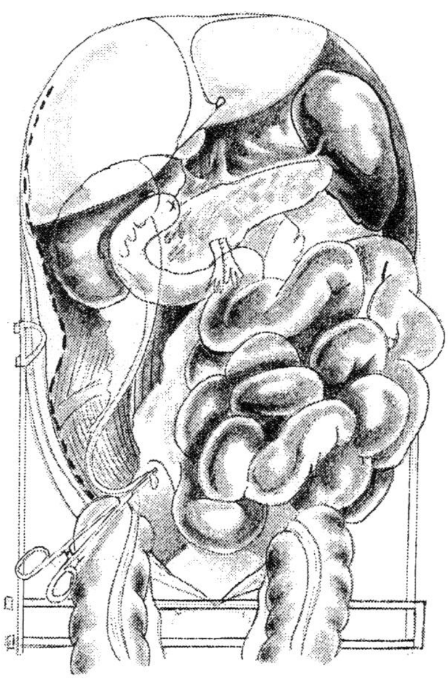

Figure 5. The ureters are tagged and kept in view during the final steps of organ procurement. The dotted line indicates the level from which lateral mobilization of the specimen is begun.

The multi-organ specimen was then mobilized medially to the spine (Fig. 6).

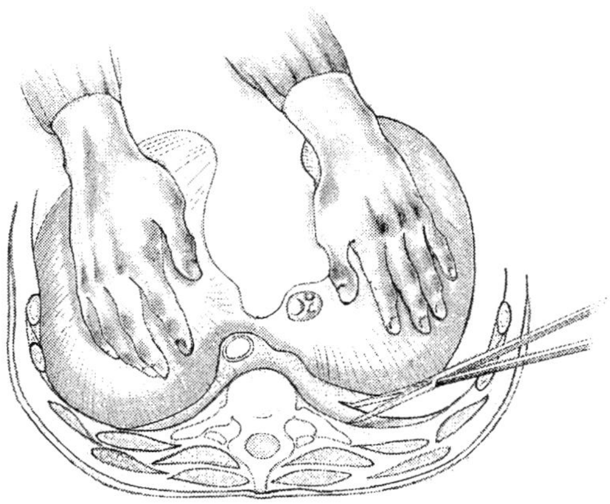

Figure 6. Lateral mobilization of the specimen

The first jejunal loop was closed and divided with the GIA stapler, the mesenteric root was transected, and the small bowel laid on the donor's legs (Fig. 7). The supraceliac and distal aorta and the proximal inferior vena cava were divided. With an assistant gently lifting the specimen, the multi-organ

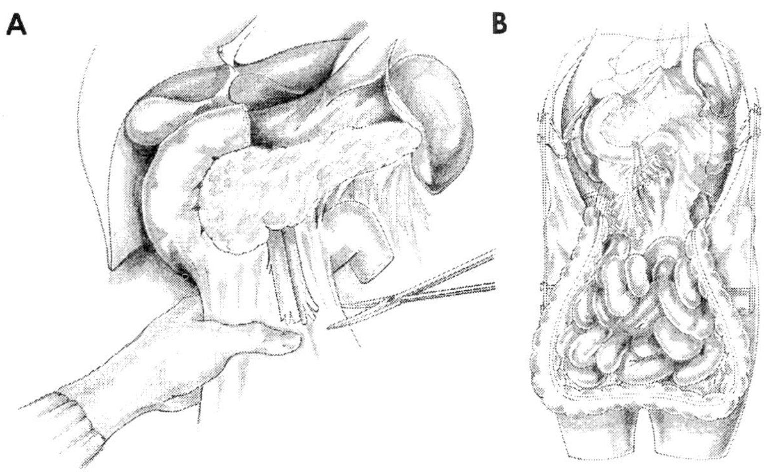

Figure 7. A: Transection of mesenteric root; B: Small bowel on donor's legs

block was removed by incising the prevertebral fascia (Fig. 8). The donor operation was completed by procurement of arterial and venous grafts. The iliac arteries and veins were procured routinely, while the carotid arteries and the internal jugular veins were procured according to the specific needs of transplant teams.

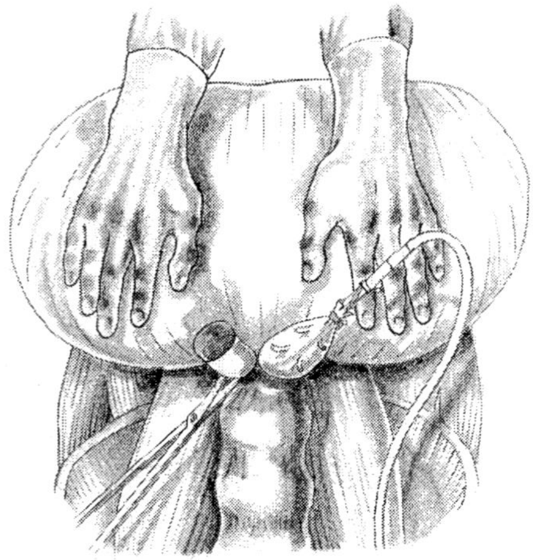

Figure 8. Removal of multiple organ specimen

BACK TABLE SURGERY

The grafts were separated on a back table working under optimal conditions of exposure and light. The specimen, kept in an ileal bag containing cold preservation solution, was placed in a basin filled with iced saline solution, and was approached from its posterior aspect. The surgeon sat on the side of the distal aorta, with an assistant settled in front of him/her.

Kidney separation

With the ureters tagged and gently retracted caudally, the aorta was incised between the paired lumbar ostia. Identification of visceral ostia facilitated subsequent maneuvers. Attention was paid to identify anomalous left renal veins crossing the aorta posteriorly. The anterior wall of the aorta was then dissected from the underlying adipose tissue, and incised longitudinally to the level of the main renal ostia. The left renal vein became hence evident between the two long aortic stripes and just below the ostium of the superior mesenteric artery. Any even small vascular ostium was gently probed before sectioning the adjacent tissues. After separating the main renal ostia from the suprarenal aorta, the proximal inferior vena cava was gently retracted caudally and dissected up to the renal veins where it was transected (Fig. 9). The left renal vein was then divided at its junction with the inferior vena cava. With the vessels always in view, it was hence possible to separate the right kidney by incising the hepatorenal ligament and the left kidney by dissecting along the adrenal gland. Dissection progressed from lateral to medial on the right side and from medial to lateral on the left side.

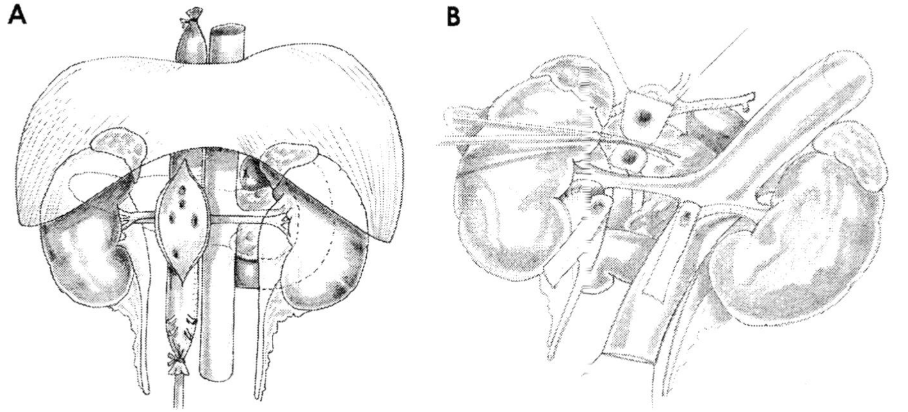

Figure 9. A: Visceral ostia are readily identified after incision of posterior aortic wall; B: Incision of anterior aortic wall and construction of Carrel patches around visceral ostia

Liver-pancreas separation

liver-pancreas detachment began with separation of the superior mesenteric artery from the celiac trunk. The celiac axis and the common hepatic artery were dissected up to the superior edge of the pancreas head. Dissection was facilitated by the fact that the tissue located posteriorly to these vessels, and hence now lying on a superficial plane, is composed exclusively of neural and lymphatic structures, and can be quickly and safely cut. The splenic artery was divided a few millimeters beyond its origin, and the proximal stump was suture-ligated. Before complete division, the distal stump was tagged with a 6/0 prolene suture, in order to facilitate subsequent identification of the vessel. Separation of the two grafts was completed by dissecting the hepato-duodenal ligament, and by sectioning the common bile duct, the portal vein and the gastro-duodenal artery above the pancreatic head (Fig. 10). The level of section

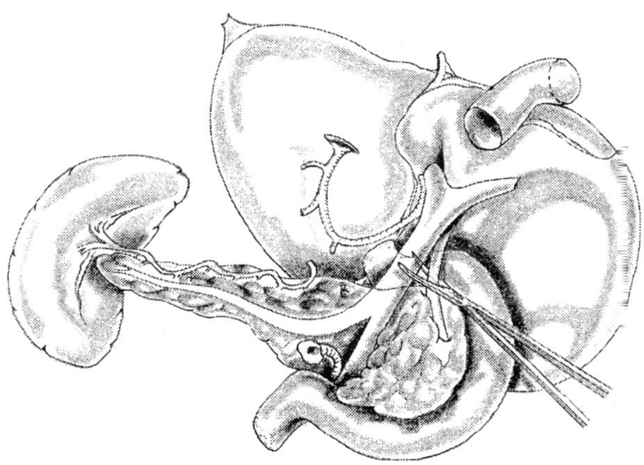

Figure 10. Section of common bile duct, portal vein and gastroduodenal artery concludes liver-pancreas separation

of the portal vein was agreed on between liver and pancreas teams, depending on individual needs and necessity for vascular reconstructions. Anomalous right hepatic arteries were easily identified during this phase, were dissected as proximally as possible, sectioned and anastomosed end-to-end to the stump of the gastro-duodenal artery with interrupted 7/0 or 8/0 prolene sutures. Alternatively, when requested by the liver team, the anomalous right hepatic artery was left in continuity with the first centimeters of the superior mesenteric artery. In this case, while sectioning vessels, attention should be paid to preserve the origin of the inferior pancreatico-duodenal artery.

Final preparation of the pancreas

Pancreas preparation was completed by selective ligature of vascular pedicles, splenectomy and extension arterial grafts. The pancreas was approached from its anterior surface. Beginning from the neck, and proceeding counterclockwise, the peripancreatic tissue was carefully dissected and ligated. The inferior mesenteric vein and the left gastric vein were carefully identified and individually ligated. Moreover, during splenectomy injury to the tail was prevented by checking its position also from the posterior aspect. Once the preparation of the body-tail was completed, attention was directed to the root of the mesentery. Dissection of the superior mesenteric vein was carried out as close to spleno-portal junction as possible, with the aim of avoiding the creation of a closed venous stump, possibly resulting from a more distal ligature. On the contrary, the superior mesenteric artery, and its branches, were ligated more distally, at the level of the inferior edge of the duodenum, in order to avoid unintentional injury to the arterial supply for the pancreas head.

Excess proximal duodenum was mobilized, closed with a GIA stapler and inverted with a 2/0 pursestring suture. The distal duodenum was mobilized from the pancreatic head, sparing a 6 to 8 cm segment of the second portion, but it was not removed at this time. As shown in Figure 11, the jejunal-duodenal

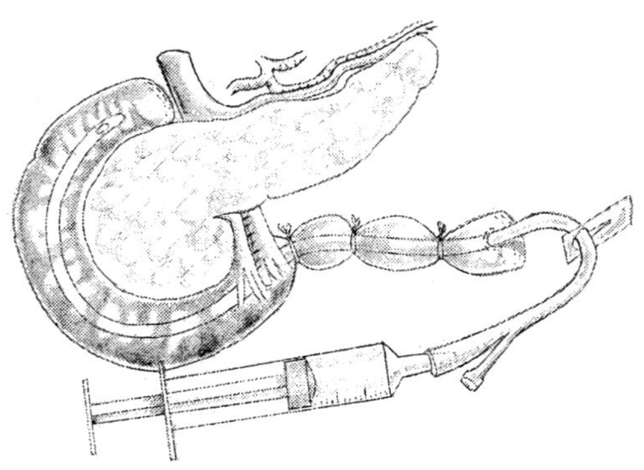

Figure 11. A Foley catheter is introduced into the second duodenal portion through the jejunal-duodenal conduit

conduit was used to introduce a large bore (24 Ch) Foley catheter into the second duodenal portion, thus creating a closed suction system useful for avoiding duodenal overdistension before drainage. Excess distal duodenum was removed at the time of duodenal anastomosis.

The final step involved the preparation of vascular pedicles of convenient length for graft implantation. The splenic and the superior mesenteric arteries were identified, and prepared by careful removal of surrounding lymphatic and ganglion tissue. The internal iliac artery was joined to the splenic artery (interrupted 6/0 polypropylene sutures) and the external iliac artery to the superior mesenteric artery (interrupted 6/0 or 5/0 polypropylene sutures). Both anastomoses were done in an end-to-end fashion, avoiding twisting or torsion of the graft limbs.

PREPARATION OF THE ISLETS

The islets were prepared by a modification of the procedures previously reported in detail [14-15]. The enzyme collagenase (Collagenase P, Boehinger-Mannheim, Mannheim, Germany) was used for digestion of the pancreas. The pancreatic duct was cannulated and the digestion solution, collagenase 1,8 mg/ml dissolved in 300 ml Hanks' balanced salt solution (HBSS, Sigma Chemicals, St. Louis, MO), was slowly injected to distend the tissue. The collagensae solution injected was approximately 3-fold in volume the weight of the pancreas. After distension, the gland was placed in a 500 ml glass beaker, and the digestion solution not used for distension was added to the beaker. This was located in a shaking water bath at 37°C, activated at 120 revolutions per minute. After 10 minutes, the pancreas was shaken with forceps for 60 seconds; then the digestate was filtered through 300 and 90 mμ mesh stainless steel filters, in sequence. The solution that passed through the filters, and the tissue entrapped on the 300 mμ mesh filter were placed back into the water bath, for further digestion. The tissue which remained on the 90 mμ mesh filter was washed with HBSS and 10% bovine serum. The same procedures of filtration, washing and settling in the HBSS solution were repeated every 8-10 minutes for up to 40-50 minutes.

For the purification procedure, 3 ml of tissue was loaded into 250 ml plastic conicals, and resuspended in 50 ml of 80% Histopaque 1.077 (Sigma) and 20% HBSS, topped with 40 ml HBSS. After centrifugation at 800 x g for 5 minutes at 4°C, the islets were recovered at the interface between Histopaque and HBSS layers. The islets were washed with HBSS by centrifugation at 800 x g for 2 minutes at 4° C, resuspended in M 199 culture medium (supplemented with 10% serum and antibiotics), and cultured at 37° C in a CO_2 incubator. The medium was changed the morning after the isolation and weekly thereafter.

INSULIN SECRETION STUDIES

Insulin secretion was assessed by static incubation experiments, as detailed previously [14-15]. After a period of preincubation of 30 minutes at 37°C in Krebs-Ringer bicarbonate solution, 0,5% albumin, pH 7,4, containing 3,3 mmol/l, batches of approximately 10 islets of equivalent size were incubated at 37°C for 45 minutes, in the Krebs-Ringer bicarbonate solution, with either 3,3 mmol/l glucose, 3,3 mmol/l glucose plus 20 mmol/l arginine, or 16,7 mmol/l glucose.

DEFINITION OF ENDOCRINE PANCREAS FUNCTION

Primary endocrine pancreas nonfunction was defined as the absence of any metabolic improvement with steady insulin requirements. Delayed endocrine pancreas function was defined as a total insulin requirement of > 30 U between post-Tx days 5, and 10 and/or > 15 U between days 11 and 15, irrespective of the insulin dose administered during the first 5 days after Tx [16].

RESULTS

Table 2 summarizes the times required for procurement, back table separation of the grafts and final preparation of the pancreas.

Table 2. Time (minutes) required for multiple organ procurement*, grafts' separation and final preparation of the pancreas

	Mean	Standard deviation
In vivo		
Normothermic dissection	19.8	5.2
Hypothermic dissection	18.2	6.4
Back table		
Kidney separation	11.6	2.3
Liver-pancreas separation	30.4	4.6
Final pancreas preparation	138.9	28.2

*Time required for in vivo dissection of thoracic organs, in situ liver split, and dissection of superior mesenteric vessels in case of small bowel procurement is not considered

In 1 donor, in heart arrest, and in 12 further donors, with impending risk of cardiac standstill, in vivo normothermic dissection was always carried out in less than 10 minutes. When thoracic organs were not retrieved, and the donor was not planned for in situ liver split, the entire in vivo procedure never required more than 60 minutes. Anesthesia was never necessary for more than 30 minutes, if the time required for preliminary dissection of thoracic organs, in situ liver split, and dissection of superior mesenteric vessels in case of procurement of the intestine is not considered.

In 20 instances the liver was not allocated to our center. Nineteen liver teams (95%) from 9 different institutions, agreed to our procurement technique, although they had no specific experience of it. Seven procurements were done entirely by our team, and the livers were subsequently shipped to their final destination. In the remaining 12 procurements a surgeon from the liver transplant team performed the entire procedure, while being assisted by a surgeon from our team. One pancreas was also procured by our team and shipped to another institution. On the whole, 10 liver transplant centers were asked to modify their habitual technique, in order to procure the pancreas according to our system: 9 teams agreed and 1 declined.

IATROGENIC INJURIES TO PROCURED ORGANS

No graft was discarded because of iatrogenic injury which occurred as a result of surgical misadventure, or failure to recognize anatomical variations. Superficial liver tears were noted in 5 grafts (2.2%), which were all procured from markedly obese donors (BMI > 35 Kg/m^2).

VASCULAR VARIATIONS

As summarized in Table 3 vascular variations were identified in 82 procurements (36.7%). The "normal" pattern of arterial liver supply, as described in textbooks, was identified in 63.2% of the donors. All vascular variations were readily identified during back-table preparation of the grafts, and no iatrogenic injury occurred.

In 6 donors selected for pancreas transplant the liver was totally (n=1) or partially supplied (n=5) by anomalous branches originating from the superior mesenteric artery. In 3 cases the anomalous right hepatic artery was divided on the back of the head of the pancreas, and anastomosed end-to-end to the stump of the gastroduodenal artery. In the remaining 3 cases, as requested by the liver team, the anomalous right hepatic artery was left in continuity with its origin from the superior mesenteric artery.

Table 3. Vascular variations in decreasing order of frequency

Type of variation	N°	%
Two renal arteries supplying one kidney	42	18.8
Accessory left hepatic artery from the left gastric artery	26	11.6
Replaced right hepatic artery from the superior mesenteric artery	21	9.4
Accessory right hepatic artery from the superior mesenteric artery	11	4.9
Three renal arteries supplying one kidney	9	4
Hepatosplenic trunk	6	2.6
Replaced left gastric artery from the left gastric artery	6	2.6
Hepatomesenteric trunk	5	2.2
Gastrosplenic trunk	4	1.7
Retroaortic left renal vein	3	1.3
Gastrohepatosplenomesenteric trunk	2	0.8
Accessory hepatic artery from the gastroduodenal artery	1	0.4
Gastrohepatic trunk	1	0.4
Hepatosplenomesenteric trunk	1	0.4
Left sided inferior vena cava	1	0.4
Splenomesenteric trunk	1	0.4
Cumulative number of vascular variations	140	-
Donors with vascular variations	82	36.7

PANCREAS AND PANCREAS-KIDNEY TRANSPLANTS

Forty-eight pancreata were transplanted simultaneously with a kidney procured from the same cadaveric donor, 6 simultaneously with a living donor kidney, and 10 alone. Cold ischemia time averaged 597 minutes for pancreata (SD: ± 128 minutes; range 360-900 minutes) and 622 minutes for cadaveric kidneys (SD: ± 156 minutes; range 201-1035).

On the whole, out of 64 pancreas transplants no clinical graft pancreatitis occurred. Three recipients developed peripancreatic fluid collections, successfully treated by either percutaneous catheter drainage (n=2) or relaparotomy (n=1). Other 3 recipients necessitated second-look surgery, because of bleeding, dehishence of duodeno-vescical anastomosis, and small bowel occlusion due to bezoar, respectively. One additional recipient, who had developed life-threatening lung fungal infection, necessitating complete withdrawal of immunosuppression, underwent allograft pancreatectomy and nephrectomy. On the whole, the rate of relaparotomy was 7.8% (5 recipients out of 64 transplants). No graft was lost due to surgical complications. One patient developed partial portal trhombosis (1/64, 1.5%), and was rescued by prompt intravenous heparinization.

Sixty-one recipients discontinued insulin assumption immediately after Tx (95.3 %), and 3 had a delayed endocrine pancreas graft function (Tab. 4).

Table 4. Parameters of early pancreatic funcion and preservation

	Mean	±SD	Range
Fasting blood sugar (mg/dl)*			
POD 1	122.7	40.6	72-191
POD 5	111.5	27.4	65-168
POD 10	98.4	17.2	78-144
Urine amylase (U/L)§			
POD 1	41,716	102,794	1,920-475,000
POD 5	28,439	22,883	1,400-88,200
POD 10	56,651	61,546	7,550-214,360
Serum amylase (U/L)			
POD 1	410.3	386.7	52-1,816
POD 5	140.6	69.8	65-392
POD 10	159.4	89.0	65-404
Serum Lipase (U/L)			
POD 1	528.3	421.3	110-2,130
POD 5	184.2	91.5	89-612
POD 10	158.3	88.3	75-423

POD: postoperative day; *61 recipients with immediate endocrine functional recovery; § 32 recipients with bladder drainage

Forty-five recipients of cadaveric kidney grafts had immediate functional recovery (90%).

Three patients with functioning grafts died from sudden death, and 1 from cerebral hemorrhage. Actuarial 1 and 3-year patient survival rates are both 91.7%.

Six-month actuarial survival rates for pancreata transplanted simultaneously with a cadaveric kidney, with a living kidney, or alone, are 86.9%,

100% and 100%, respectively. Equivalent figures for kidneys procured from cadaveric and living donors are 87% and 100%, respectively.

ISLET CELL TRANSPLANTS

A total of 3 islet cell injections were done in a single recipient over a 6 week period. After the last injection basal and stimulated C-peptide productions had increased markedly, with a concurrent reduction of daily insulin administration of about 70% compared to pre-transplant requirements. However, despite the clearly improved metabolic profiles, without recurrence of the frequent hypoglicemic attacks that had plagued the pre-transplant period, the patient never became truly insulin independent.

ISLET CELL ISOLATION AND VIABILITY STUDIES

The actual and equivalent number of islets yielded from 96 prancreata were 330,655 (± SD: 62,730; range 199,600 – 461,300) and 326,440 (± SD: 62,750; range 180,300 –440,900) before purification, and 313,210 (± SD: 59,740; range 190,700 –440,200) and 287,060 (± SD: 98,380; range 166,200 – 390,600) after purification, respectively. The purity of islets, roughly estimated by dithizone staining, ranged from 40 to 80%. Insulin secretion studies confirmed the in-vitro viability of the islets, showing the capability of the islets to sense varying scretagogues for up to 1 month from isolation (Tab. 5).

Table 5. In-vitro insulin release (ng/ml) from human pancreatic islets in response to varying secretagogues up to 4 weeks of culture. Number of replicates is given in parentheses

	Insulin release			
	Fresh islets	**1 w**	**2 w**	**4 w**
Stimulation				
3.3 mmol/l glucose	2.3±0.1 (8)	3.3±0.3 (14)	5.1±0.6 (10)	5.9±1.5(10)
16.7 mmol/l glucose	8.6±1.7 (9)**	10.6±1.3 (9)**	11.7±0.9 (8)*	11.6±1.4 (10)*
16.7 mmol/l glucose+	16.5±2.9 (8)§	13.9±2.4 (10)§	13.9±1.9 (10)§	23.5±4.8 (8)§

1, 2 and 4w: weeks of culture
*: $p < 0.05$ vs 3.3 mmol/l glucose
**: $p < 0.02$ vs 3.3 mmol/l glucose
§: $p < 0.05$ vs 16.7mmol/l glucose

DISCUSSION

Despite the clearly beneficial effects of pancreas transplant on the quality of life of diabetic patients [17-19], and the continuously growing evidence of its possible life-saving effect in the long-term period [20-25], many fewer pancreata are procured than are actually needed [26].

The safety of combined liver-pancreas procurement has been clearly established [9, 27-28] and, at least in theory, the majority of liver donors should be also pancreas donors. Shortage of suitable donors can only partially explain the reduced number of pancreas transplants compared to those of the liver, even if this organ is currently procured from elderly donors [29]. However, it cannot account for the extremely different rates of pancreas procurement, ranging from 0 to more than 70% [30], among various regions and nations. Annually, many more pancreas transplants are done in the United States of America than in Europe [31]. Italy ranks among the last positions in this particular standing, with only 43 pancreas transplants done during the year 2000 (approximately 0.6 pancreas transplants per million inhabitants), despite the availability of 821 donor organs (14.2 donor organs per million inhabitants). On the whole, the national Caldes index for pancreas procurement was 5.7% ranging from 0, in 10 out of 19 procurement regions, to 25% (www.sanita.it/trapianti). Thus, differently from any other organ, pancreas shortage does not exist, yet there is a significant organ wastage. No single reason can explain this dismal result. Unwillingness to share a donor kidney with the pancreas, even despite mandatory payback policies, is among the possible explanations, and has certainly hampered the development of pancreas transplant in our country. Fear of compromising the quality of the liver and/or making liver grafting more technically demanding or at risk of vascular complications because of shortened vascular pedicles, or necessity for vascular reconstructions, may be other possible explanations. More in general, however, there still seems to be an incomplete awareness of transplant needs in diabetic patients when compared to other recipient categories, despite the remarkable incidence and prevalence of diabetes in Italy [32]. Consequently, in our Country pancreas transplant programs have been so far developed on the basis of local voluntary enterprises, rather than as a consequence of nationally agreed programs.

The Pisa pancreas transplant program was initiated in January 1996. Initially, we decided to select for pancreas transplant only young (< 40 years) stable donors whose procurement was planned in large hospitals with sufficient facilities and experience to meet the needs of a rather complex operation such as pancreas procurement. Indeed, like other authors [33-36] we had decided to adopt a "conventional" procurement technique, with in situ dissection of hilar structures, coeliac axis and superior mesenteric vessels before perfusion. With this policy we were able to perform 2 pancreas transplants over a 2-year period.

Consequently, we decided to develop a technique suitable for pancreas procurement under any operative condition, which should not be influenced by donor characteristics. In March 1998, we performed the first pancreas transplant with a graft procured with the technique described in this paper. During the subsequent 45 months up to December 2001 we transplanted 64 pancreata. An additional graft was also procured and shipped to another transplant center. According to Kapur's criteria [26], 35 out of 64 pancreas donors (54.7%) can be classified as marginal pancreas donors. Probably, the extreme hemodynamic instability of the majority of them would not have allowed a conventional procurement. At least, implementation of the procurement technique described herein allowed us to optimize the use of available resources as is witnessed by the sharp increase of our activity between 1996 (1 transplant per year) and 2001 (35 transplants per year). The development and application of this technique has certainly been facilitated by the fact that in Pisa the same team performs liver, pancreas and kidney transplants. As a consequence, not only do we not have any competition with other abdominal teams, but also every surgeon is fully committed to maximize the use of all available resources. Thanks to this situation, procurement of all abdominal organs by one team is currently a reality in our region, and has greatly facilitated procurement organization and coordination. As first reported by Starzl [7], the rapid technique has been welcomed enthusiastically by transplant coordinators, thoracic teams and operating room staff, who currently identify it as the "Pisa's technique".

When the liver was not allocated to us, 19 out of 20 liver procurement teams agreed to change their habitual techniques in our favour. In seven instances, the liver surgeon preferred not to be directly involved in the procurement, while in the remaining 13 operations he or she was willing to try the en-bloc technique. Despite the fact that none of them had ever seen the technique before, all were able to procure all abdominal organs expeditiously, while being assisted by one of us. If on one hand these figures demonstrate the willingness of the majority of liver teams to share a donor with the pancreas, on the other, they underline the clear safety of our method, that was almost unanimously trusted simply after a brief discussion of the technique.

The concept of rapid organ cooling and abdominal evisceration is not new to procurement surgery [5, 7, 11, 13, 37-41]. To the best of our knowledge, the first description of such techniques was made as early as 1969, and referred to procurement of kidneys [37]. Björkén described the first en-bloc technique employed for pancreas procurement from non heart-beating donors in 1976 [38]. Subsequently, with the acceptance of the concept of brain death, and the availability of heart-beating donors, these techniques fell into abeyance. Indeed, during the early years of the modern era of organ transplant, donors were almost invariably young individuals with a high degree of hemodynamic stability. The favorable type of donor and the concurrent necessity of reducing cold ischemia times, because of the still incomplete development of preservation solutions, facilitated the diffusion of procurement techniques aimed at complete or near-complete graft preparation before perfusion [8]. The only exceptions to this rule were dictated by contingent difficulties such as donor instability [5] or local regulations, such as those in force in Russia, allowing procurement of abdominal organs only after heart retrieval [39]. In 1992 Nakazato and co-workers revived the idea of rapid organ cooling with en-bloc procurement, and underlined its advantages in hemodynamically stable donors [13]. Subsequently, other authors have confirmed the suitability of this approach, especially in the case of pancreas procurement [11, 40-41]. These techniques have a number of practical advantages, such as reduced operative times and costs, standardization, reduced risk of iatrogenic graft injuries and improved team coordination. Moreover, from a physiologic point of view, rapid en bloc techniques are more conducive to the success of organ transplant, since they allow organ procurement and preservation in a pristine condition. On the contrary, techniques that entail meticulous in vivo dissections have prolonged operative times, increased logistic necessities (e.g. intraoperative support), and may enhance team competition. Destabilization of a frail donor may be the most evident consequence [5]. However, warm ischemic injury, resulting from unintentional vascular occlusion [3], or arterial spasm [10], may be a more silent, but equally undesiderable, complication. An additional risk is the possibility of iatrogenic injuries, especially in the case of variations in the vascular anatomy of liver supply [42-43]. On the whole, the final outcome of "conventional" abdominal organ procurement is probably more influenced by the experience and ability of the operating surgeon, rather than by the safety of the technique itself. Indeed, after procurements done with "conventional" techniques, de ville de Goyet and co-workers reported an incidence of liver injuries ranging from 8.7% [11], for locally procured grafts, to 23.1% (44), for shipped organs. On the contrary, no iatrogenic injury occurred in 109 consecutive livers procured by the same group with a quick en-bloc technique [11]. Similarly in our series of 223 procurements only superficial tears were noted in a total of 5 livers (2.2%), and no vascular pedicle was injured despite the quite remarkable number of vascular variations encountered. The fact that this result was obtained in a totally unselected series of donors, including extremely obese and hemodynamically unstable donors, underlines the extreme simplicity and absolute safety of this technique. Indeed, any relevant decision can be deferred to the back-table when any single step is standardized and dissection is greatly facilitated by excellent exposure, absence of bleeding and complete hypothermic protection of graft viability. The posterior approach to the multi-organ specimen, although clearly nonconventional, is a corner-stone of this procedure. Although some practice is required before becoming familiar and confident with it, early identification of vascular ostia before attempting any dissection ensures safe organ separation under any operative condition, irrespectively of vascular variations. Sharing of donors among different transplant teams is also facilitated since division of vascular pedicles can be agreed on more easily. We have noted that the length of the portal vein left with the liver is clearly increased when the organs are separated on the back-table, compared to the cases in which the same manoeuvre is done in situ.

In 2 instances the liver, the pancreas, the small bowel and the kidneys were procured from the same donor, to be implanted into different recipients. The procedure was first done on January 20, 2001 and, although the operating surgeons had no direct experience with a similar procurement, the unique safety and flexibility profiles of the technique described herein allowed expeditious procurement of all grafts, with excellent transplant outcomes. Prior to this experience, simultaneous recovery of liver, pancreas and small bowel for transplant to different recipients has been described only by one team [45]. Although both techniques rely on a sound knowledge of the vascular anatomy of the upper abdomen, that is on a remarkable experience in pancreatic and liver surgery, they demonstrate that simultaneous procurement of liver, pancreas and intestine is feasible and safe.

Although the superiority of exclusively aortic perfusion of abdominal organs has not been proven yet, it seems, at least, that it does not compromise the outcome of hepatic transplants [3, 41, 46]. Lower transaminase peak values with equivalent rates of good graft function, have indeed been obtained with livers flushed only through the aorta, as compared to grafts perfused simultaneously through the portal vein and the aorta [3, 41, 46]. Experimental data support these findings [6, 47], and show how rapid hepatic cooling may directly produce parenchymal damage that worsen after reperfusion [48]. Definition of the optimal route for liver perfusion would probably require a large prospective randomized trial, with standardization of perfusion techniques and stratification of grafts according to their quality. Exclusively aortic flush, however, is clearly not detrimental for the liver, and should be preferred in the case of pancreas procurement since it provides indirect portal perfusion, without the risk of pancreatic outflow hyperpressure [11].

In conclusion, the procurement technique presented herein is quick, simple, safe, standardized, flexible and at least as effective as "conventional" procedures. Since one team can procure all abdominal organs, this technique may facilitate organization and reduce costs of multiorgan procurement. In our experience, it has allowed a clear increase in the number of pancreas transplants.

REFERENCES

1. Mackersie RC, Bronsther Ol Shackford SR. Organ procurement in patients with fatal head injuries. The fate of the potential donor. *Ann Surg* 1991; 213: 143-50

2. Douzdjian V, Gugliuzza KG, Fish J. Multivariate analysis of donor risk factors for pancreas allograft failure after simultaneous pancreas kidney transplantation. *Surgery* 1995; 118: 73-81

3. de Ville de Goyet J, Hausleithner V, Malaise J, Reding R, Lerut J, Jamart J, Barker A, Otte JB. Liver procurement without in situ portal perfusion. A safe procedure for more flexible multiple organ harvesting. *Transplantation* 1994; 57: 1328-32

4. Gubernatis G, Oldhafer K, Rohwer K, Fieguth HG, Körner MM, Vogelsang F, Schott W, Haverich A, Körfer R, Pichlmayr R. Regional organ procurement teams for abdominal and thoracic organs provide a rapid and personal service for organ donation in peripheral hospitals. *Transplant Proc* 1997; 29: 1484-6,

5. Starzl TE, Iwatsuki S, Shaw BW Jr, Gordon RD. Orthotopic liver transplantation in 1984. *Transplant Proc* 1985; 17: 250-8.

6. Christophi C, Morgan B, McInnes I. A comparison of standard and rapid infusion methods of liver preservation during multi-organ procurement. *Aust N Z J Surg* 1991; 61: 692-4.

7. Starzl TE, Miller C, Broznick B, Makowka L. An improved technique for multiple organ harvesting. *Surg Gynecol Obstet* 1987; 165: 343-8.

8. Rosenthal JT, Shaw BW Jr, Hardesty RL, Griffith BP, Starzl TE, Hakala TR. Principles of multiple organ procurement from cadaver donors. *Ann Surg* 1983; 198: 617-21.

9. Sollinger HW, Vernon WB, D'Alessandro AM, Kalayoglu M, Stratta RJ, Belzer FO. Combined liver and pancreas procurement with Belzer-UW solution. *Surgery* 1989; 106: 685-91

10. D'Alessandro AM, Stratta RJ, Southard JH, Kalayoglu M, Belzer FO. Agonal hepatic artery vasospasm: demonstration, prevention and possible clinical implications. *Surg Gynecol Obstet* 1989; 169: 324-8.

11. de Ville de Goyet J, Reding R, Hausleithner V, Lerut J, Otte JB. Standardized quick en bloc technique for procurement of cadaveric liver grafts for pediatric liver transplantation. *Transpl Int*, 1995; 8: 280-5.

12. van Wezel HB, van der Vliet JA, Hordijk W, Haase-Kromwijk B, Barendregt WB, Boll APM, van Goor H. A regional explantation team: a big step forward organisation of organ procurement. *Transplant Proc* 1997; 29: 1487-8.

13. Nakazato PZ, Concepcion W, Bry W, Limm W, Tokunaga Y, Itasaka H, Feduska N, Esquivel CO, Collins GM. Total abdominal evisceration: an en bloc technique for abdominal organ harvesting. *Surgery* 1992; 111: 37-47.

14. Giannarelli R, Coppelli A, Marchetti P, Tellini C, Del Guerra S, Lupi R, Lorenzetti M, Masiello P, Carmellini M, Mosca F, Lencioni C, Navalesi R. Preparation and long-term culture of isolated human pancreatic islets. *Transplant Proc* 1998; 30: 384-5.

15. Marchetti P, Giannarelli R, Cosimi S, Masiello P, Coppelli A, Viacava P, Navalesi R. Massive isolation, morphological and functional characterization and xenotransplantation of bovine pancreatic islets. *Diabetes* 1995; 44: 375-81.

16. Troppmann C, Gruessner AC, Papalios BE, Sutherland DER, Matas AJ, Benedetti E, Gruessner RW. Delayed endocrine pancreas graft function after simultaneous pancreas-kidney transplantation. Incidence, risk factors and impact on long term outcome. *Transplantation* 1996; 61: 1323-30.

17. Zehrer CL, Gross CR. Quality of life of pancreas transplant recipients. *Diabetologia* 1991; 34 (suppl 1): s145-9.

18. Nathan C, Fogel H, Norman D, Russell PS, Tolkoff-Rubin N, Delmonico F, Auchincloss H Jr, Camuso J, Cosimi AB. Long-term metabolic and quality of life results with pancreatic renal transplantation in insulin-dependent diabetes mellitus. *Transplantation* 1991; 52: 85-91

19. Hathaway DK, Hartwig MS, Milstead J, Elmer D, Evans S, Gaber AO. Improvements in quality of life reported by diabetic recipients of kidney-only and pancreas-kidney allografts. *Transplant Proc* 1994; 26: 512-4.

20. Navarro X, Kennedy WR, Loenson RB, Sutherland DE. Influence of pancreas transplantation on cardiorespiratory reflexes, nerve conduction and mortality in diabetes mellitus. *Diabetes* 1990; 39: 802-6.
21. Tibell A, Solders G, Larsson M, Brattstrom C, Tyden G. Superior survival after simultaneous pancreas and kidney transplantation compared with transplantation of a kidney alone in diabetic recipients followed for 8 years. *Transplant Proc* 1997; 29: 668
22. Smets YF, Westendorp Rg, van der Pijl JW, de Charro FT, Ringers J, de Fister JW, Lemres HM. Effect of simultaneous pancreas-kidney transplantation on mortality of patients with type-1 diabetes mellitus and end-stage renal failure. *Lancet* 1999; 353 (9168): 1915-9.
23. Tydén G, Bolinder J, Solders G, Brattström C, Tibell A, Groth CG. Improved survival in patients with insulin-dependent diabetes mellitus and end-stage diabetic nephropathy 10 years after combined pancreas and kidney transplantation. *Transplantation* 1999; 67: 645-8.
24. Becker BN, Brazy PC, Becker YT, Odorico JS, Pintar TJ, Collins BH, Pirsch JD, Leverson GE, Heisey DM, Sollinger HW. Simultaneous pancreas-kidney transplantation reduces excess mortality in type 1 diabetic patients with end-stage renal disease. *Kidney Int* 2000; 57: 2129-35.
25. Tydén G, Tollemar J. Bolinder J. Combined pancreas and kidney transplantation improves survival in patients with end-stage diabetic nephropathy. *Clin Transplant* 2000; 14: 505-8.
26. Kapur S, Bonham A, Dodson SF, Dvorchik I, Corry RJ. Strategies to expand the donor pool for pancreas transplantation. *Transplantation* 1999; 67: 284-90.
27. Dunn DL, Morel P, Schlumpf R, Mayoral JL, Gillingham KJ, Moudry-Munns KC, Krom RA, Gruessner RW, Payne WD, Sutherland DE, Najarian JS. Evidence that combined procurement of pancreas and liver grafts does not affect transplant outcome. *Transplantation* 1991; 51: 150-7.
28. Delmonico FL, Jenkins RL, Auchincloss H Jr, Etienne TJ, Russel PS, Monaco AB, Cosimi AB. Procurement of a whole pancreas and liver from the same cadaveric donor. *Surgery* 1989; 105: 718-23.
29. Filipponi F, Roncella M, Boggi U, Pietrabissa A, Romagnoli J, Urbani L, Biancofiore G, Mosca F. Liver transplantation in recipients over 60. *Transplant Proc* 2001; 33: 1465-6.
30. Stratta RJ, Bennet L. Pancreas undereutilization in the United States: analysis of United Network for Organ Sharing data. *Transplant Proc* 1997; 29: 3309-10
31. International Pancreas Transplant Registry. Newsletter 2000 August 31; Volume 12 Number 1.
32. Muntoni M, Songini M, Sardinian Collaborative Group for Epidemiology of IDDM. High incidence rate of IDDM in Sardinia. *Diabetes Care* 1992; 15: 1317-22.
33. Stratta RJ, Taylor RJ, Spees EK, Langnas AN, Marujo WC, Li S, Ozaki C, Ranjan D, Duckworth RM, Shaw BW Jr. Refinements in cadaveric pancreas-kidney procurement and preservation. *Transplant Proc* 1991; 23: 2320-2.
34. Johnson CP, Roza AM, Adams MB. Simultaneous liver and pancreas procurement - a simplified method. *Transplant Proc* 1990; 22: 425-6.
35. Nghiem DD. A technique for concomitant whole duodenopancreatectomy and hepatectomy for transplantation in the multiple organ donor. *Surg Gynecol Obstet* 1989; 169: 257-8.
36. Bandlien KO, Mittal VK, Toledo-Pereyra LH. Procurement and workbench procedures in preparation of pancreatic allografts. Factors essential for a successful pancreas transplant. *Am Surg* 1988; 54: 578-81.
37. Ackermann JR, Snell ME. Cadaveric renal transplantation: a technique for donor kidney removal. *Br J Urol* 1968; 40: 515-21.
38. Björkén C, Lundgren G, Ringdén O, Groth CG. A technique for rapid harvesting of cadaveric renal and pancreatic grafts after circulatory arrest. *Br J Surg* 1976; 63: 517-9.
39. Moisiuk YG, Tarabarko NV, Dolbin AG, Gorbunov VV, Shumakov VI. A modified technique for rapid combined heart, pancreas and kidney harvesting. *Transplant Proc* 1991; 23: 2326

40. Imagawa DK, Olthoff KM, Yersiz H, Shackleton CR, Colquhoun SD, Shaked A, Busuttil RW. Rapid en bloc technique for pancreas-liver procurement. Improved early liver function. *Transplantation* 1996; 61: 1605-9.
41. Pinna AD, Dodson FS, Smith CV, Furukawa H, Sugitani A, Fung JJ, Corry RJ. Rapid en bloc technique for liver and pancreas procurement. *Transplant Proc* 1997; 29: 647-8.
42. Ferla G, Colledan M, Doglia M, Fassati LR, Gridelli B, Rossi G, Caccamo L, Gatti S, Galmarini D. Back table surgery for liver grafts. *Transplant Proc* 1988; 20: 1003-4.
43. Todo S, Makowka L, Tzakis AG, Marsh JW Jr, Karrer FM, Armany M, Miller C, Tallent MB, Esquivel CO, Gordon RD, Iwatsuki S, Starzl TE. Hepatic artery in liver transplantation. *Transplant Proc* 1987; 19: 2406-11.
44. Lerut J, Reding R, de Ville de Goyet J, Baranski A, Barker A, Otte JB. Technical problems in shipped hepatic allografts: the UCL experience. *Transpl Int* 1994; 7: 297-301.
45. Abu-Elmagd K, Fung J, Bueno J, Martin D, Madariaga JR, Mazariegos G, Bond G, Molmenti E, Corry RJ, Starzl TE, Reyes J. Logistics and technique for procurement of intestinal, pancreatic and hepatic grats from the same donor. *Ann Surg* 2000; 232: 680-7.
46. Boillot O, Benchetrit S, Dawahra M, Porcheron J, Martin X, Fontaumard E. Early graft function in liver transplantation: comparison of two techniques of graft procurement. *Transplant Proc* 1993; 25: 2626-7.
47. Filipponi F, Oleggini M, Romagnoli P, Fossati N, Pardini P, Mosca F. Exclusively aortic cold flushnig for liver procurement from hemodynamically stable donors. An experimental study in the pig. *G Chir* 1996; 17: 59-63.
48. Otto G, Wolff H, Uerlings I, Gellert K. Preservation damage in liver transplantation. Influence of rapid cooling. *Transplantation* 1986; 42: 122-4.

CHAPTER 27

REPLACEMENT THERAPY IN ACUTE LIVER FAILURE

Giorgio Splendiani, Valentina Mazzarella*, Carlo Meloni*, Giuseppe Tisone, Franco Pisani, Silvia Cipriani, Stefano Pollicita, Carlo Umberto Casciani.
*Department of Surgery, University of Rome "Tor Vergata" and *CNR Institute , Rome, Italy*

Abstract
Acute liver failure is generally a fatal disease, although mortality is highly dependent on etiology. Renal failure is a common complication in patients with severe liver disease, and may be due to pre-renal causes, acute tubular necrosis, hepatorenal syndrome and chronic renal disease associated with the underlying chronic liver disease. Orthotopic Liver Transplantation (OLTx) has become the accepted treatment of choice for patients with advanced liver disease; dialytic treatment may be useful in treating renal complication, and to gain time either for liver regeneration or for the acquisition of a donor liver. Among the natural toxic causes of ALF, Amanita Phalloides poisoning (APP) is one of the most frequent. Managing patients suffering from APP may be very challenging; furthermore, treatment must be started in time to be effective. In this study we report our experience on replacement therapy in ALF due to APP.

We retrospectively evaluated 6 patients suffering from APP and hospitalized within our Intensive Care Unit, by assessing different kinds of treatment: two different dialytic techniques, namely Continuous Renal Replacement Therapy (CRRT) and Charcoal Plasmaperfusion-(CPP), and Orthotopic Liver Transplantation (OLTx).

Three patients treated with CRRT+CPP, one patient treated with CRRT only, and the patient treated with OLTx recovered. One patient, undergoing CRRT only, died after 14 days of treatment. During the CRRT+CPP treatment no relevant complication occurred. The transplanted patient received dialytic treatment for 17 days after transplantation, in order to support renal function impairment and to favor liver function recovery.

In conclusion, we can say that the clinical management of patients suffering from APP requires a multiple disciplinary intervention, therefore it is recommended to treat these patients in a specialized dialysis department in collaboration with an organ transplantation team. In the near future we wish to associate to dialytic treatment with a bioartificial liver device, which could bridge the time to liver transplantation.

A.*M. Farinon (ed.), Advances in Abdominal Surgery 2002*, 385-392.

INTRODUCTION

Acute Liver Failure (ALF) is a clinical syndrome with multiple organ involvement, resulting from abrupt loss of hepatic function. It is defined as the onset of encephalopathy and coagulopathy within 6 months from the beginning of liver disease, and can be divided into fulminant hepatic failure within 8 weeks, and subfulminant hepatic failure within 26 weeks. Clinical manifestations include encephalopathy, jaundice, bleeding, metabolic disturbances, renal failure with oliguria, hypotension and signs of portal hypertension. The mortality rate is very high, ranging between 70 and 95% as reported in literature [1], and the most frequent causes of death are cerebral edema, bleeding and infections.

Many different causes may lead to ALF but in the majority of cases it is due to viral infections. Among the natural toxic causes, mushroom poisoning and herbal tea poisoning are the most frequent. Acute mushroom poisoning caused by Amanita Phalloides (AP) is still frequent in Italy, particularly in certain regions, with a total reported incidence of about 2000-3000/year [2]. Despite improvement in intensive care management, the mortality rate ranges from 11 to 51% [3].

In this study, we report our experience of Amanita phalloides poisoning (APP) management, by different dialytic techniques and orthotopic liver transplantation (OLTx).

MATERIALS AND METHODS

We retrospectively evaluated 6 patients suffering from APP and hospitalized within our Intensive Care Unit, by assessing different kinds of treatment. Patients' clinical data are summarized in Table 1. Five of them were subjected to dialytic treatment, while one patient required prompt OLTx.

Table 1. Patients' clinical data.

Pts	Age	Sex	Treatment
CL	75	F[1]	CRRT[2]+CPP[3]
AC	56	F	CRRT+CPP
FG	63	M[4]	CRRT+CPP
SA	27	F	CRRT
SV	59	M	CRRT
IN	30	F	OLTx[5]

[1]F: Female; [2]CRRT: Continuous Renal Replacement Therapy; [3]CPP: Charcoal Plasma Perfusion; [4]M: Male; [5]OLTx:Orthotopic Liver Transplantation

As far as the dialytic treatment is concerned, we treated 2 patients with Continuous Renal Replacement Therapy (CRRT) only, and 3 patients with CRRT plus Charcoal Plasmaperfusion (CPP). All dialyzed patients were connected to a Hospal Prisma device set on Continuous Venovenous Hemofiltration (CVVH) mode. A dual-lumen catheter inserted in the femoral vein obtained vascular access and polysulfonic dialyzers were used. The dialytic protocol was established as follows: QB=100 ml/min, QF=2000 ml/hr, continuous heparinization by 500 UI/hr, length of session 24 hrs/day. In 3 patients treated with CRRT+CPP, a plasmatic separator (Hospal Plasmaflo) conveyed the plasma to a second circuit, made of a charcoal absorbent cartridge (Detoxil-3) connected to the lateral exit site of Plasmaflo by the venous limb. In these patients we adopted the following dialytic protocol: QB=50-60 ml/min, QP=1100 ml/hr (18.3 ml/min), continuous heparinization by 500 UI/hr, length of session 3 hrs/day. Transmembrane pressure shouldn't be more than 60 mmHg in order to separate plasma.

As regards the patient treated by OLTx, selection criteria adopted were based on those developed at the Hopital Beaujon in Clichy (Tab. 2) [4].

Table 2. Selection criteria for liver transplantation adopted at Hopital Beaujon in Clichy

	Pts <30 yrs	**Pts >30 yrs**
Encephalopathy grade	3 or 4	3 or 4
Factor V level	<20%	<30%

RESULTS

Patients' outcome is summarized in Table 3. Three patients treated with CRRT+CPP recovered, as well as one patient treated with CRRT only, and the patient treated with OLTx. One patient only undergoing CRRT died after 14 days of treatment while during the CRRT+CPP treatment no relevant complication occurred. One patient entered the urgent OLTx waiting list, and received transplant after 3 days from AP ingestion. This patient received dialytic treatment for 17 days after transplantation in order to support renal function impairment and to favor liver function recovery. The long hospitalization time was due to poisoning complications, particularly to the neurological peripheral complications (peripheral axon damage and cochlear nerve injury).

Table 3. Patients' outcome

Pts	Hospital days	Dialysis hours	Time between ingestion and hospitalization	OLTx	Outcome
CL	7	105 CRRT[7]+15 CPP[8]	48 hrs	No	R[9]
AC	5	84 CRRT+12 CPP	36 hrs	No	R
FG	9	147 CRRT+21 CPP	24 hrs	No	R
SA	4	72 CRRT	12 hrs	No	R
SV	14	336 CRRT	24 hrs	No	D[10]
IN	53	48 CRRT pre OLTx 144 CRRT+10 HD post OLTx	24 hrs	Yes	R

[6]OLTx: Othotopic Liver Transplantation; [7]CRRT: Continuous Renal Replacement Therapy; [8]CPP: Charcoal Plasma perfusion; [9]R: Recovery; [10] D: Death

DISCUSSION

Many different causes may lead to ALF and an etiology-related therapy is virtually impossible, except for ALF due to acetamoniphen intoxication and herpes virus infection, treated respectively with acetylcysteine and acyclovir administration. In managing patients suffering from ALF, treating and preventing complications is very important in order to gain time for liver regeneration or to bridge the time to OLTx. Standard therapeutical approaches include: careful monitoring of the fluid balance, in order to avoid worsening of the encephalopathy and portal hypertension and the development of cerebral oedema; renal replacement therapy when renal function cannot be preserved; mechanical ventilation to manage an eventual respiratory failure; the administration of gastroprotective medications to prevent gastrointestinal bleeding; selective bowel decontamination (avoiding nephrotoxic antibiotics) for the prevention of possible infections; administration of neomycin, lactulose, medium chain fatty acids and branched chain aminoacids, to improve encephalopathy and nutritional status.

Among the natural toxic causes of ALF, mushroom poisoning is one of the most frequent. Amanita Phalloides (AP) is a poisonous mushroom containing α-amanitin, which inhibits cellular RNA-synthase leading to tissural damage. After 6-24 hours from ingestion, toxins actively destroy hepatic and renal tissues but no relevant clinical sign appears. In the following 24 hours vomiting, hematic diarrhea and abdominal pain appear. After apparent improvement, the poisoned subject shows the clinical signs of severe hepatic and renal failure, which shortly leads to the patient's death if it's not promptly and adequately treated. In Italy 200 death cases per year are due to mushroom poisoning (50%

mortality rate), which may occur all the year round with a peak of incidence during the Autumn. The characteristic of familiarity is frequently observed in affected subjects, or in people who had a meal together.

Different therapeutic options have been used in the treatment of APP, but nevertheless the mortality rate ranges from 11 to 51% [3]. This variability is due to several factors, such as the kind of therapeutical approach, the total amount of the ingested toxic substance, and the patient's clinical status before poisoning, particularly the hepatic function. Renal function impairment is a prognostic factor, too.

The role of various treatment modalities is debatable. APP requires that the patient be treated in ICU, using artificial support devices until transplantation, necessary to replace liver and renal function when irreparably impaired by toxic factors.

Available therapeutical approaches are different, but they are all based on the possibility of replacing impaired renal and hepatic functions. Hemodialysis is the first choice replacement therapy in renal failure but it's not so easy to reproduce the entire complex enzymatic and biosynthetic functions of the liver in an artificial way. Anyway, it's possible to purify the blood of toxic molecules, which are no longer metabolized by the liver, by performing conventional or alternative dialytic treatment, thus favoring hepatic cells' regeneration [5]. Two factors must be considered in choosing the dialytic technique: the molecular weight of the substances to remove and their percentage of protein binding. In ALF we need to remove middling and big molecules, mostly bound to plasma proteins. For this reason, it would be suitable to choose techniques such as plasmapheresis and charcoal hemoperfusion and dialyzers with a high permeability to middle-sized molecules, such as polysulphone and polyacrilonytrile. Plasmapheresis allows us to completely remove from the patient the plasma containing the toxic substances, and to substitute it with new fresh plasma, or by polyelectrolytic solutions and/or solutions containing albumin. In this way the metabolic overload may be significantly improved and encephalopathy may partially regress [6]. Hemoperfusion allows a good removal of substances with a high molecular weight and eventually bound to plasma protein by direct contact with absorbent molecules, such as microparticles of activated charcoal, showing a much more elevated purifying capacity than traditional hemodialysis. In treating our patients we used continuous renal replacement therapy (CRRT) in continuous veno-venous hemofiltration (CVVH) mode, and a variant of plasmaperfusion, that is plasmaperfusion-hemofiltration (CVVH-CPP). In this kind of technique the plasma is obtained by a cell-separator flowing through a charcoal cartridge for 3 hours (charcoal plasmaperfusion-CPP), and then a 20 hours' duration CVVH session was performed. In this way, we carried out a long-lasting treatment, which provided good hemodynamic stability and improved patients' survival. In fact, among 5 treated patients, only one patient, treated with CRRT only, died after 14 days of treatment (but we noticed a significant improvement in encephalopathy anyway), while the other 4 recovered.

In case the hepatic injury is sudden, and too serious to allow adequate hepatocytes regeneration and liver-function recovery, in spite of dialytic support, the only therapeutic chance is liver transplantation (OLTx). In Europe ALF represents 11% and in Italy 5.5% of the pathologies requiring OLTx; 20% of patients suffering from fulminating or subfulminating hepatitis survive anyway without undergoing OLTx [4]. Several prognostic scores have been developed in order to provide indication criteria for OLTx. The most commonly used are the Clichy criteria [7-8] and the King's College criteria [8-9]. We used the Clichy criteria, based upon the presence and degree of mental alteration (hepatic encephalopathy grade 3 or 4), and the impairment of coagulation (factor V level 30% below normal in patients more than 30 years old, or 20% below normal in patients less than 30 years old) independent of the etiology. Further approaches have been proposed in order to provide selection criteria, like echographic evaluation of the reduction in size of the liver [10], liver biopsy to assess the extension of hepatic necrosis, measurement of intracranial pressure or cerebral perfusion pressure [11], and others. However, it seems doubtful that a single parameter could provide an objective indication to OLTx. Anyway the selection criteria for transplantation used in the published European series are by no means standardized, and furthermore the patients reported are not always comparable [4]. For this reason, it is necessary to develop objective and standardized indication criteria for OLTx. In our Center we performed 11 OLTx in emergency for fulminating hepatic failure (9 due to viral hepatitis B, 1 due to undefined toxic substances and 1 due to Amanita phalloides poisoning)

Recently, a new kind of therapeutical approach, the bioartificial liver support (BLS), has come under assessment, and it may help to bridge the time to transplantation. BLS is a hybrid device that includes functioning hepatocytes contained in the extra capillary space, and multiple hollow fiber capillaries that pass through a sealed housing. Patient's blood or plasma flows through the capillaries and exchange of metabolic products occurs. At present, three kinds of BLS are available, although they are still undergoing clinical assessment: namely, the bioartificial liver (BAL), the extra corporeal liver assist device (ELAD) and the Berlin extracorporeal liver support system (BELS). The first one consists of primary porcine hepatocytes separated from patient's plasma, flowing within capillary space. Molecular exchanges occur by diffusion, between intra and extracapillary compartments. It also comprises an in-line plasma-oxygenation system to fulfill hepatocytes oxygen demand, and a cellulose coated charcoal column in order to protect cells against toxic substances in the plasma. The ELAD is made of hepatocytes derived from a well-differentiated human hepatoblastoma cell-line. Whole blood perfusion is used and so systemic heparinization is required. The BELS contains porcine hepatocytes and consists of sets of interwoven capillaries, with separate sets for plasma inflow and outflow, and molecular exchanges occur in the extracapillary space. It also includes a separate capillary system for hepatocytes oxygenation, providing a superior oxygenation capacity, similar to the physiological situation [12]. These kinds of devices are able to produce therapeutical levels of plasma proteins, with an albumin synthesis rate of about 5g/die, and also to synthesize urea and glucose. So there is the possibility to act favorably on hepatic coma, also improving mental state and reactivating enzymatic systems responsible for the correct hematoencephalic barrier functioning. At present our study group is involved in a research program to test BAL capacity to keep alive both animals and humans (suffering from ALF, while waiting for a suitable graft, or affected with primary rejection and waiting for a new graft). We use bioreactors made of animal hepatocytes included in a hydrogel matrix, but predisposed for the subsequent use of human hepatocytes from non-neoplastic cellular lines.

CONCLUSIONS

The clinical management of patients suffering from APP requires multiple-disciplinary intervention, therefore it is recommended that these patients be treated in a specialized dialysis department, in collaboration with an organ transplantation team. In the near future we wish to associate dialytic treatment with a bioartificial liver device, which could substitute hepatic function in patients waiting for liver transplantation.

REFERENCES

1. Meerman J, Zijlstra JG, Schweizer JJ, Verwer R, Sloof MJH and Haagsma EB. Acute Liver Failure: spontaneous recovery or transplantration? *Scand J Gastroenterol* 1997; 32 Suppl 223: 55-59.

2. Splendiani G, Zazzaro D, Di Pietrantonio P, Delfino L, Tullio T. Continous renal replacement therapy and charcoal plasma perfusion in Amanita mushroom poisoning. *Artif Organs* 2000; 24(4): 305-308.

3. Mydlik M, Derzsiova K, Klan J, Zima T. Hemoperfusion with α-amanitin: an in vitro study. *Int J of Artifl Organs* 1997; 20(2): 105-107.

4. Bismuth H, Samuel D, Castaing D, Williams R, Pereira SP. Liver transplantation in Europe for patients with acute renal failure. *Semin Liver Dis* 1996; 16(4): 415-425.

5. Gazzard BG, Weston MJ, Murray-Lyon IM, Flax H, Record CO, Williams R, Portmann B. Charcoal hemoperfusion in the treatment of fulminant hepatic failure. *Lancet* 1974; 1(7870): 1301-1307.

6. Ouchi K, Asanuma Y, Owada Y, Koyama K, Sato T. Comparison of three liver support systems with patients: RP6-HD, plasma perfusion over multile sorbents and plasma exchange. In: *Plasmapheresis: new trends in therapeutical applications*. ISAO Press 1983; 215-222.

7. Bernuau J, Godeau A, Poynard T, Dobois F, Lesage G, Yvonnet B et al. Multivariate analysis of prognostic factors in fulminant hepatitis B. *Hepatology* 1986; 6: 648-651.
8. Fischer L, Sterneck M, Rogiers X. Liver transplantation for acute liver failure. *Eur J Gastroenterol Hepatol* 1999; 11: 985-990.
9. O'Grady JG, Alexander GJ, Hayllar KM, Williams R. Early indicators of prognosis in fulminant hepatic failure. *Gastroenterology* 1989; 97: 439-445.
10. Van Thiel DH. When should a decision to proceed with transplantation actually be made in cases of fulminant or subfulminant hepatic failure; at admission to hospital or when a donor organ is made available? *J Hepatol* 1993; 17: 1-2.
11. Lidofsky SD, Bass NM, Prager MC, Washington DE, Read AE, Wright TL et al. Intracranial pressure monitoring and liver transplantation for fulminant hepatic failure. *Hepatology* 1992; 16: 1-7.
12. Dowling DJ, Mutimer DJ. Artificial liver support in acute liver failure. *Eur J Gastroenterol Hepatol* 1999; 11: 991-996.

COLOR PLATES

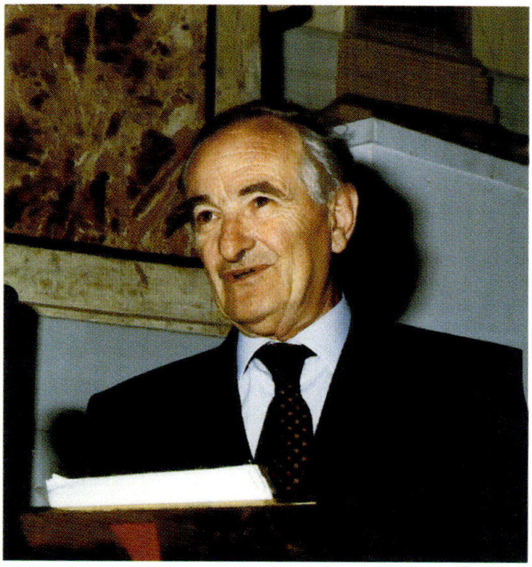

To the memory of Professor Everardo Zanella for his distinguished contribution to surgical sciences (Dedication p. v)

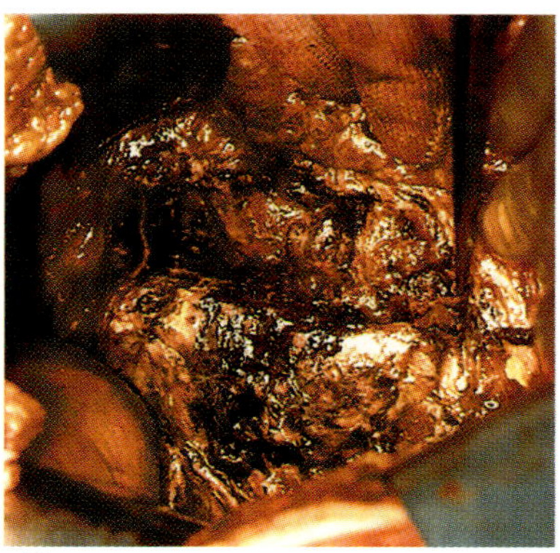

C

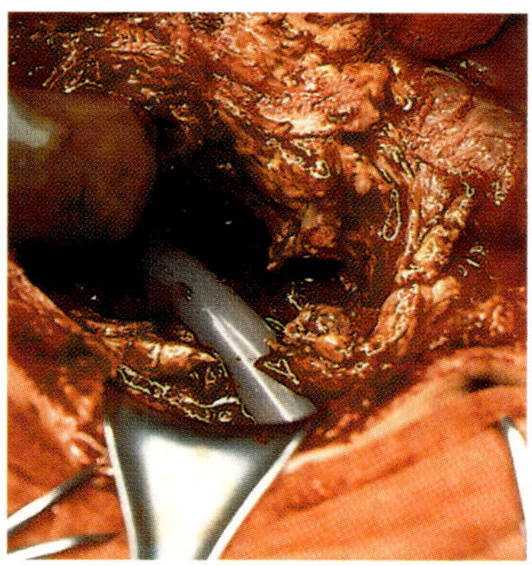

D

Figures 3 C,D. Ultrasound findings are confirmed by targeted surgical exploration (C) followed by drainage positioning (D) (Personal experience). *Ch.2, p. 29.*

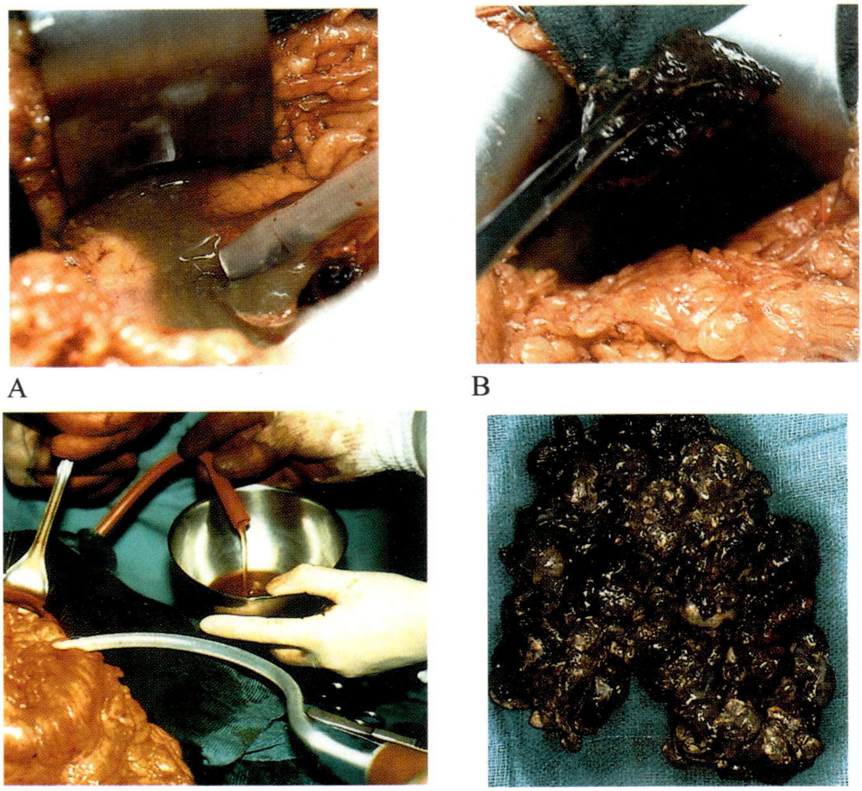

A B C D

Figures 4. Intraoperative sequence of surgical treatment of infected pancreatic necrosis: the abdomen is opened and an abundant amount of purulent material is removed (A); then necrosectomy is performed (B) and tubes are positioned for postoperative drainage (C). Detail of removed I.N. (D) (Personal Experience). *Ch.2, p. 31.*

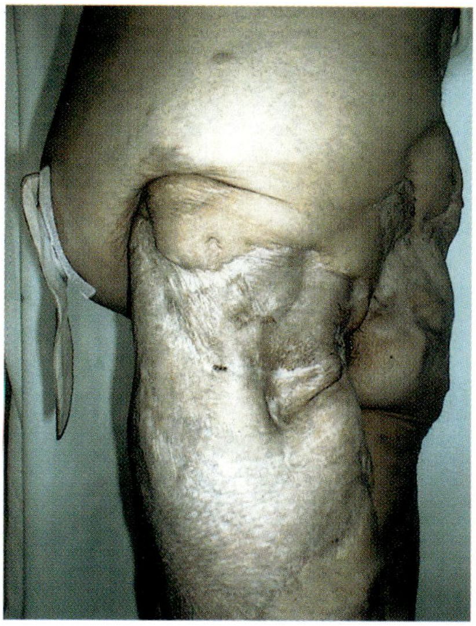

Figure 2. Pelvic trauma following automotive accident. *Ch.20, p.293.*

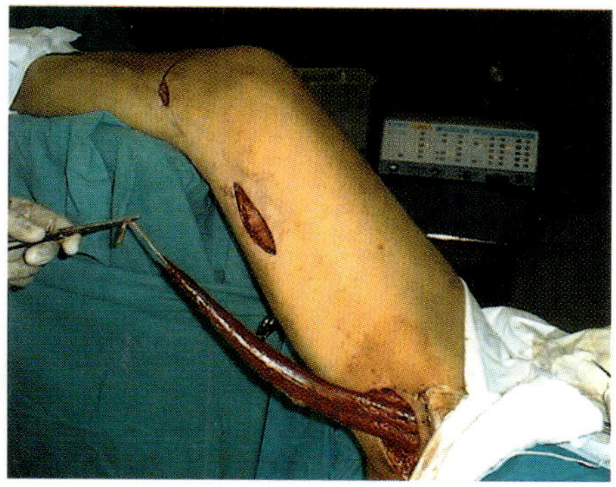

Figure 4. Gracilis mobilization. *Ch.20, p.294.*

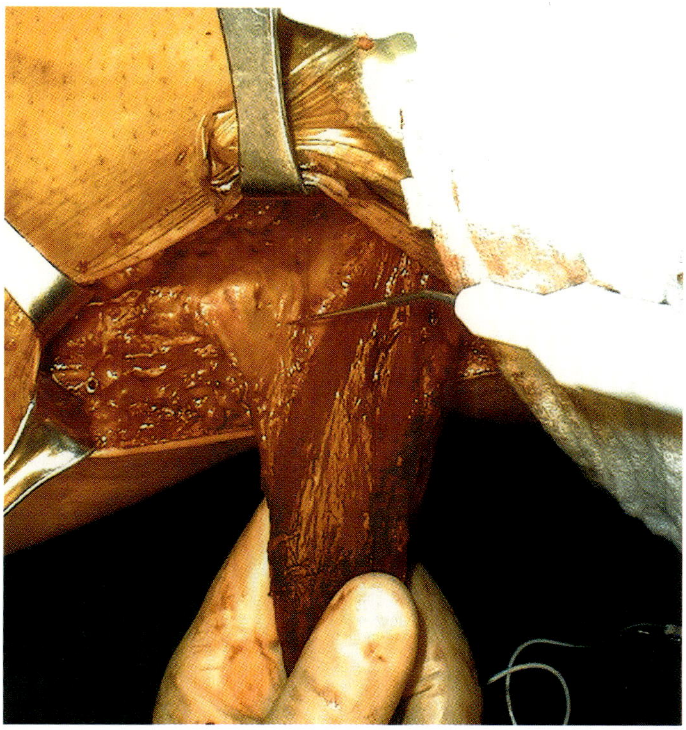

Figure 5. Nerve identification. *Ch.20, p.294.*

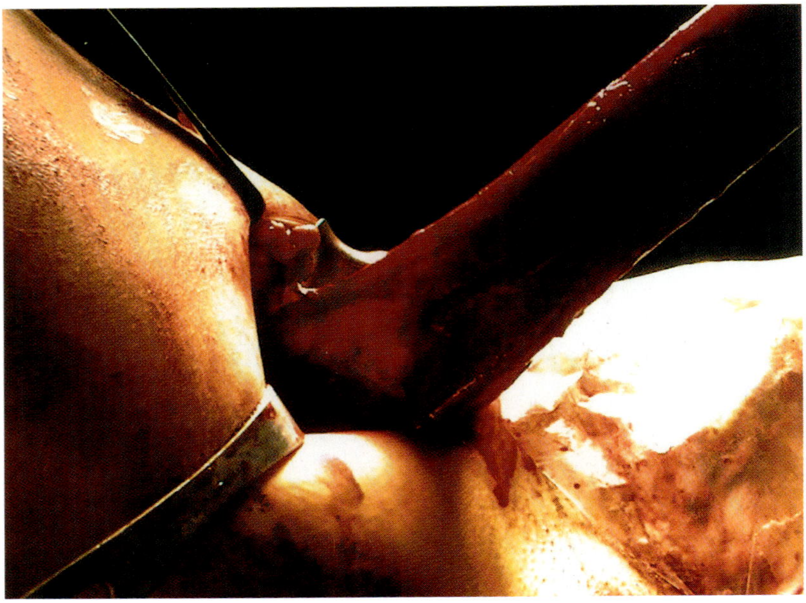

Figure 6. *Nerve entry. Ch.20, p.295.*

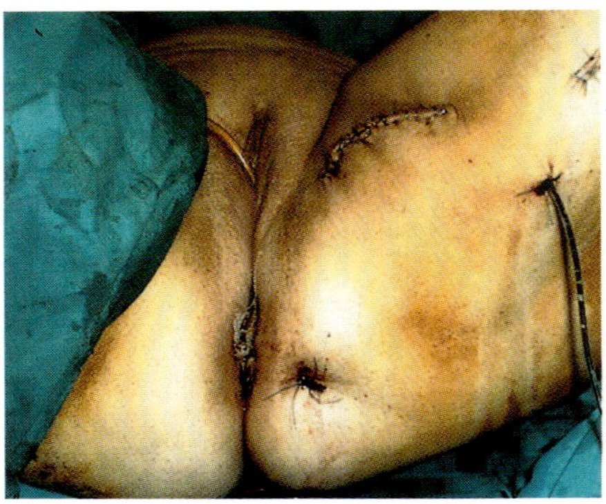

Figure 10. End of gp. *Ch.20, p.297.*

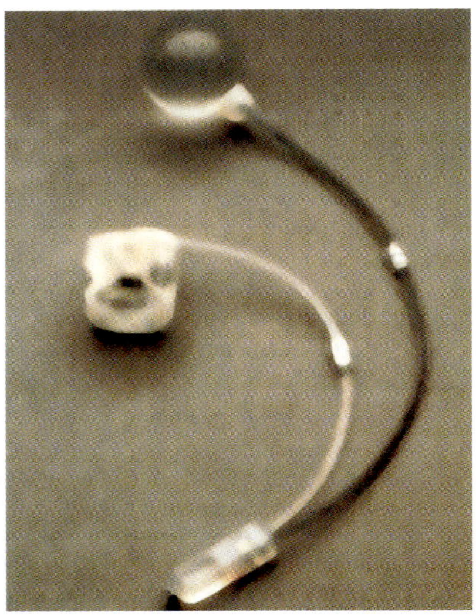

Figure 1. The Artificial Bowel Sphincter *Ch.21, p. 304.*

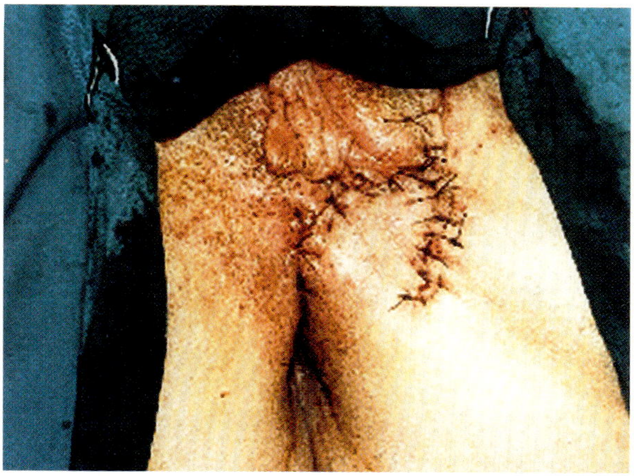

Figure 5. Rotating skin flap for perineal repair. *Ch.21, p.309.*

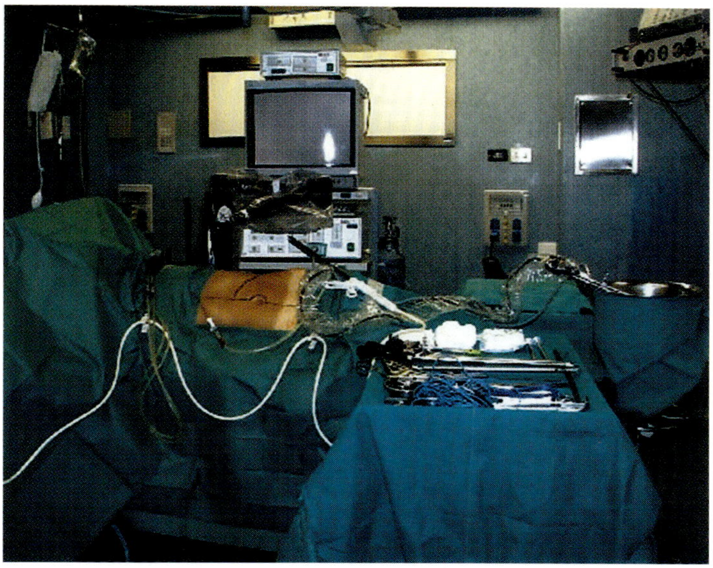

Figure 1. Operative setting for Hand-Assisted distal pancreatectomy using the Omniport device and a robotic visualization system. *Ch.24, p.341.*

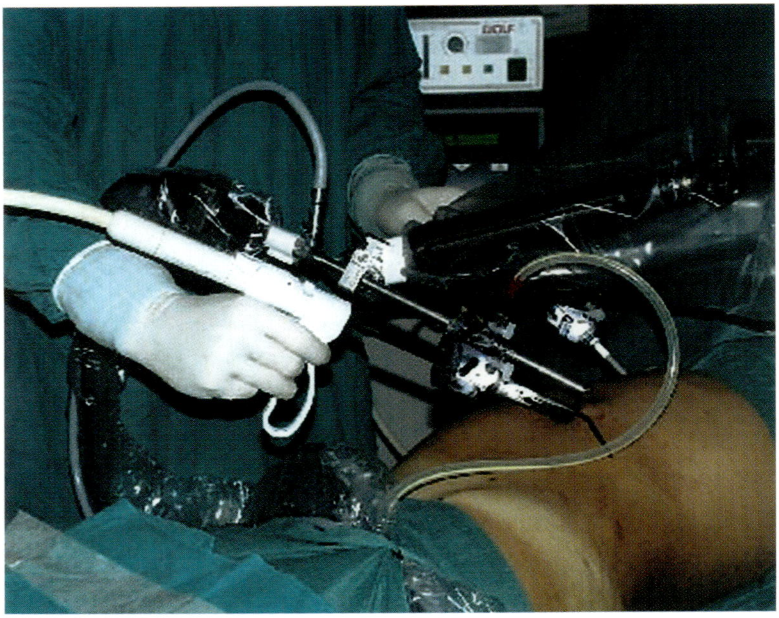

Figure 2. The robotic visualization system AESOP 3000 allows the performance of laparoscopic distal pancreatectomy in "solo-surgery". *Ch.24, p.342.*

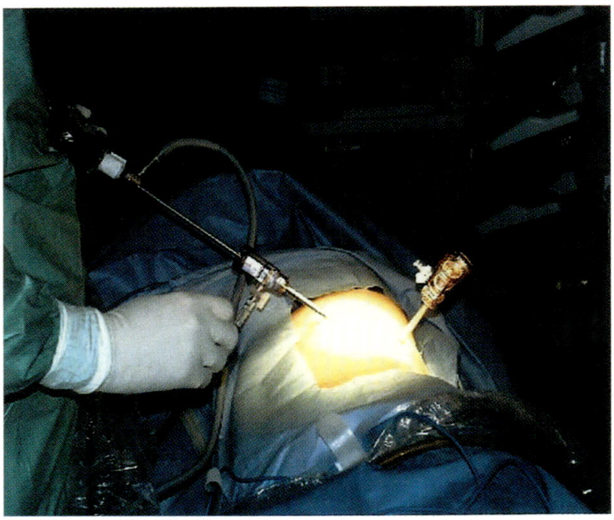

Figure 3. Positioning of trocars for thoracoscopic splanchnicectomy. *Ch.24, p.344.*

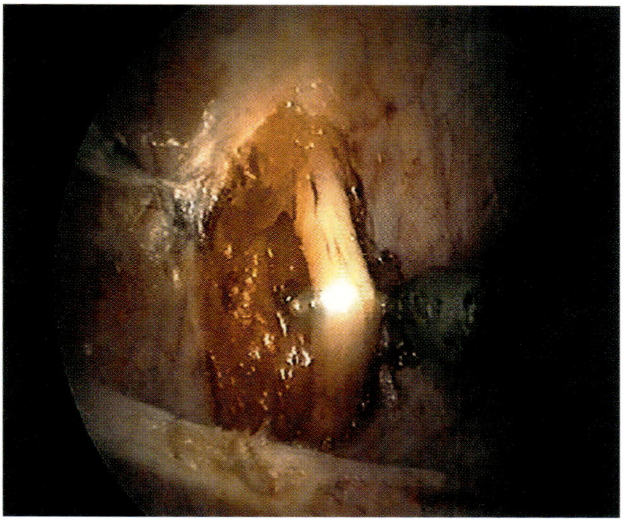

Figure 4. The greater splanchnic nerve is identified and then sectioned. *Ch.24, p.344.*

Author Index

Subject Index